SURGERY OF THE MALE REPRODUCTIVE TRACT

CLINICS IN ANDROLOGY

E.S.E. HAFEZ, *series editor*

VOLUME 2

1. J.C. Emperaire, A. Audebert, E.S.E. Hafez, eds., Homologous artificial insemination. 1980. ISBN 90-247-2269-1.
2. L.I. Lipshultz, J.N. Corriere Jr., E.S.E. Hafez, eds., Surgery of the male reproductive tract. 1980. ISBN 90-247-2315-9.
3. E.S.E. Hafez, ed., Descended and cryptorchid testis. 1980. ISBN 90-247-2299-3.
4. J. Bain, E.S.E. Hafez, eds., Diagnosis in andrology. 1980. ISBN 90-247-2365-5.
5. G.R. Cunningham, W.-B. Schill, E.S.E. Hafez, eds., Regulation of male fertility. 1980. ISBN 90-247-2373-6.
6. E.S.E. Hafez, E. Spring-Mills, eds., Prostatic carcinoma: biology and diagnosis. 1980. ISBN 90-247-2379-5.
7. S.J. Kogan, E.S.E. Hafez, eds., Pediatric Andrology. 1981. ISBN 90-247-2407-4.

series ISBN 90-247-2333-7

SURGERY OF THE MALE REPRODUCTIVE TRACT

edited by

L.I. LIPSHULTZ
Houston, Texas

J.N. CORRIERE, Jr.
Houston, Texas

and

E.S.E. HAFEZ
Detroit, Michigan

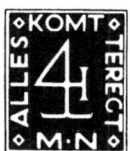

1980

MARTINUS NIJHOFF PUBLISHERS
THE HAGUE / BOSTON / LONDON

Distributors:

for the United States and Canada

Kluwer Boston, Inc.
190 Old Derby Street
Hingham, MA 02043
USA

for all other countries

Kluwer Academic Publishers Group
Distribution Center
P.O. Box 322
3300 AH Dordrecht
The Netherlands

Library of Congress Cataloging in Publication Data   CIP

Main entry under title:

Surgery of the male reproductive tract.

   (Clinics in andrology; v. 2)
   Includes index.
   1. Generative organs, Male – Surgery. I. Lipshultz, Larry I. II. Corriere, J.N. III. Hafez, E.S.E., 1922-
IV. Series. [DNLM: 1. Genitalia, Male – Surgery. W1 CL831AD v. 2 / WJ700 S961]
RD586.S93   617'.463   80-12297

ISBN-13 : 978-94-009-8851-4   e-ISBN-13 : 978-94-009-8849-1
DOI : 10.1007 / 978-94-009-8849-1

TABLE OF CONTENTS

List of Contributors   VII

Foreword   IX

I. ANATOMY AND PHYSIOLOGY OF THE MALE REPRODUCTIVE TRACT

1. Embryology and Functional Anatomy of Male Reproductive Organs   5
    E.S.E. HAFEZ

II. DISORDERS OF SPERMATOGENESIS AND EJACULATION

2. Orchiopexy and the Use of a Testicular Prosthesis for the Undescended Testicle   31
    J.N. CORRIERE, JR.

3. Epididymovasostomy for Epididymal Obstruction   38
    H. FENSTER and M.G. MCLOUGHLIN

4. Scrotal Exploration, Testis Biopsy and Vasography for Testicular Failure   47
    D.J. MEHAN

5. Internal Spermatic Vein Ligation for Varicocele   55
    L. DUBIN and R.D. AMELAR

6. Bladder Neck Reconstruction for Retrograde Ejaculation   62
    A.D. JENKINS and S.S. HOWARDS

III. DISORDERS OF ERECTION, EMISSION AND VAGINAL PENETRATION

7. Urethroplasty for Hypospadias   69
    J.N. CORRIERE, JR.

8. Genital Reconstruction of Anomalies of the Genitalia other than Hypospadias   79
    W.J. CROMIE and J.W. DUCKETT, JR.

9. Genital Reconstruction for Traumatic and Infectious Diseases   98
    W.S. MCDOUGAL

10. The Inflatable Penile Prosthesis for Treatment of Erectile Impotence   114
     F.B. Scott and I.J. Fishman

11. Grafts and Prostheses for Peyronie's Disease   125
     E. Houttuin and I.S. Hawatmeh

12. Corporal Shunts for Priapism   135
     H.W. Schoenberg and J. Banno

13. Vasectomy   143
     J.E. Davis

14. Vasovasostomy   157
     S.S. Schmidt

IV. Gender Reassignment

15. Orchiectomy, Penectomy, Vaginoplasty for the Male Transsexual   169
     L.I. Lipshultz

V. Benign Disorders of the Male Accessory Glands

16. Prostatectomy for Benign Prostatic Hyperplasia   177
     S.G. Mulholland and J.R. Dalton

17. Epididymectomy, Seminal Vesiculectomy and Hydrocelectomy for Epididymitis, Seminal
     Vesiculitis and Hydrocele   195
     M.A. Silvert and T.H. Stanisic

VI. Oncological Surgery

18. Penectomy and Groin Dissection for Carcinoma of the Penis   215
     T.R. Malloy and A.J. Wein

19. Orchiectomy and Retroperitoneal Node Dissection for Carcinoma of the Testicle   226
     T.J. Rohner, Jr. and E.J. Sanford

20. Total Prostatectomy for Carcinoma of the Prostate   237
     J.G. Gregory

21. Combined Radiotherapy for Carcinoma of the Prostate   251
     W.G. Guerriero

Index   263

LIST OF CONTRIBUTORS

Richard D. Amelar, M.D. Professor of Clinical Urology, New York University School of Medicine ,New York, New York, USA

Joseph Banno, M.D., Chief Resident in Urology, University of Chicago Hospitals and Clinics, Chicago, Illinois, USA

Joseph N. Corriere, Jr., M.D., Professor and Director of Urology, Division of Urology, Department of Surgery, University of Texas Medical School at Houston, Texas Medical Center, Houston, Texas, USA

William J. Cromie, M.D., Associate Professor of Surgery, University of Pennsylvania Medical School, Philadelphia, Pennsylvania, USA

John R. Dalton, M.D., Assistant Professor of Urology, Thomas Jefferson University, Philadelphia, Pennsylvania, USA

Joseph E. Davis, M.D., Clinical Professor of Urology, New York Medical College, New York, New York, USA

Lawrence Dubin, M.D., Professor of Clinical Urology, New York University School of Medicine, New York, New York, USA

John W. Duckett, M.D., Associate Professor of Urology, University of Pennsylvania School of Medicine, Philadelphia, Pennsylvania, USA

Howard Fenster, M.D., Clinical Instructor in Surgery, Division of Urology, University of British Columbia, Vancouver, B.C., Canada

Irving Fishman, M.D., Instructor in Urology, Baylor College of Medicine, Houston, Texas, USA

John G. Gregory, M.D., Director of the Program in Urology, Department of Surgery, Section of Urology, St. Louis University School of Medicine, St. Louis, Missouri, USA

William G. Guerriero, M.D., Associate Professor of Urology, Baylor College of Medicine, Houston, Texas, USA

E.S.E. Hafez, Ph.D., Professor, Gynecology/Andrology and Reproductive Physiology, Wayne State University School of Medicine, Detroit, Michigan, USA

Ibrahim S. Hawatmeh, M.D., Fellow, Department of Surgery, Section of Urology, St. Louis University School of Medicine, St. Louis, Missouri, USA

Erik Houttuin, M.D., Associate Professor of Surgery in Urology, Department of Surgery, Section of Urology, St. Louis University School of Medicine, St. Louis, Missouri, USA

Stuart S. Howards, M.D., Professor of Urology, University of Virginia School of Medicine, Department of Urology, Charlottesville, Virginia, USA

Alan D. Jenkins, M.D., University of Virginia School of Medicine, Department of Urology, Charlottesville, Virginia, USA

Larry I. Lipshultz, M.D., Associate Professor of Urology, Division of Urology, Department of Surgery, University of Texas Medical School at Houston, Texas Medical Center, Houston, Texas, USA

W. Scott McDougal, M.D., Associate Professor of Surgery (Urology), University Hospital, Case Western Reserve Medical School, Cleveland, Ohio, USA

M.G. McLoughlin, M.D., Chairman, Division of Urology, University of British Columbia, Vancouver, B.C., Canada

Terrence R. Malloy, M.D., Clinical Associate Professor of Urology, University of Pennsylvania Medical School, Philadelphia, Pennsylvania, USA

Donald J. Mehan, M.D., Associate Clinical Professor of Urology, St. Louis University School of Medicine, St. Louis, Missouri, USA

S. Grant Mulholland, M.D., Professor and Chairman, Department of Urology, Thomas Jefferson University, Philadelphia, Pennsylvania, USA

Thomas J. Rohner, Jr., M.D., Professor of Surgery, Chief, Division of Urology, The Milton S. Hershey Medical Center, The Pennsylvania State University College of Medicine, Hershey, Pennsylvania, USA

Edgar J. Sanford, M.D., Associate Professor of Surgery (Urology), The Milton S. Hershey Medical Center, The Pennsylvania State University College of Medicine, Hershey, Pennsylvania, USA

Stanwood S. Schmidt, M.D., Research Associate, Department of Urology, University of California School of Medicine, San Francisco, California, USA

Mark A. Silvert, M.D., Assistant Professor of Surgery/Urology, University of Arizona, Health Sciences Center, Tucson, Arizona, USA

Harry W. Schoenberg, M.D., Chairman, Department of Urology, University of Chicago Hospitals and Clinics, Chicago, Illinois, USA

F. Brantley Scott, M.D., Professor of Urology, Baylor College of Medicine, Houston, Texas, USA

Thomas H. Stanisic, M.D., Assistant Professor of Surgery/Urology, University of Arizona, Health Sciences Center, Tucson, Arizona, USA

Alan J. Wein, M.D., Associate Professor of Urology, University of Pennsylvania School of Medicine, Philadelphia, Pennsylvania, USA

FOREWORD

In the last decade, physicians have witnessed a growing awareness of and concern with diseases of the male reproductive tract. Stimulated by this interest, a refinement and re-evaluation of existing surgical techniques for treatment of male reproductive disorders has been concurrently appreciated. Rapid progress in this area has resulted primarily from a cooperative effort from those specialists in the areas of microsurgery, medical and surgical oncology, endocrinology and neurophysiology, pathology, immunology, genetics and biochemistry.

As the surgical treatment of diseases and abnormalities of the male reproductive system has expanded, so have the articles describing these often innovative techniques; unfortunately the journals and texts reporting these operations have likewise exploded in number. Because of the widely scattered publication of this andrological surgery, we thought it relevant to present for the first time, a single text which might collate current surgical techniques involving treatment of the many disease processes involved in modern management of abnormalities of the male reproductive system.

It is hoped that this monograph will serve in part as a reference for those interested in reviewing modern surgical trends in a relatively new area of genitourinary surgery. It is also hoped that this publication will serve as a stimulus to surgeons concerned with male reproductive disorders to intensify their personal research attempts to develop better therapy for diseases referable to the male reproductive system. It is finally hoped that this publication will stimulate critical analysis of what we feel are currently accepted surgical modes of therapy and to better promote a general interchange of clinical information referable to these disorders.

Those who have provided the text and illustrations for this volume have contributed a significant amount of work, and we hope that they feel their material has been well used. The editors also wish to thank Mr. Jeffrey Smith of Martinus Nijhoff for his cooperation during the production of this volume, Harriet Lowenthal for editorial assistance, Homer Tolan for manuscript preparation, and Jackie Blain for proofing, indexing, and final preparation.

July, 1980

Houston, Texas

Detroit, Michigan

L.I. LIPSHULTZ
J.N. CORRIERE, JR.
E.S.E. HAFEZ

SURGERY OF THE MALE REPRODUCTIVE TRACT

I. ANATOMY AND PHYSIOLOGY OF THE MALE REPRODUCTIVE TRACT

1. EMBRYOLOGY AND FUNCTIONAL ANATOMY OF MALE REPRODUCTIVE ORGANS

E.S.E. HAFEZ

I. EMBRYOLOGY

A. Gonad and Duct System

The fetal testes develop in close association with the mesonephros (Figure 1). The coelomic epithelium which covers the mesonephric ridge thickens and forms a primary blastema that includes the primordial germ cells. The formation of an indifferent gonad showing no sexual differentiation takes place between growth stages 5 mm and 15 mm, a period which corresponds to the 5th and 6th weeks of gestational age. During the 6th week of fetal life, the gonad differentiates into either a testis or an ovary. In the testicular anlage the primary blastema becomes separated from the coelomic epithelium by a primitive tunica albuginea, forming a medullary blastema which immediately differentiates into testicular cords and interstitial tissue (Wartenberg 1978). In the ovarian anlage the first ingrowth of the primary blastema terminates.

The germ cells themselves do not have any influence on the sexual differentiation of the gonad. The two primordia (cortex and medulla) seem to guide the gonad in different directions, the male or the female. The gonadal blastema represents a pool for the different groups of somatic cell precursors: Sertoli cells, Leydig cells and peritubular cells. In order to provide the lower part of the testicular anlage and its already formed testicular cords with somatic cells, strands of blastemal cells (rete blastema) connect the upper with the lower part of the testis. Actually these strands are not precursors of the rete testis, which does not develop before the 5th month of fetal life. The embryonic origin of Sertoli cells is uncertain.

During embryonic life (7 cm crown-rump length), 37 to 40 lateral tubules evaginate from right to left

lateral walls of the primitive urethra. They grow outward backwards giving rise to 2 lateral lobes which form most of adult prostate. Middle (medial) lobe develops from a group of 7 to 12 tubules in the floor of urethra proximal to ejaculatory ducts and orifice of bladder. During the 3rd month of gestation, 4-11 tubules from the floor of urethra distal to colliculus seminalis form posterior lobe; ducts and alveoli of posterior lobe grow backwards behind ejaculatory ducts but remain bands of fibro-elastic ventral lobe in this.

Inductors: The Wolffian and Mullerian systems are present by the 8th week of fetal life (Figure 2). The former will give rise to the epididymis, ductus deferens, and seminal vesicles, and will atrophy in the female. The latter forms the uterus, the oviducts and the superior part of the vagina in the female, and will atrophy in the male. In the adult vestigial remnants from one or the other of the atrophic systems are present: in the male remnants of the Mullerian system are the appendix of the testis and prostatic utricle.

Evidently there are one or more inductors capable of directing the development, whereas the ovary is not essential for differentiation in a female sense. It is probable that there are more masculinizing substances formed by the fetal testis, one responsible for the development of the Wolffian ducts, another responsible for the atrophy of the Mullerian system, and a third substance for male differentiation of the external genitals. The inducing substances which determine the masculinization of the Wolffian ducts seem to act only locally.

B. Male Accessory Organs

Primordia of seminal vesicles arise in 13-week

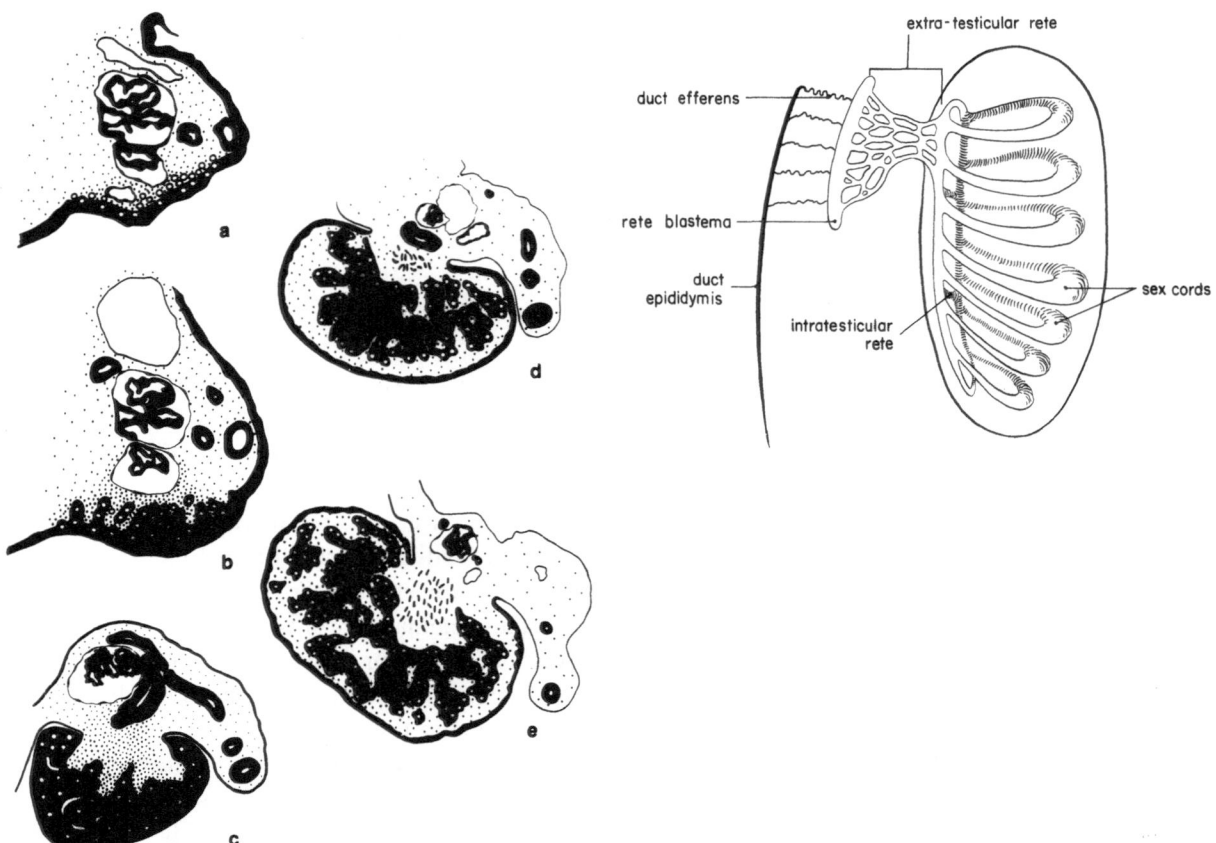

Figure 1. Top: Diagrammatic illustration showing the early development of the human indifferent gonad (a-c) and testis (d-e). a. Cross-section through the urogenital fold, representing a developmental stage of 6-8 mm (day 30 to 34 ovulation age OA): The genital ridge is slightly bordered by low invaginations (arrows), the coelomic epithelium contains some primordial germ cells which are concentrated below the epithelium. Note close relationship to themesonephric structures. b. 12-15 mm (day 35 to 36 OA): The coelomic epithelium is spissated and forms a primary gonadal blastema. c. 18-20 mm (day 39 to 40 OA): The gonad formed from an undifferentiated blastema protrudes into the coelomic cavity. It is still attached to the mesonephric region by means of a wide mesogonadium. Müllerian and Wolffian ducts are displaced laterally within the mesonephric fold. d. 21 mm (day 42 OA approx.): Medullary blastema is separated from the superficial epithelium and forms platelike testicular cords. In the hilar region strands of epitheloid cells (rete blastema) connect the mesonephric structures and the intratesticular cords. e. 28 mm (day 49 OA approx.): The medulla still consists of platelike strands rather than testicular cords (or tubuli). The so-called rete blastema fills the center of the medulla (magnif. a-b 110×, c 85×, d-e 65×) (after Wartenberg 1978). Bottom: Line drawing showing development of sex cords and testicular rete.

fetuses as an evagination of the caudal wall of each of the paired mesonephric (Wolffian) ducts near the urogenital sinus. At the site of evagination, the mesonephric duct becomes dilated to form an ampulla. The saccular evagination of the wall forms the seminal vesicle, whereas the site of evagination divides the mesonephric duct into: a) different duct (vas deferens) and b) ejaculatory duct. The mesonephric duct between the origin of the seminal vesicle urethra gives rise to the ejaculatory duct. Seminal vesicles complete prenatal development in 7-month fetuses. The fetal prostate is under the constant influence of maternal, placental and fetal hormones. Squamous metaplasia within the fetal prostatic epithelium and growth of the stroma are attributed to estrogens whereas secretory activity presumably is androgen-dependent (Zondek and Zondek 1975). The presence of prostate glands in normal females of certain species and the similarities between the male and female prostates in many of these animals, indicates that the Y chromosome is unnecessary for organogenesis and histogenesis of the prostates in these females (Price 1975).

Glandular portions of the prostate originate from that portion of the cloacal endoderm, the 'primitive posterior, urogenital sinus' or (prostatic urethra)

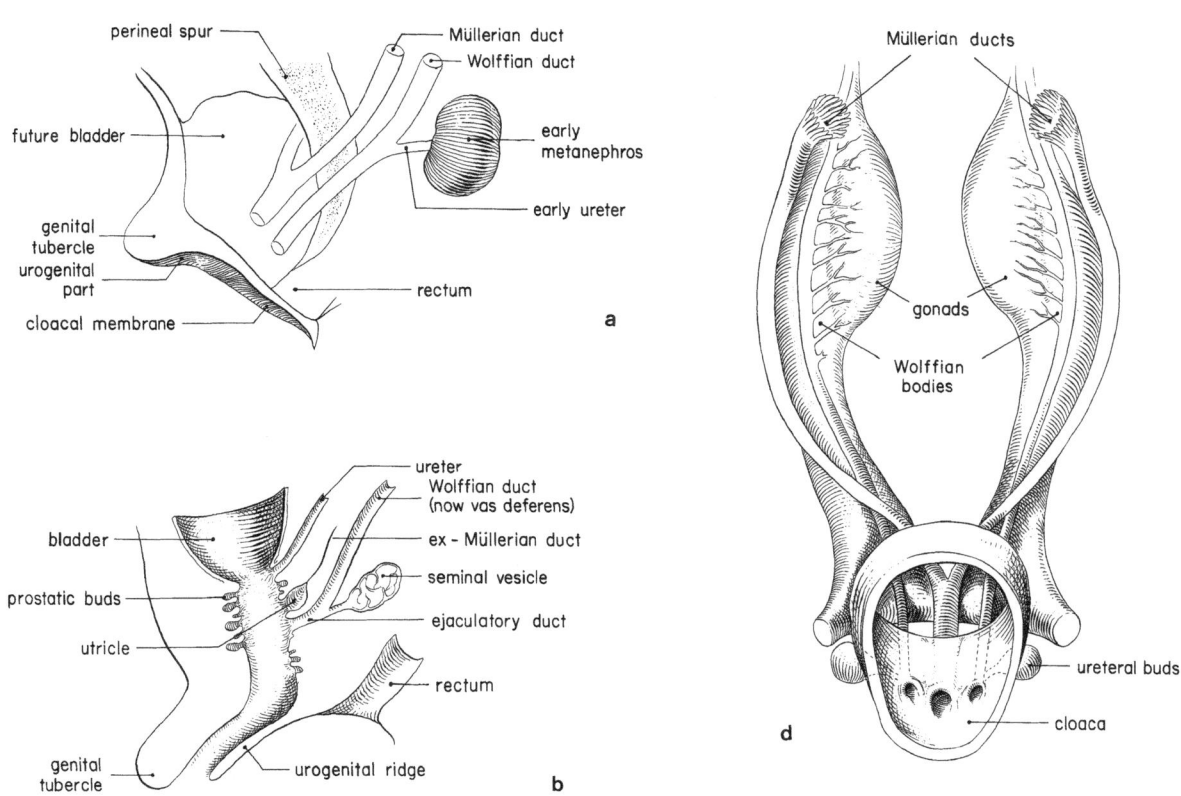

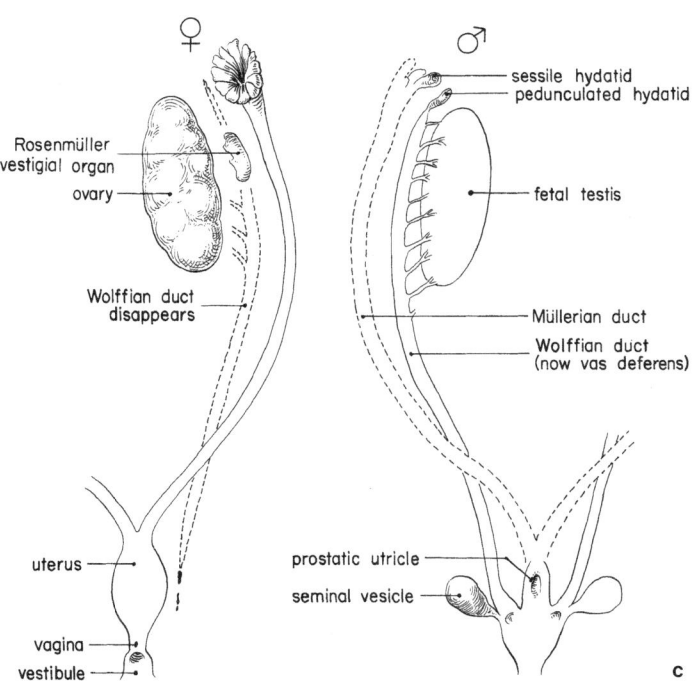

Figure 2. a, b. Anatomical relationships of genito-urinary duct system of the human fetus. c, d. Fetal differentiation of male and female reproductive organs (c); details of Müllerian and Wolffian ducts in relation to ureteral buds and cloaca (d).

which evaginates from the urethra into the mesenchyme at 13th week of gestation: five groups of epithelial buds grow from the primitive urethra and form 5 lobes which fuse during the second half of gestation and are no longer perceptible.

C. External Genitalia

The external genitalia originate at the genital eminence located on the median ventral surface of the body of the developing embryo. The eminence develops into the genital tubercle and eventually into the penis (Figure 3). The urethral groove, a midline invagination of the ectoderm of the cloacal membrane within the proctodeum, is formed in 5 week fetuses (Jirasek 1971). The urogenital sinus opens into the caudal portion of the groove. Lateral and parallel to the groove, on the inferior surface of the genital tubercle, two urethral folds and two labioscrotal swellings arise. The latter form the scrotal pouch, whereas the line of closure over the urethral groove becomes the perineal raphe. At 8-9 weeks (30-44 mm), there is no sex difference in the external genitals.

At the end of the seventh week of fetal development, the genital tubercle grows rapidly and forms the corpora cavernosa as paired mesenchymal columns within the shaft of the penis. As the penis develops, the pelvic portion of the urogenital sinus becomes the membranous portion of the male urethra (Jirasek 1971). Masculinization of the male fetuses is under the influence of androstenedione and testosterone produced by testicular interstitial Leydig cells (Jirasek et al. 1969).

At the end of the twelfth week, the urethra is completely developed and extends from the uro-genital sinus in the proctodeum to the end of the penis, the so-called urethral plate. Beginning at the base of the penis, the urethral folds fuse at their edges to close off the urethra and urogenital sinus. The fused edges of the folds form the perineal raphe. The corpus spongiosum arises from the masses of mesenchyme around the penile urethra.

The scrotal swellings gradually enlarge and migrate to the midline in front of the anus and join and fuse to form the scrotum. Their fused edges form the scrotal raphe.

During the development of the urethra, the prepuce develops over the glans penis from a fold of skin from the ventrodistal epithelium in the glans region of the genital tubercle. This fold of epithelium eventually invaginates and forms the preputial cavity which separates the prepuce from the surface of the glans penis. The invaginated epithelium is solid initially, but eventually canalizes and develops into the glandular portion of the penile urethra.

The homologies of male accessory glands, external genitalia and urethra are summarized in Table 1.

II. ANATOMY

The anatomical relationships among the various male reproductive organs are illustrated in Figures 4, 5 and 6, and are summarized in Table 2. The structural characteristics and histological features of these organs are shown in Table 3. Detailed

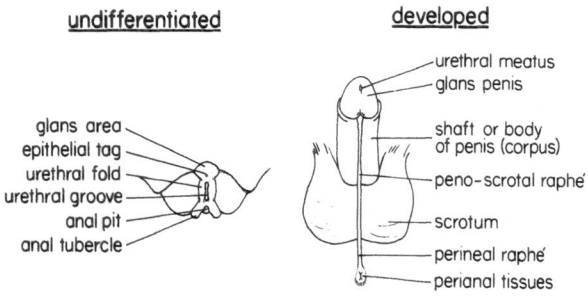

Figure 3. Diagrammatic illustration of undifferentiated and developed human penis.

Table 1. Homologues of male accessory glands, external genitalia and urethra (from Spring-Mills and Hafez 1980).

Male	Female
Cowper's glands	Bartholin's glands opening on labia majora within vestibule
Prostate	Skene's para-urethral ducts
Seminal vesicle	Canals of Gartner extending from broad ligament to vestibule of vagina
Glans penis	Glans clitoridis
Prepuce	Prepuce
Shaft (corpus) of penis	Corpus of clitoridis
Peno-scrotal raphe	Labia minora
Scrotum	Labia majora
Perineal raphe	Perineal raphe
Penile urethra	Vestibule
Prostatic urethra	Entire urethra

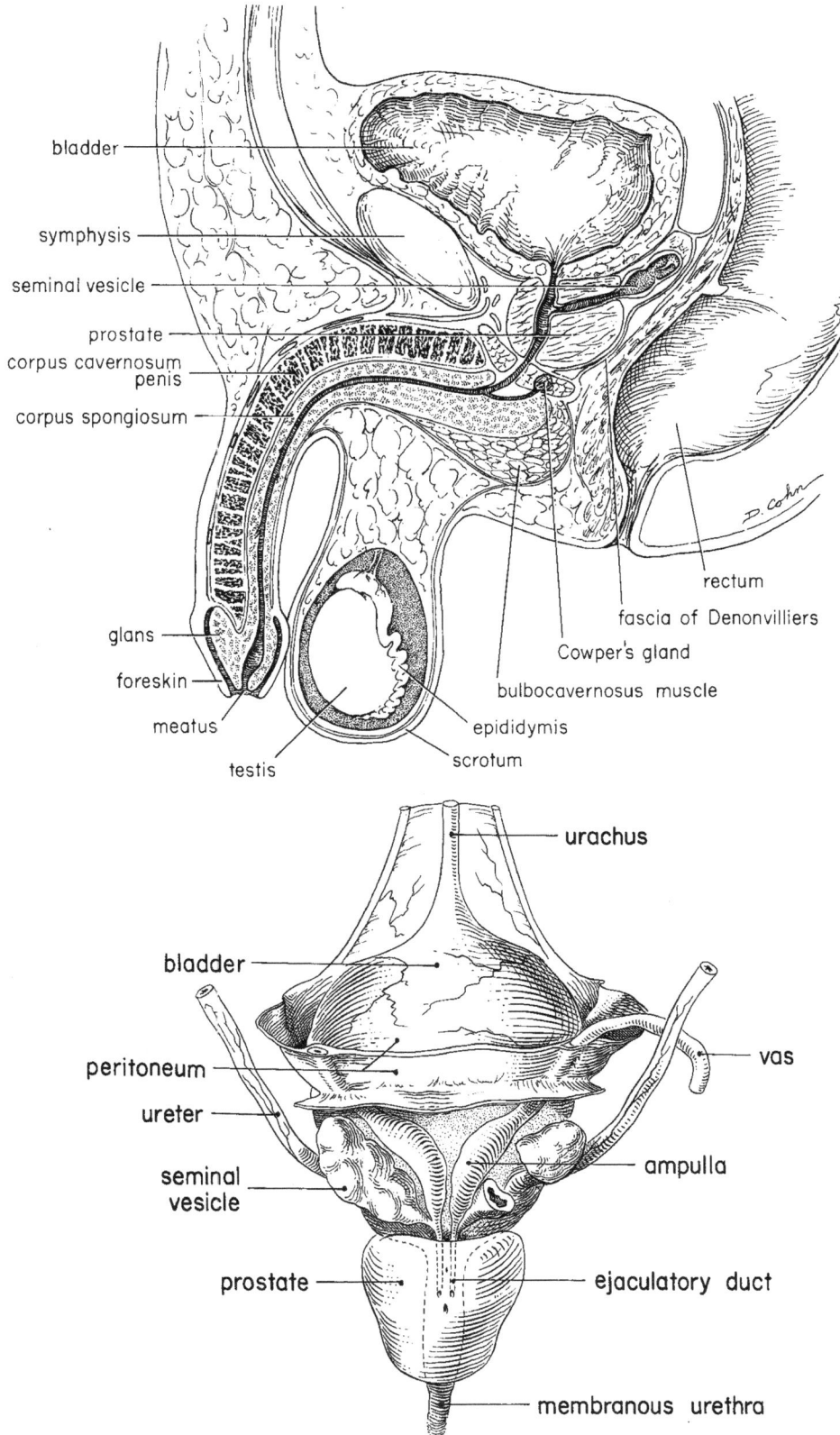

Figure 4. Male reproductive system and certain pelvic structures (sagittal view) (after Spring-Mills and Hafez 1980). Bottom: Anatomical relationships of prostate, seminal vesicles, urinary bladder and vas deferens.

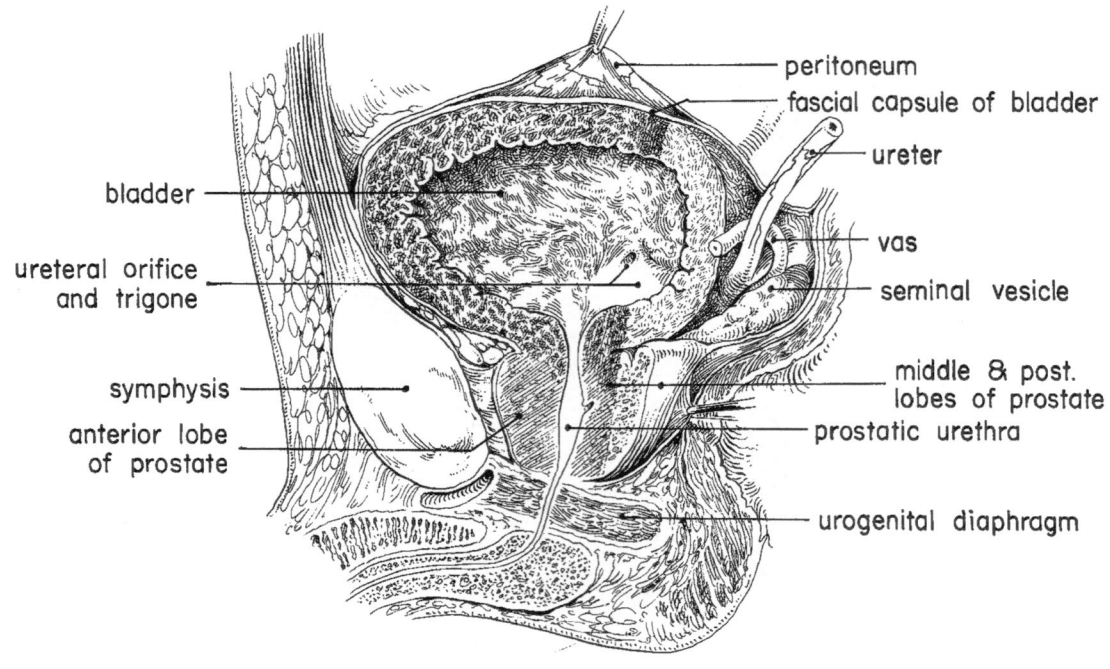

bladder

ureteral orifice
and trigone

symphysis

anterior lobe
of prostate

peritoneum

fascial capsule of bladder

ureter

vas

seminal vesicle

middle & post.
lobes of prostate

prostatic urethra

urogenital diaphragm

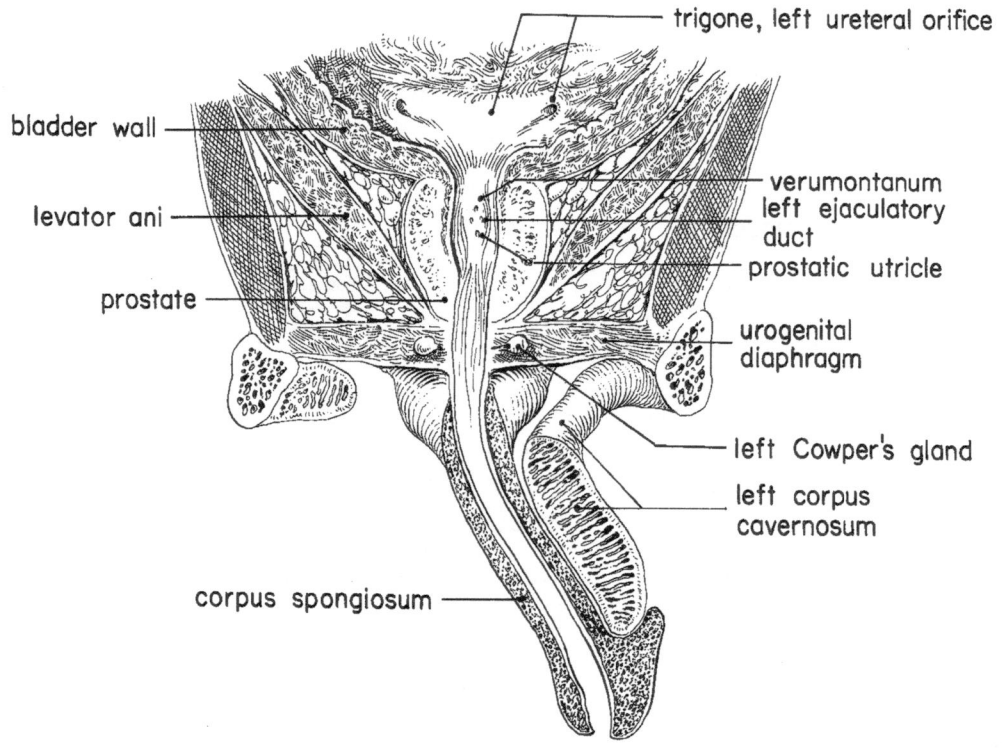

trigone, left ureteral orifice

bladder wall

levator ani

prostate

verumontanum

left ejaculatory
duct

prostatic utricle

urogenital
diaphragm

left Cowper's gland

left corpus
cavernosum

corpus spongiosum

Figure 5. Line drawings showing anatomical relationships of trigone prostate and related organs.

discussion of the functional anatomy of the penis is given below.

The size of the seminal vesicles is variable and in normal patients the size of the seminal vesicles is proportional to that of the ampullae. Large vesicles are usually associated with large ampullae and well developed pelvic organs are usually associated with large epididymis.

Like the ureter, the vas deferens dilates after obstruction. This dilatation is evident as early as 3 weeks postoperatively and appears to reach a maximum 1 year after vasectomy (Schmit 1959, 1978). Knowledge of the extent of this dilatation is important in performing vas anastomosis and in developing devices to rejoin the vas. The degree of dilatation varies between individuals but is usually similar on both sides in the same man. In a series of 22 cases, the lumen of the testicular side of the vas after vasectomy occasionally is dilated to a diameter slightly above 2 mm, without increase in the overall external diameter (Brueschke et al. 1974).

A. Penis

The penis contains the urethra, 3 cylinders of erectile tissue (two lateral corpora cavernosa and a median corpus spongiosum), connective tissue, blood vessels, lymphatics and nerves. The corpora cavernosa comprise the bulk of the penis. Posteriorly, they diverge and attach to the rami of the pubis and ischium. Distally, they end approximately 2 cm from the end of the penis. Each cylinder is surrounded by the tunica albuginea, a thick fibrous sheath containing an outer longitudinal and an inner circular layer of collagenous fibers. The pectiniform septum, a tough fibrous tissue, forms a common median partition between the two corpora cavernosa; and it is pierced by slitlike openings which allow the cavernous spaces of each corpus cavernosum to communicate (Spring-Mills and Hafez 1980). Connective tissue trabeculae extend from the tunica albuginea into each cylinder. The intervening spaces form the endothelium-lined blood sinusoids. Because of the arrangement of the trabeculae, the cavernous spaces are largest in the center of each cylinder. Each corpus cavernosum is covered by an ischiocavernosus muscle. The bulb of the urethra is covered by the bulbocavernosus muscle.

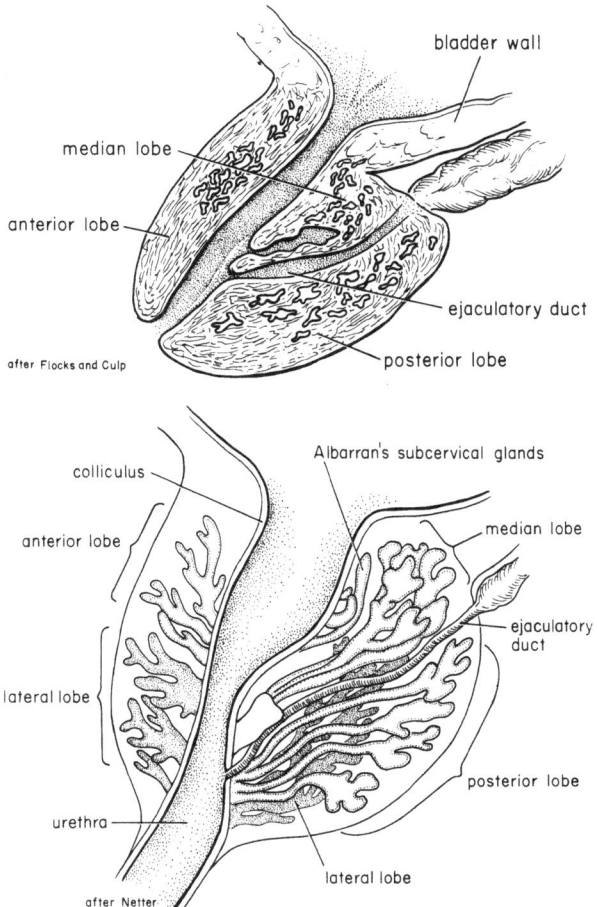

Figure 6. Top: Section in the prostate showing the anterior, median and posterior lobe in relation to the ejaculatory duct (after Flocks and Culp 1967). Bottom: Section through the prostate to show Albarran's subcervical glands, and the ducts of the anterior, lateral and posterior lobe as they connect with the urethra (after Netter).

The corpus spongiosum (corpus cavernosus urethrae) surrounds the male urethra and lies in a groove on the ventral surface of the penis beneath the corpus cavernosum. Proximally the corpus spongiosum forms the bulb which abuts the inferior layer of the triangular ligament. Distally, the corpus spongiosum forms the glans penis. The glans penis covers the ends of the corpora cavernosa, extending farther back on the dorsal than on the ventral surface. The urethral meatus lies at the top of the glans penis. The region behind the base of the glans is the corona penis. The tunica albuginea surrounding the corpus spongiosum is much thinner than that surrounding the corpora cavernosa. In addition, its trabeculae are thinner and more elastic.

Table 2. Anatomical relationships of male reproductive organs (from Brueschke et al. 1974; Batra and Lardner 1976).

Organ	Anatomical relationships
Vas deferens	Extends from tail epididymis to neck of seminal vesicle; ascends posterior border of testis on the medial side of epididymis, passes the external inguinal ring and travels along the inguinal canal to level of internal ring, terminal segment of the vas is dilated forming the ampulla at base of prostate, vas deferens fuses with neck of seminal vesicle to form ejaculatory duct which passes through prostate to open into floor of prostatic urethra at colliculus seminalis at internal inguinal ring. vas deferens leaves spermatic cord. curves around lateral side of inferior epigastric blood vessels, crosses external iliac blood vessels to enter pelvis where vas deferens descends on medial side of the obturator nerves and blood vessels, crosses in front of ureter to posterior surface of bladder.
Ampulla	Terminal part of dilated vas deferens modified to form the ampullae, passes along inner border of seminal vesicles. Right and left ampulla-vesicle complexes are separated by a V-shaped surface; this 'triangle' with a lower prostatic tip, corresponds to middle part of 'trigone' of bladder which overlaps widely above.
Seminal vesicle	Its posterior surface is most accessible by clinical examination if index finger is 12 to 15 cm long; or under pathological conditions. Surface of vesicle is situated higher than upper border of prostate. Lateral border has no important visceral relations, but related to prostatic venous plexuses subject to hemorrhage by careless surgery, stretched out summit of seminal vesicles forms a very acute angel at end of the ampullae forming ejaculatory duct, in posterior view, they lie behind posterior wall of bladder, between bladder and rectum, which undergo periodic size changes causing periodic pressure on the seminal vesicles as adjacent hollow organs are emptied; defecation exerts pressure on seminal vesicles, which may cause some pain or spermatorrhea during defecation.
Prostate	Located below bladder orifice above urogenital diaphragm; majority of its upper surface is continuous with bladder wall; Denonvillier's (rectovesicle) fascia covers posterior surfaces of prostate and seminal vesicles, separates these organs from anterior wall of rectum.
Bulbo-urethral glands of Cowper	Portions of gland lie within urogenital diaphragm lateral and posterior to membranous urethra.
Ejaculatory ducts	Two ejaculatory ducts located between middle lateral lobes of prostate; as they converge, they decrease in diameter and in very close proximity to each other within the floor of prostatic urethra, they pass through prostate and open onto the floor of the urethra at level of colliculus seminalis.
Urethra	18-20 cm long, it has three regional segments: Prostatic urethra, next to the bladder is only 3-4 cm long; floor of prostatic urethra contains numerous orifices representing the terminations of prostatic ducts and elevated urethral crest. Pocket or utricle within the crest originates during embryogenesis from fused ends of Mullerian ducts. Directly below utricle are openings of ejaculatory ducts, one orifice located on each side of urethral floor; membranous urethra, between prostate and penis, 1 cm long, is surrounded by muscles and other components of urogenital diaphragm. Urethra within the penis ('cavernous urethra', or 'bulbous urethra') refers to upper third; 'pendulous' or 'penile urethra' refers to remainder of duct.
Ureter	Related to anterior surface of seminal vesicle, in its last centimeter and intramural part; anterior surface of seminal vesicle is throughout its extent related to bladder, from which it is separated only by a thin layer of fibro-muscular connective tissue into which enters the lower end of ureter.

Table 3. Structural characteristics of the male reproductive organs.

Organ	Structural characteristics
Testis	a. Seminiferous tubules: whole seminiferous system consists of one tube, which explains the possibility of radiological examination of its lumen using opaque material. Tubules are made of stratified epithelium of about 5-8 layers of cells having different morphologies, limiting and irregular lumen tubules contain sustentacular cells (Sertoli cells) and various types of germ cells, i.e. spermatogonia, primary and secondary spermatocytes, spermatids, spermatozoa. b. Sertoli cells: elongated and irregular in shape, attached to basement membrane of tubules, lamellae-shaped processes radiate from cellular trunk and extend laterally between maturing germinal cells surrounding them. c. blood testis barrier: junctional complexes divide Sertoli cells into two compartments: a basal (external) and apial (adluminal). Interstitial tissue formed of a ground substance containing blood and lymphatic vessels, clusters of Leydig cells, nerves, fibroblasts, macrophages, mast cells, collagen and elastic fibers; Leydig cells situated primarily along blood vessels; capillary wall is thick and does not contain fenestrae characteristic of many endocrine organs.
Epididymis (from Holstein 1969, 1976)	Caps the testis, unrolled is about 3-6m long; consists of a single tube folded on itself. Several segments are distinguished morphologically: there is a proximodistal decrease in width of lumen, with narrowest portion at transition of corpus and cauda, the remaining cauda sections have a wide lumen. Epithelium consists of two cell types: principal cells and basal cells; principal cells are high columnar elements, the perikarya of which are classified into zones according to number and relative distribution of cell organelle; morphological characteristics of principal cells vary along the different sections of epididymis. Basal cells are spherical and occur randomly between more numerous principal cells; they do not extend toward luminal surface of epithelium. Epididymal lumen contains immature germ cells, and fragments of cells such as nuclei, organelles, or membranes.
Vas deferens	Junction between epididymis and vas deferens is abrupt. Vas contain 3 concentric coats: mucosa, muscularis and adventitia. Mucosa is pseudostratified epithelium similar to epididymis: clear cells disappear and principal cells increase in height, some stereocilia, in cross sections lumen has irregular contour. Epithelium contains a discontinuous layer of small, round or pyramidal basal cells and thin columnar cells extending from basal lamina to lumen; principal cells have stereocilia on apical surface and coated invaginations of apical plasmalemma between their bases; small coated vesicles may be involved in uptake of materials from lumen. Mitochondria rich cells may be involved in acidification of seminal plasma or transport of electrolytes, hydrogen ions and water across mucosa, 'pencil cells' appear to be dead or dying columnar epithelial cells without any important function, muscularis, 1-1.5 mm thick, contains 3 layers of musculature, inner and outer muscle layers are longitudinally arranged, middle layer is circularly arranged; proportion of longitudinal to circular musculature and overall thickness of muscularis varies from epididymal to urethral end of vas.
Seminal vesicles	Very variable in size and may be spherical, tubular, or branched in appearance; mucosa – each gland consists of a single tube, coiled upon itself and containing several irregular recesses, coils and convolutions apparent in cross section; proximal extremity of tube tapers and joins vas deferens to form ejaculatory duct. Mucosa is made of complex folds, honeycomb in shape (due to numerous foldings forming recesses of variable sizes which open into a large central cavity) containing pseudostratified columnar or simple columnar epithelium with pronounced variation in appearance depending on age and hormonal status. Superficial cells contain granules and clumps of lipochrome pigment which first appears at puberty, yellow viscous secretions appear in histological sections as coagulated, netlike deeply staining masses.
Ampullary glands	Tubules enclosed by a capsule of connective tissue, formed from vas deferens near its junctions with urethra; mucosal folds of gland form irregular branching which anastomose forming partitions and invaginations which extend to the muscularis.

continued on page 14

Table 3 continued.

Organ	Anatomical relationships
Prostate	Largest male accessory gland; size of a chestnut; 3.8 cm in diameter, 29 gm in weight, made of 5 lobes: a) posterior lobe located posterior to urethra deferential canal; b) middle (median) lobe between urethra deferential canal; c) largely vestigial anterior lobe containing 8 or 10 alveoli located anterior to urethra; d) two lateral lobes on either side of urethra which contain ducts that empty into sides of the verumontanum. A thin fibro-elastic capsule surrounds prostate, giving rise to septa which extend inward forming lobes; fibromuscular attachments between capsule and recto-prostatic fascia and fascia of levator ani. Contains 30-50 branching tubulo-alveoli or succular glands which vary greatly in size and morphology; 16-32 excretory ducts; highly folded epithelium often forms papillae which project into lumen which is dilated with secretions; saccular recesses. cystic dilations of alveoli and ducts are common, two types of epithelial cells predominate: a) columnar secretory cells containing a moderate number of mitochondria, apical Golgi apparatus and densely packed secretory vacuoles; b) basal columnar cells, polygonal in shape, lack secretory vesicles and contain few mitochondria, poorly developed endoplasmic reticulum, Golgi apparatus, and ribosomes, smooth muscle cells, fibroblasts, abundant collagen and elastic fibers which give characteristic elasticity to gland are used to distinguish normal prostate from abnormal during physical examination.
Bulbo-urethral glands	Two yellowish brown glands, each the size of a pea, located dorsal to bulb of penis; partially or completely embedded in muscles of the urogenital diaphragm, branched tubulo-alveolar glands on either side of membranous portion of the urethra, lined with simple low cuboidal to columnar epithelium; epithelium varies in shape with age and functional activity, in each gland a thin connective tissue capsule sends septa into interior to divide gland into lobes and lobules, septa are 1-3 mm thick, contain collagen, elastic and reticular fibers, skeletal and smooth muscle fibers. Excretory duct, 3 to 4 cm long, enters bulbus, runs parallel to urethra in which it opens.
Urethral glands (Littre's)	Some urethral glands are simple outpocketings of the urethral mucosa, whereas others contain a globular secretory segment connected to the urethra by a short duct; glands open into cavernous portion of urethra.
Subcervical urethral glands of Albarran	Small glands above verumontanum (colliculis seminalis) which are formed from urethral diverticula, glands extend radially into periurethral connective tissue and smooth muscle of internal sphincter of bladder, but they are ontogenetically and functionally distinct from glands of the prostate proper.
Preputial glands	On the prepuce and neck of penis – modified sebaceous glands.
Ejaculatory duct	Folded mucosa is lined by an epithelium similar to that of ampullar simple columnar or pseudostratified columnar containing many yellow pigment granules. The walls of the ducts contain only connective tissue. In the terminal regions close to the urethra, cavernous vascular spaces are present in the wall and the epithelium may become 'transitional'.
Spermatic cord	Surrounded by tunica vaginalis, contains vas deferens, spermatic (testicular) artery, veins of pampiniform plexus, surrounding artery, lymphatic vessels and sympathetic nerves of testis and epididymis, and internal creamaster muscle which elicits 'creamasteric reflex' when the thigh is stroked.

The cavernous spaces are small and quite uniform in size. The glans contains a dense venous plexus but no tunica albuginea. The erectile tissue of the glans penis is composed only of convolutions of large veins; therefore, the glans penis does not become as rigid as the shaft of the penis does during erection.

The base of the penis lies within the perineum between the inferior layer of the triangular ligament and Colle's fascia (Figure 7). Fascia derived from Scarpa's and dartos fasciae cover the entire penis. The three cylinders of erectile tissue are covered by subcutaneous tissue devoid of adipose tissue but containing many smooth muscle fibers.

The skin covering the penis is very thin and is reduplicated over the glans penis as a fold, the prepuce, which is continuous with the urethral outlet. The inner surface of the prepuce is moist, nonkeratinizing and resembles a mucous membrane. The skin of the penis contains sweat glands and sebaceous glands of Tyson which are not associated with hair follicles. Very fine hairs are present at the base of the penis.

The erectile tissue within the penis is a labyrinth of irregular blood sinuses or spaces. The sinuses, supplied by capillaries and afferent arterioles, are drained by venules. When the penis is flaccid, the spaces contain little blood and appear as narrow clefts. The trabeculae of erectile tissue form the partitions between adjacent sinuses. They are composed of collagen, elastic and smooth muscle fibers as well as numerous fibroblasts. The surfaces of the trabeculae are covered with endothelium continuous with the lining of the afferent and efferent blood vessels. During erection, the sinuses become engorged with blood.

B. Vascular Supply

The internal iliac or hypogastric artery supplies most of the pelvic wall and pelvic organs. It gives rise to both the superior and inferior vesical arteries which bring arterial blood to the vas deferens and the globus minor of the epididymis (Brueschke et al. 1974). The veins of the spermatic cord after leaving the mediastinum of the testis form the pampiniform plexus. The plexus, in turn, contains at least three groups of veins. The middle group gives rise to the veins of the vas deferens which course with the vas and anastomose with other veins in the pelvis.

The vascular supply of the prostate is primarily derived from the inferior vesical artery, a branch of the anterior trunk of the internal iliac (hypogastric) artery (Figure 8) (Duclos et al. 1972). The inferior

vesical artery also supplies the seminal vesicle, base of the bladder and the vas deferens. The middle hemorrhoidal and internal pudendal arteries which enter the base of the prostate at the vesicoprostatic junction also bring blood to the gland. The veins constitute, around the ampullae and the seminal vesicles, remarkable venous plexuses which anastomose with the prostatic and pelvic plexuses.

1. Penis. The terminal branches of the internal pudendal artery, the deep and the dorsal arteries, supply blood to the penis. The deep arteries (arteria profunda) of the penis originate from the internal pudendal artery at the urogenital diaphragm. They pass through the inferior layer of the triangular ligament and eventually into the corpora cavernosa. Even before these arterial branches enter the erectile tissue, the intimal lining of the blood vessels forms ridges which protrude into the lumen. The trabecular branches of the deep arteries (helicine arteries), are spiralling arterioles. Their media is unusually thick and, as in the case of the larger arterial branches before they enter the erectile tissue, the helicine arteries contain subintimal longitudinal ridges of connective tissue and smooth muscle fibers. The convolutions in the spiralling arteries flatten during erection. Helicine arteries 65-80 μm in diameter travel in the longitudinal trabeculae of

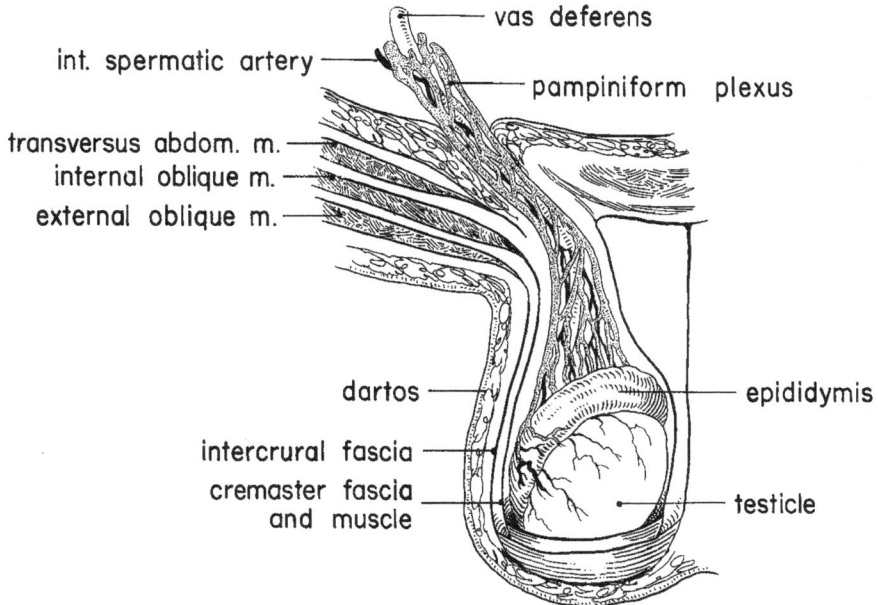

Figure 7. Musculature of the scrotum and adjacent anatomical connections (adapted from the literature).

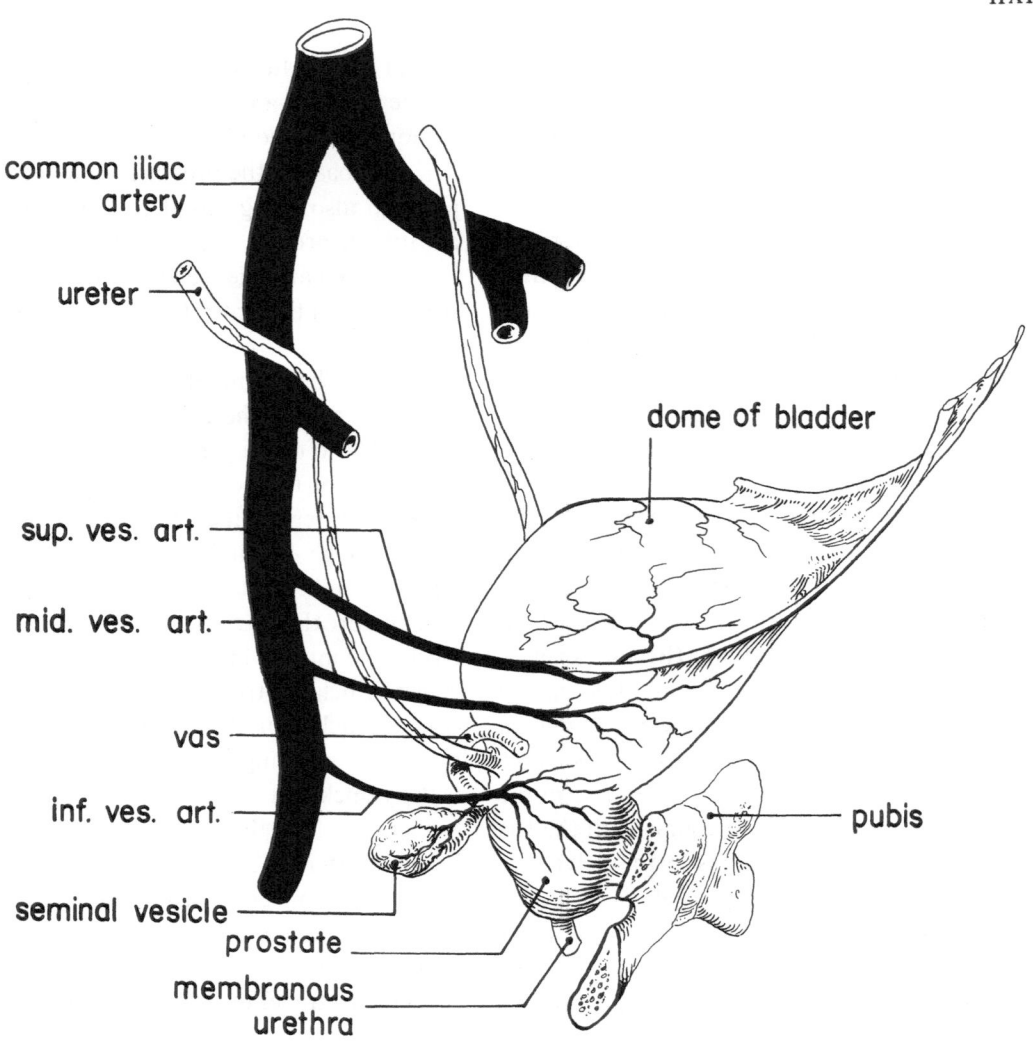

common iliac
artery

ureter

dome of bladder

sup. ves. art.

mid. ves. art.

vas

inf. ves. art.

pubis

seminal vesicle
prostate
membranous
urethra

Figure 8. Vascular supply of the prostate and bladder (adapted from the literature).

the corpora cavernosa and open directly into the sinuses (Spring-Mills and Hafez 1980).

The dorsal arteries (dorsalis penis) also pass through the inferior layer of the urogenital diaphragm and then travel between the corpora cavernosa en route to the dorsal surface of the penis. On the dorsal surface, the dorsal arteries run deep to the fascia and lateral to the deep dorsal vein of the penis. The dorsal arteries supply the skin and the fibrous sheath of the corpora cavernosa penis. Branches of the dorsal arteries pass into the sheath and anastomose with the deep arteries of the penis. When the penis is flaccid only a small amount of blood enters the sinuses and the major fraction of the blood comes from the dorsal artery. A bulbar artery supplies the corpus spongiosum.

The veins of the penis belong to two groups: a superficial and a deep group (Figure 9). The superficial group drains the foreskin and skin; however, most of the blood leaves the penis through the deep veins which drain the glans penis and the corpora cavernosa. All the major branches of the deep veins (vena profunda penis) have very thick muscular walls. They originate within and just beneath the albuginea, especially the posterior regions of the erectile tissue, from the junction of the branched postcavernous venules which have no smooth muscle in their walls. The initial set of veins draining the corpora cavernosa penis empty into larger caliber vessels with funnel-shaped valves which retard the egress of blood. The walls of these veins are so thick that at first glance they may be mistaken for arteries. Columns of longitudinal smooth muscle fibers in the subendothelium impart

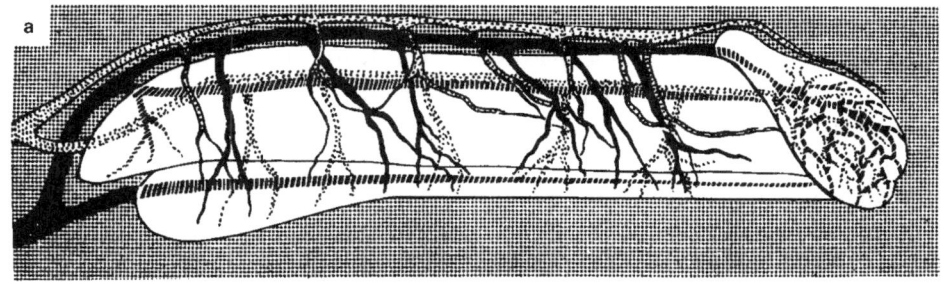

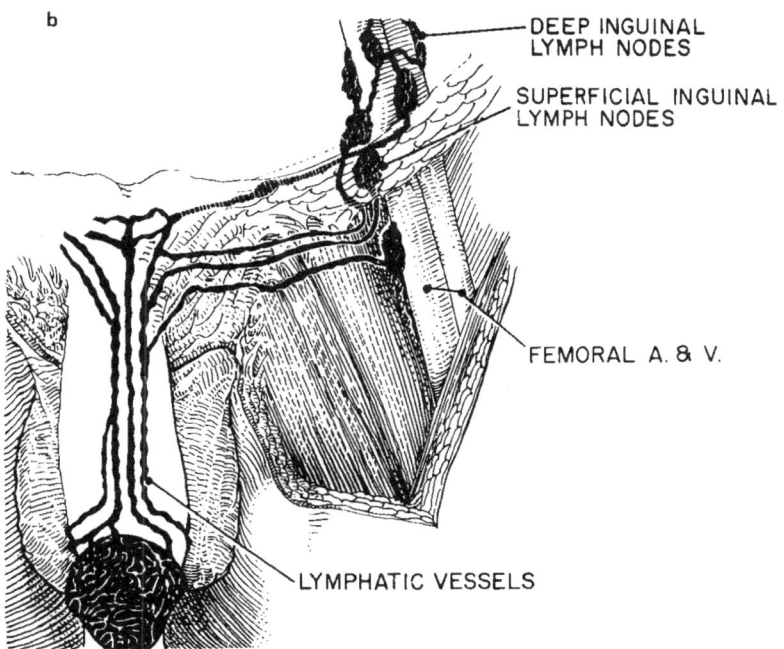

Figure 9. Vascular and lymph supply of the penis. a. The veins of the penis are composed of a superficial and a deep group. The superficial veins drain the foreskin and skin of the penis, run backward in the subcutaneous tissue and empty into the external pudendal vein. The deep veins lie beneath the deep fascia of the penis and drain the glans penis and the corpora cavernosa. They course backward through the suspensory ligament of the penis and the arcuate pubic ligament to empty into the pudendal plexus. b. The lymphatics of the penis are composed of two main groups. Those from the skin empty into the superficial and deep inguinal nodes, whereas those from the glans and corpora empty into the deep inguinal and external iliac nodes (after Flocks and Culp 1967).

an irregular contour to the lumen. Ultimately the deep veins empty into the pudendal plexus.

Blood from the corpus spongiosum, surrounding the urethra, is drained primarily by the dorsal veins (vena dorsalis penis). The terminals of these vessels originate from the lacunae and exit by piercing the albuginea.

2. Prostate. The prostate is supplied by two groups of arteries a) an external capsular group which shows little change with age and hyperplasia; and b) an internal group, the urethral group, which enlarges with age and with hyperplasia. The latter group is of clinical significance in relation to transurethral prostatic resection and in local repair following this operation for two reasons: a) its anatomic arrangement – the urethral group of arteries penetrates at the prostatic-vesicle junction and then turns distally in a course more or less parallel to the urethral surface, and b) its ultimate destination – this group of arteries forms the main source of blood supply to the hypertrophied portion of the prostate (Flocks and Culp 1967).

The prostatic veins form a plexus around the base of the gland, especially on the anterior and lateral surface. This plexus receives branches of the deep dorsal vein of the penis, the pudendal and vesical venous plexuses. Ultimately the prostatic plexus terminates in several small veins which join the internal iliac (hypogastric) veins. The veins in and near the capsule of the prostate are of unexpectedly large caliber (Spring-Mills and Hafez 1980). If and when these veins are accidentally transacted during transurethral resection, severe systemic infection and/or intravascular hemolysis can arise if the irrigating fluid is not isotonic or sterile.

C. Lymph Supply

The lymphatic vessels of the epididymis and vas deferens end in the external iliac nodes (Pabst 1970; Pabst and Lippert 1970). The lymphatic drainage from the prostate primarily enters the internal iliac (hypogastric) and presacral nodes. Lymphatics from the prostate may drain into the sacral, vesical

and external iliac lymph nodes (Figure 10).

The lymphatics form plexuses, which lead into the lymph nodes of the pelvic wall. Lymphatics from the skin of the penis drain into the superficial and deep inguinal nodes. Lymphatics from the glans penis and corpora empty into the deep inguinal and external iliac nodes.

D. Nerve Supply

The male reproductive tract receives sympathetic and parasympathetic innervation through the pelvic ganglia (Figures 11, 12). The sympathetic fibers come from the twelfth thoracic and upper lumbar segments of the spinal cord. They descend to the presacral area. Below the aortic bifurcation they form the superior hypogastric plexus, which divides at the first level of the sacrum into two hypogastric nerves (Spring-Mills and Hafez 1980).

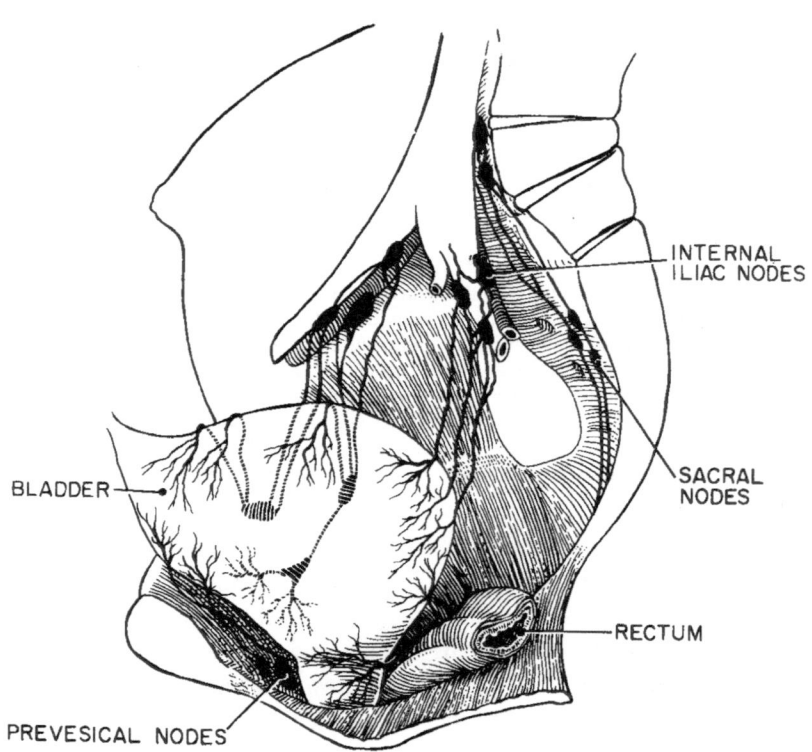

Figure 10. Lymph supply. The lymphatics of the bladder accompany the veins. They begin in the submucosal layer of the bladder wall and collect in increasingly larger channels until they join the lymphatic plexus at the base of the bladder or empty directly into the internal iliac lymph nodes at the bifurcation of the aorta. The lymph channels from the anterior wall of the bladder may empty into the external iliac nodes while some of the lateral lymphatics course along the hollow of the sacrum to the presacral nodes (after Flocks and Culp 1967).

Branches of the superior and inferior hypogastric plexus supply the prostate and seminal vesicles. Fibers from the inferior hypogastric plexus also give rise to periureteral nerve loops which supply the ejaculatory ducts and pass down the vas deferens to the epididymis.

The spermatic cord, epididymis, vas deferens and testis are innervated by the superior, middle and inferior spermatic nerves. The middle spermatic nerves, which are derived from the superior hypogastric plexus, join the vas deferens at the internal inguinal ring. The inferior spermatic nerves, derived chiefly from the inferior hypogastric nerve plexus, also innervate the vas deferens and epididymis.

A few preganglionic and many postganglionic fibers innervate individual smooth muscle cells of the vas deferens. Most of the postganglionic fibers are adrenergic (Baumgarten et al. 1971).

1. Accessory Glands. The accessory glands are innervated by several types of sensory nerve endings in the connective tissue and free nerve endings in the epithelium. The autonomic innervation is parasympathetic and sympathetic (hypogastric nerve) from the pelvic plexus. If the plexus is resected or the sympathetic chain above is interrupted, there is no reflex release of the glandular secretions. Stimulation of the hypogastric nerves causes peristaltic contraction of the vas deferens, seminal vesicles and prostate, whereas stimulation of the parasympathetic system of the administration of pilocarpine activates prostatic secretions (Blacklock 1976).

2. Penis. The nerve supply of the penis comes from the pudendal nerve and the pelvic autonomic plexus. The pudendal nerve supplies motor function to the bulbocavernosus and ischiocavernosus

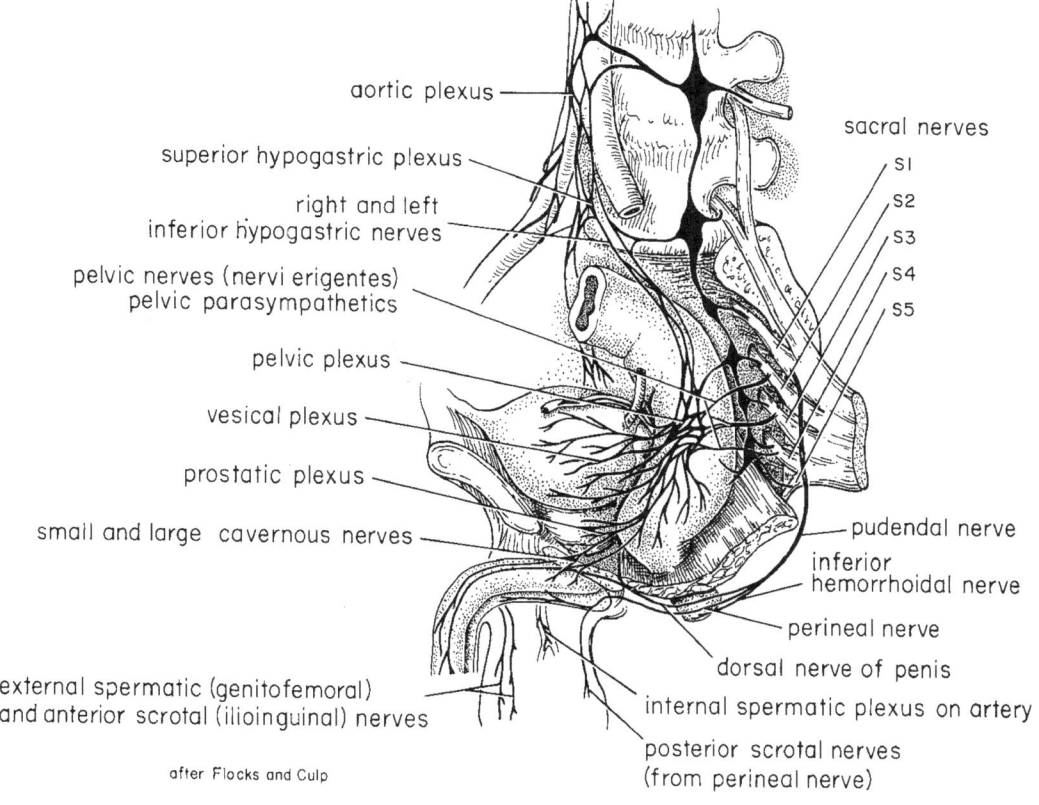

aortic plexus

superior hypogastric plexus

right and left
inferior hypogastric nerves

pelvic nerves (nervi erigentes)
pelvic parasympathetics

pelvic plexus

vesical plexus

prostatic plexus

small and large cavernous nerves

external spermatic (genitofemoral)
and anterior scrotal (ilioinguinal) nerves

after Flocks and Culp

sacral nerves
S1
S2
S3
S4
S5

pudendal nerve
inferior
hemorrhoidal nerve
perineal nerve
dorsal nerve of penis
internal spermatic plexus on artery
posterior scrotal nerves
(from perineal nerve)

Figure 11. Nerve supply of the bladder and some pelvic organs. The sympathetic fibers reach the bladder from the first, second and third lumbar segments through the presacral nerve which passes to the hypogastric ganglions located in front of the fifth lumbar and first sacral vertebrae between the two common iliac arteries (B). The sacral autonomic nerves are carried by the nervi erigentes to the hypogastric plexus which acts as a relay station for both the sympathetic and parasympathetic stimuli. From the hypogastric plexus the post-ganglionic fibers of both the sacral and lumbar outflow proceed to the detrusor muscle and trigone of the bladder. The afferent fibers of the bladder travel along the sympathetic chain to the posterior roots of the first and second lumbar nerves and along the sacral autonomic nerves into the sacral posterior nerve roots (after Flocks and Culp 1967).

muscles, the muscles of the urogenital diaphragm and the external sphincter (sphincter urethrae). The skin of the penis, perineum and posterior aspect of the scrotum are innervated from the pudendal nerve. Corpuscles of Meissner occur in the papillae of the skin of the prepuce and the glans. Genital corpuscles are found in the dermis of the glans and the mucosa of the urethra, whereas Vater-Pacini corpuscles occur along the dorsal vein, in the connective tissue of the glans and under the tunica albuginea of the corpora cavernosa.

The smooth muscle surrounding the corpora cavernosa and the arterioles within the trabeculae of the penis are innervated from the pelvic autonomic plexus via the hypogastric and prostatic plexus.

III. PHYSIOLOGY

During fetal development, puberty and old age the male reproductive organs undergo a remarkable developmental and involutionary change. For example, during the third trimester, the prostate enlarges because of maternal gonadal and gonadotropic hormones, then atrophies a few days after birth and does not fully develop until puberty. Atrophic changes recur with advancing age – usually during the fifth decade – and affect different parts of the gland in various ways. The median lobe, the glands of Albarran and the two lateral lobes often enlarge and undergo nodular hyperplasia. The fact that nodular hyperplasia generally arises in those regions and malignant tumors in the so-called outer glands or posterior lobe suggests there may be functional diversity within the prostate (Franks 1974).

At puberty, the hormones secreted by the testis, activated by the pituitary gland, induce maturation of the accessory organs. Castration, hypophysectomy or androgen deficiency produce atrophy and cessation of secretion during postpubertal life, whereas, estrogens produce atrophy of the glands in most postpubertal boys. Androgen replacement therapy will reverse the atrophy (postpubertal) or restore normal maturation of the prepubertal glands. Pituitary gonadotropins, however, usually affect accessory glands only when functional testi-

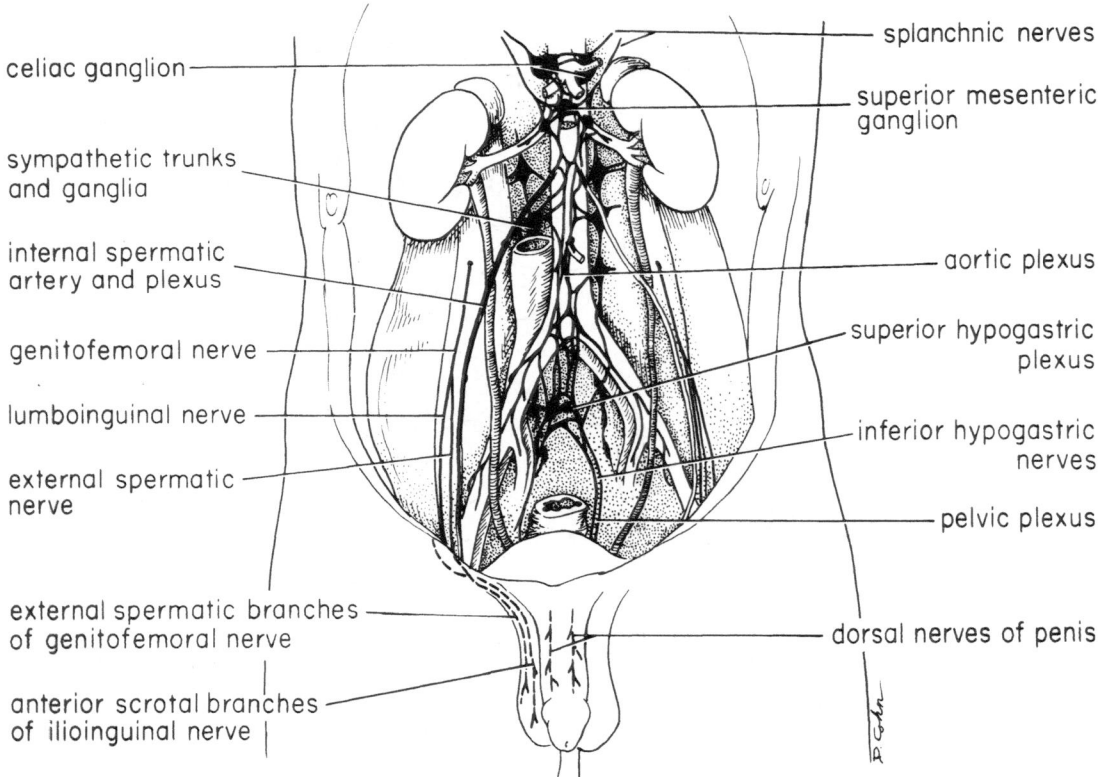

celiac ganglion

splanchnic nerves

superior mesenteric ganglion

sympathetic trunks and ganglia

internal spermatic artery and plexus

aortic plexus

genitofemoral nerve

superior hypogastric plexus

lumboinguinal nerve

inferior hypogastric nerves

external spermatic nerve

pelvic plexus

external spermatic branches of genitofemoral nerve

dorsal nerves of penis

anterior scrotal branches of ilioinguinal nerve

Figure 12. Innervation of male accessory sex organs (after Spring-Mills and Hafez 1980).

cular tissue is present or the gonadotropins are given together with testosterone (Franks 1974; Flocks 1974). The development of the accessory organs reflects the endocrine activity of the patient, rather than his sexual capacities which are not necessarily equivalent.

The physiological functions of the male reproductive organs (Table 4) are controlled by various regulatory mechanisms (Table 5, Figures 13, 14). Several biochemical components of the secretions of seminal vesicles and prostate are used as biochemical markers for the diagnosis of functional activities of these glands (Table 6).

A. Erection

The physiological mechanisms of erection involve:

a) the closure of arterio-venous anastomoses between the deep artery of the penis and the peripheral venous return; b) the constriction of penial arterioles which facilitate the entry of blood into the corpora cavernosa; and c) the simultaneous constriction of efferent penial veins which prevent blood from leaving the cavernosa. As the helicine arteries open and their intimal ridges flatten, the lacunae of the cavernous spaces fill with blood. In the corpora cavernosa the large central sinuses compress the small peripheral spaces as well as the veins on the lateral surfaces of the penis between tunica albuginea and Buck's fascia. Therefore, blood flow is restricted, and blood accumulates in the corpora cavernosa under increased pressure causing the erectile tissue to become rigid. When a critical amount of blood (i.e. 20-50 ml/min) flows

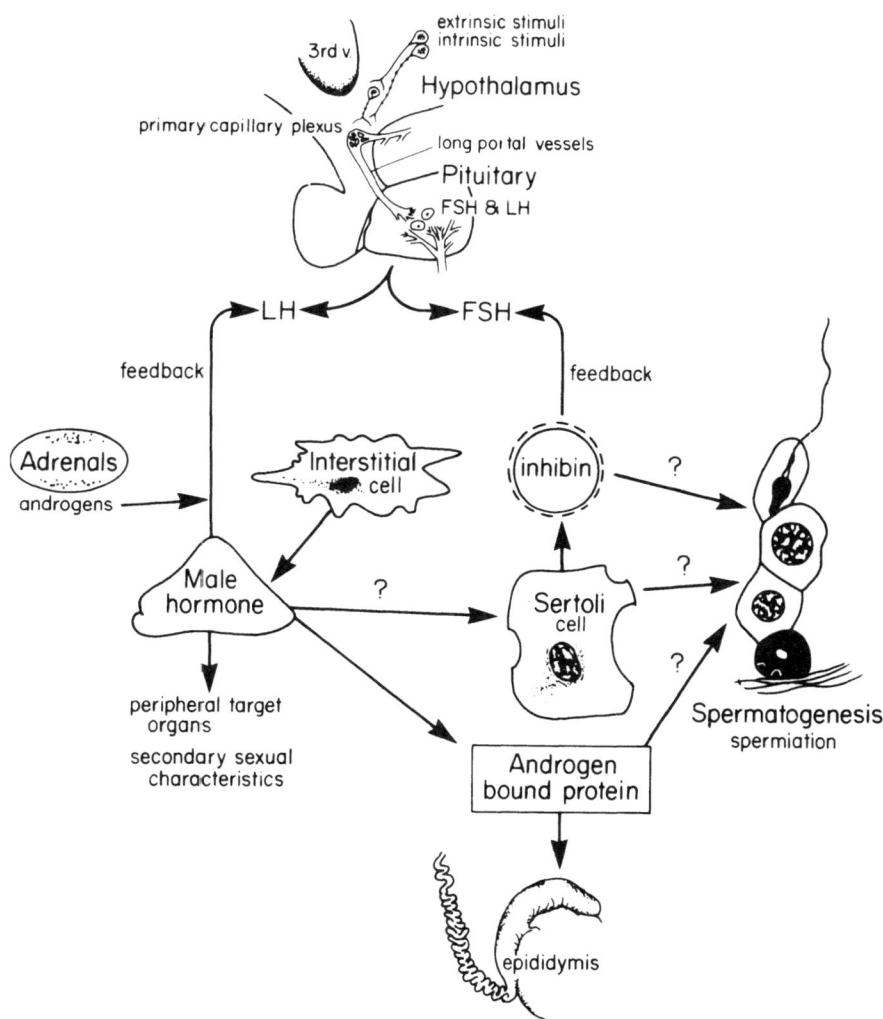

Figure 13. Hormonal control of reproductive function in the male.

Table 4. Physiological functions of male reproductive organs.

Organ	Functions
Testis	1. Spermatocytogenesis: cellular division which reduces DNA content of cells to one half of somatic cells, spermatid haploid cells: 2. Spermogenesis: spermatid undergoes 4 major metamorphic changes (Golgi, cap, acrosomal, and maturation phase) to form spermatozoa; 3. myoid cells: contraction of tubules; 4. Sertoli cell a) secretion of fluid into lumen of seminiferous tubules, b) synthesis of proteins, c) phagocytosis of degenerating germ cells and residual bodies, d) facilitate release of spermatozoa in lumen, e) facilitate movement of germ cells from base of tubule to lumen, f) metabolism of steroids, g) formation of blood-testis barrier; 5. Leydig cells: steroidogenesis – biosynthesis of 5 pregnenolone from cholesterol occurs in Leydig cell mitochondria; newly formed 5-pregnenolone can be stored in the mitochondria or transported to the smooth endoplasmic reticulum, to be converted to 3-Byl-sulfate conjugate and/or to successive steps of steroidogenesis.
Epididymis	Sperm are stored in tail of epididymis where lumen of duct is widest and internal milieu is conducive for sperm survival; about half of the sperm which enter the head of the epididymis disintegrate before reaching its tail; tail of the epididymis contains some 70% of sperm in male tract; increasing motility during epididymal transport reflects maturational processes associated with sperm fertilizability; maturation of epididymal sperm may involve progressive changes in flexibility and patterns of movement of their flagella. Testiculo-epididymal secretion is continuous, it progresses along the epididymal duct and the vas deferens which ensures the transport of sperm by their motility and it then accumulates in the ampulla of the vas deferens.
Vas deferens	Sperm transport through the vas deferens at ejaculation and during sexual rest; physical pressure exerted by the accumulation of epididymal spermatozoa force the sperm into and through the vas deferens; the vas may contract spontaneously during sexual rest. During sexual rest many spermatozoa stored in the epididymis are transported through the vas during ejaculation by coordinated contractions presumably controlled by release of norepinephrine from the nerve endings in its wall. Vas deferens may be involved in the maintenance and regulation of sperm viability and metabolism and overall integrity of the male reproductive system. The lumen of the vas varies greatly in size even from one vas to the other within the same individual. The ability of the vas to stretch and to change the diameter of its lumen is important since approx. 100 to 500 million spermatozoa can pass through the vas at one time. 60-70% of the spermatozoa within a normal ejaculate come from the epididymis and proximal part of the vas and these spermatozoa are contained within 50-60% of the total ejaculate volume. Sperm transport through the vas deferens may involve a peristaltic mechanism, seminal fluid may be delivered by the vas into prostatic urethra within 12 seconds. Vas can synthesize testosterone and other steroids from acetate; these steroids may depress the respiratory metabolism of spermatozoa.
Ampulla	Contraction of the ampulla causes expulsion of spermatozoa; motor reflexes play a role in the initiation of contractions of various muscles of the anterior perineum. The high pressure obtained in the dilated urethra forces open the striated sphincter and spermatozoa are released.
Seminal vesicle	Secretions, accumulated in interior of gland, are excreted during ejaculation by the contraction of two layers of muscularis connected to a plexus of nerve fibers and sympathetic ganglia. Secretions, 0.8 to 1.3 ml in volume, make up 70% of the ejaculate and can be collected by digital massage of gland. Secretions are continuous but may occur in 'spurts' for the glandular cells do not have a very active basal rhythm. Seminal vesicles are depleted in a single ejaculate as judged by the fructose test. During sexual excitement, the seminal vesicles become extremely tense, and undergo contraction; during coitus secretion is intensely stimulated under influence of neural stimuli. At emission, the contents of the vas deferens are discharged into the posterior urethra via the ejaculatory duct without first entering the seminal vesicle as occurs during sexual rest. During ejaculation, the seminal vesicles undergo 6-10 peristaltic contractions discharging secretions into the urethra; levator ani contractions facilitate the emission of secretion. Prostaglandin originates from the seminal vesicles, and their concentration. Seminal vesicles are not a storage depot for spermatozoa. Last fraction of the ejaculate contains primarily seminal vesicle secretions; very few immotile or quality spermatozoa which may have been transported into the gland during sexual rest (the longer the period of sexual rest, the larger the number of spermatozoa that accumulate in the seminal vesicles). Seminal vesicle fluids, ejaculated last, may serve to flush spermatozoa from the urethra. Secretions, rich in fructose citric acid, provide nutritive supplies

Organ	Structural characteristics
	and energy to ejaculated spermatozoa. Fructose is metabolized by the mitochondria in the middle piece of the spermatozoa which liberate energy required for sperm motility. Vesicular fluid contains certain 'protective agents' e.g., proteinase inhibitors which presumably preserve sperm activity by stabilizing sperm membranes preventing the release of active acrosomal enzymes. Gland produces proteinase inhibitors, e.g., antichymotrypsin, other low molecular weight inhibitors found in semen.
Prostate	0.5-2 ml of prostatic secretions (continual state of activity) are transported directly from the excretory ducts into the urethra via the openings on the right and left sides of the colliculus seminalis (verumontanum or prostatic utricle). The smooth muscle surrounding the entire gland is involved in seminal emission. Secretions account for some 30% of the ejaculate. The presence of specific compounds together with the absence of fructose is used as biochemical marker to differentiate prostatic from seminal vesicle contributions to the seminal plasma. Secretions contain diastase, beta glucuronidase, proteolytic enzymes, fibrinolysin, citric acid, acid phosphatase, choline, cephalin, cholesterol, magnesium and zinc. Essentially all the citric acid and zinc within seminal plasma originates in the prostate. Acid phosphatase is also a principal constituent, but it is not yet known how unique any of the acid phosphatases are to the prostate. Clear viscid, mucus-like secretions are discharged during erection and possibly during orgasm; secretions ejaculated prior to spermatozoa may lubricate the urethra. Secretions may not be essential for reproduction; they contribute several metabolites to the seminal plasma to facilitate fertilizability and coagulation/liquefaction of semen, e.g., fibrinolysin, coagulase and other coagulum-lysing enzyme secretions promote sperm survival by reducing acidity of the urethra. Secretions contribute certain metabolites (e.g., albumin) to seminal plasma which stimulates and enhances motility of epididymal and washed, ejaculated spermatozoa. Acid phosphatase, in secretions, by hydrolyzing phosphorylcholine to choline is directly concerned with sperm metabolism.
Bulbo urethra	Clear, viscid, mucus-like secretions are discharged during erection and possibly during orgasm; secretions, rich in sialoprotein, are emptied into first part of the cavernous urethra. Secretions, ejaculated prior to spermatozoa, may lubricate the urethra.

into the cavernosa, an erection could occur independent of a blockage in venous return (Newman et al. 1964). It is also possible to assume that other factors such as parasympathetic activity for closing the AV complexes and increasing flow of blood into the sinuses and sympathetic activity for constricting the arterioles in the remainder of the penis are required in addition to the critical volume.

Using corpus cavernosography Fitzpatrick (1975) reported that in the flaccid state venous return from the glans penis takes about one minute, while the transit time from the corpora cavernosa takes up to ten minutes. The anatomic differences between the venous system of the glans penis and corpora cavernosa seem to be responsible for the difference in drainage times. By making serial cavernosograms, the entire venous network of the penis is outlined. Each corpus cavernosum communicates with the other via medial septal apertures and their associated blood vessels. The cavernosum also communicates with the glans penis and the circumflex venous drainage system which originates on the under surface of each cavernosum and passes along the lateral surfaces of the penis between the tunica albuginea and Buck's fascia. These veins end

at bulbous junctions between the circumflex and dorsal or circumflex and ventral veins. Since the venous blood from the glans penis is returned rapidly and does not drain through the circumflex system, it is possible that the cavernosum venous system impedes venous drainage and thereby might play a role in maintaining erection. Elderly men with unsustained erections have little venous drainage through the circumflex system and little blood trapped within the cavernous sinuses.

The penial vasculature has various anatomical characteristics which assist in maintaining erection by delaying venous return from the corpora cavernosa, e.g. the funnel-shaped valves of the deep dorsal veins (Fitzpatrick and Cooper 1975). Men with well sustained erections have competent deep dorsal vein valves just distal to the suspensory ligament whereas in aged men with unsustained erections the presence and competency of the deep dorsal valves is diminished. The overall lag in venous return circulation at the time of erection may be attributed to the complicated circumflex venous network, the sluggish action of the deep dorsal vein valves and to the retention of a critical volume of blood within the cavernosa (Fitzpatrick 1975).

The increase in blood flow into the corpus cavernosum during erection is accompanied by an increased venous return from the penis. Thus, a venous-return blocking mechanism for either the initiation or maintenance of erection may be unnecessary.

B. Ejaculation

Ejaculation involves the emission or transport of semen into the urethra, the propulsion of semen out of the urethra during orgasm and closure of the bladder neck. Normal ejaculation depends upon an intact autonomic nervous system. Afferent stimuli from the glans penis travel over the pudendal nerve into the spinal cord and on into the cerebral cortex. Efferent fibers, in turn, travel through the antero-

lateral column to the thoracolumbar sympathetic outflow at the spinal sympathetic ganglia T_{12} - L_3. This sympathetic output stimulates smooth muscle contraction and probably peristalsis within the vas deferens, which, in turn, propels semen from the tail of the epididymis to the ampulla of the vas deferens. In addition, the sympathetic impulses cause the smooth muscle within the ampulla of the vas,

Table 5. Physiological mechanisms which regulate testicular function.

Organ	Mechanisms
Brain	Exteroceptive factors
	Sensory modalities
Hypothalmus	Monoamines (Dopamine, norepinephrine)
	Gonadotropin releasing hormones
Pituitary	FSH, LH, Growth Hormone, Prolactin
Sertoli cells	Inhibin, androgen bound protein
Interstitial cells in testis	Androgens, estrogens, other steroids, binding proteins

Table 6. Some biochemical components of the secretions of seminal vesicles and prostate.

Seminal vesicle	Prostate
Ascorbic acid*	Acid phosphatase*
Citric acid (traces)	Albumin
Fructose*	α-amylase
Inorganic phosphorous	Beta glucuronidase
Lactoferrin	Cephalin
Phosphorylcholine	Cholesterol
Prostaglandins	Choline
Protein	Citric acid*
Proteinase inhibitors	Diastase
Sodium	Fibrinolytic enzymes
	Inositol
	Magnesium
	Plasminogen activator
	Proteolytic enzymes
	Seminin
	Sodium
	Spermine
	Zinc*

* Used as biochemical marker for diagnosis of functional activity of gland.

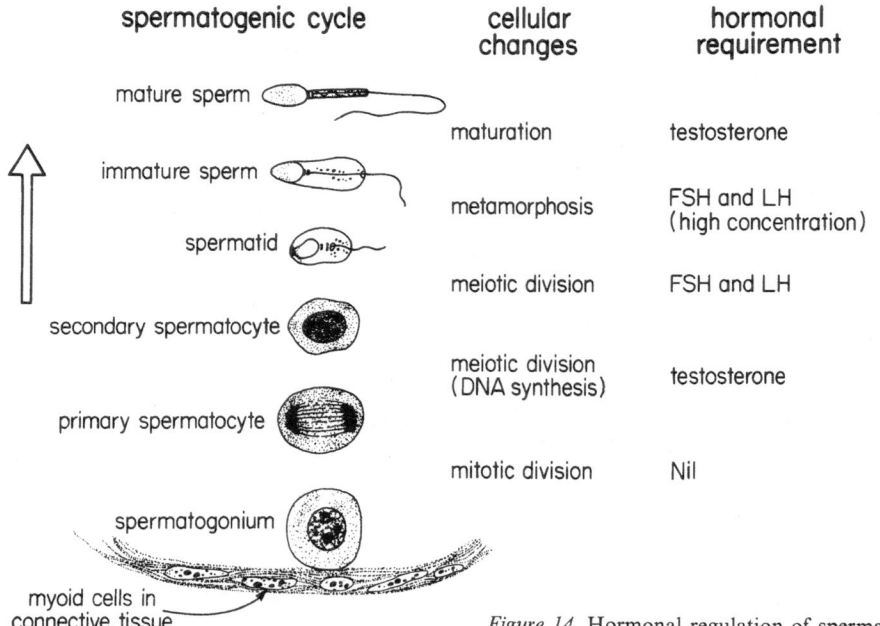

spermatogenic cycle	cellular changes	hormonal requirement
mature sperm	maturation	testosterone
immature sperm	metamorphosis	FSH and LH (high concentration)
spermatid	meiotic division	FSH and LH
secondary spermatocyte		
primary spermatocyte	meiotic division (DNA synthesis)	testosterone
spermatogonium	mitotic division	Nil
myoid cells in connective tissue		

Figure 14. Hormonal regulation of spermatogenesis.

prostate, seminal vesicles and the neck of the bladder to contract. Secretions of the seminal vesicles and prostate are then released in the ejaculatory duct (Figure 15). This results in the transport or emission of semen into the posterior urethra.

Efferent impulses from the sacral parasympathetics initiate clonic contraction of the bulbocavernosus, ischiocavernosus and other muscles of the pelvic floor, lower extremities and trunk. These responses in conjunction with the complete closure of the bladder neck culminate in ejaculation.

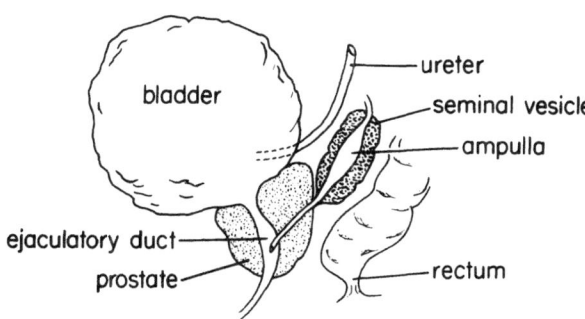

Figure 15. Anatomical relationship of the ureter, bladder, seminal vesicle, prostate and ejaculatory duct (redrawn from Becker 1967).

IV. CONGENITAL ANOMALIES AND PATHO-PHYSIOLOGY

Unilateral and bilateral anomalies of the male reproductive organs include:

1) ectopic sites of the testes in relation to the external ring (Figure 16);
2) various types of congenital obstructive azoospermia (Figure 17);
3) congenital remnants from which a spermatocele may arise (Figure 18);
4) various types of hydrocele (Figure 19);
5) distension due to a localized lesion or severe infection, e.g., pyospermatocyst;
6) amputation of the vas deferens or seminal vesicle;
7) atrophy of a seminal duct;
8) communication with an extra-vesicular lesion; and
9) deferential, ampullary or vesicular calcifications, several congenital and acquired anomalies may be detected by proper palpation during routine physical examination, e.g. lipomas, fibromas,

leiomyomas, hemangiomas, lymphangiomas, neurilemmomas, adenomatoid tumors, teratomas, agenesis, atresia and duplications of the spermatic cords and vas deferens and certain diseases of the prostate, seminal vesicle, spermatic cord and urethra.

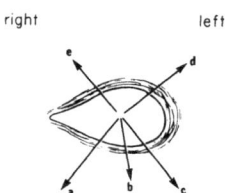

Figure 16. Ectopic sites of the testes in relation to external ring.
a. Scrotal (normal).
b. Perineal.
c. Femoral.
d. Superficial inguinal.
e. Pubic. From Girgis and Hafez 1980.

Most obstructive lesions of the vas deferens are not found on the duct itself, but at its origin or at its termination, i.e., on the tail of the epididymis or its origin in the ampulla. Mechanical lesions of the vas deferens include hernia, cysts of spermatic cord, undescended testis, varicoceles, surgery including ligature or reanastomosis. Congenital absence of vas may be accompanied by absence of seminal vesicle and atrophy of the epididymis.

The occurrence of sperm granuloma, testicular degeneration and the development of auto-immunity post-vasectomy, in cases of congenital absence of the vas or as sequelae to Bilharzial infections all indirectly illustrate the overall importance of the vas deferens in the normal homeostasis of the male reproductive system (Hackett and Waterhouse 1973; Heidger and Sawatzke 1977).

Normal seminal vesicles usually are not palpable. They become palpable, hard, and indurated during chronic infection and advanced carcinoma. The walls of the vesicles become thickened and fibrous in consistency during these diseases. Seminal vesiculitis from gonorrheal, tuberculous or nonspecific infections may result in abscess formation. When tuberculosis is present, the vesicles are filled with caseous material and this, in turn, may lead to partial or total calcification of the vesicles. All of these conditions, therefore, produce enlargement of the seminal vesicles and characteristic alterations in consistency of the glands.

X-ray cinematography has been used with contrast dyes to study the seminal vesicles before and during ejaculation (Mitsuya et al. 1960). Dye injected into the vas deferens at sexual rest flows into the seminal vesicles, then into the bladder via the ejaculatory ducts. This is primarily due to the inactivity of the bladder sphincter at sexual rest. When the bladder sphincter is damaged, retrograde ejaculate, seminal plasma and spermatozoa are transported during ejaculation into the bladder.

The viscid, yellowish secretions are characterized by the presence of an unusually high level of fructose (315 mg/100 ml), the concentration of which is used as a biochemical marker to indicate the functional activity of the seminal vesicles.

Since the seminal vesicles are of the same embryonic origin as the vas deferens, the congenital absence of the vas is associated with the absence of the seminal vesicles. This is of clinical significance

to differentiate azoospermia (complete absence of spermatozoa) due to testicular abnormalities from that due to bilateral congenital absence of the vas deferens. In the latter case, semen contains no fructose. Only small amounts of citric acid are present in the seminal vesicles, most of it being produced in the prostate.

During collection of vesicular fluid by massage of the gland, it is difficult to avoid the contamination of the vesicular fluid with the ampullary, prostatic and urethral secretions. Sampling of vesicular fluid by the massage of the seminal vesicle gives mainly prostatic fluid, since the index finger only rarely reaches the seminal vesicle.

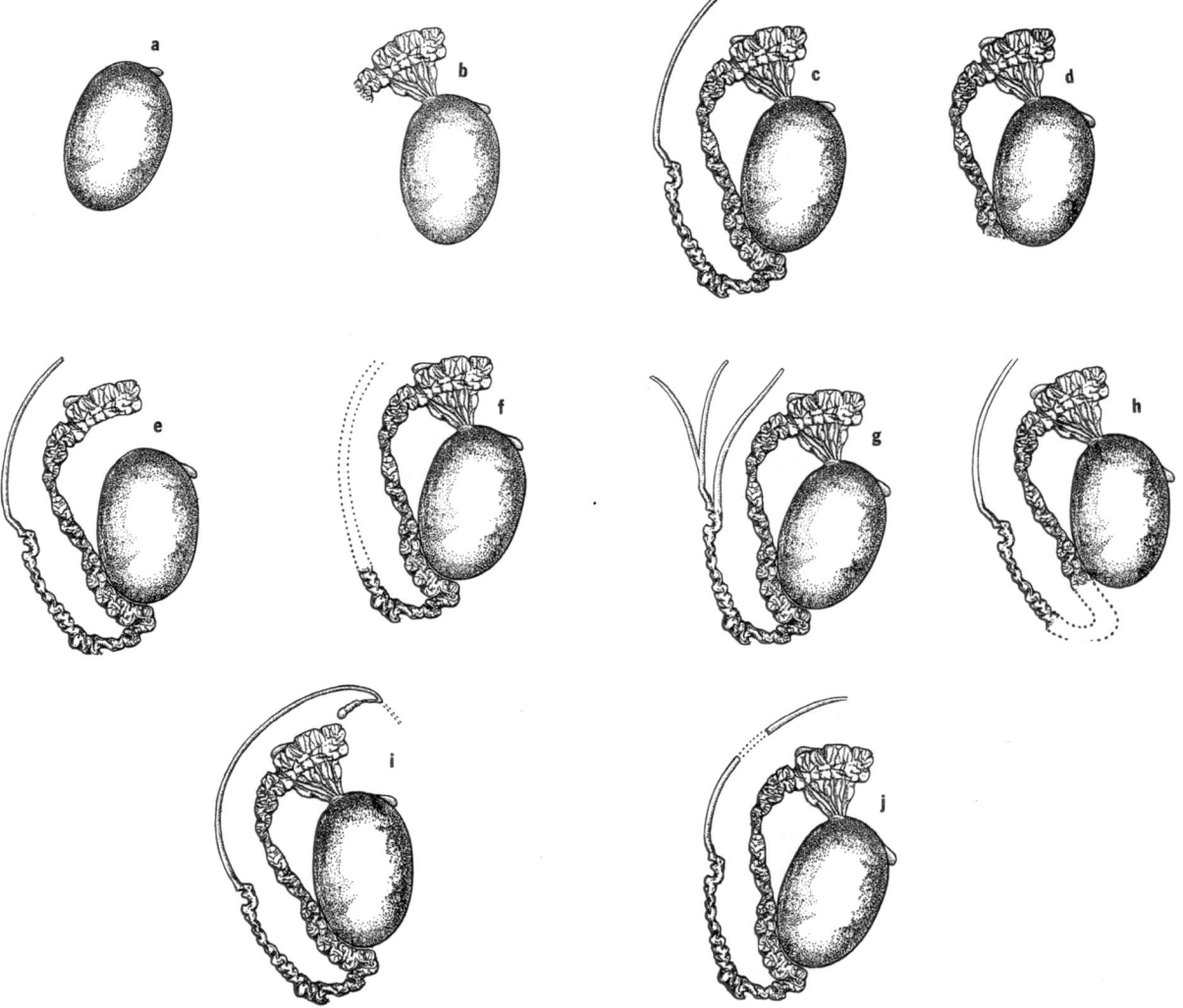

Figure 17. Types of congenital obstructive azoospermia. a. Absence of the whole epididymis and vas deferens. b. Absence of body and tail of epididymis and of the vas deferens. c. Lack of communication between head and body of the epididymis. d. Absence of the vas deferens. e. Lack of communication between testes and epididymis. f. Partial absence of the vas deferens (dotted). g. Vas deferens dividing and ending blindly. h. Lack of canalization or communication between tail of the epididymis and vas deferens. i. Atresia, lack of canalization or absence of the ejaculatory duct. j. Atresia or lack of canalization along course of the vas. From Girgis and Hafez 1980.

Prepubertal castration produces underdevelopment of seminal vesicle and secretory failure; whereas postpubertal castration causes atrophy of epithelium, which can be rejuvenated by exogenous androgens.

The mobility of the prostate is restricted in advanced carcinoma because of extension of the tumor through the capsule. Prostatic massage and microscopic examination of the gland's secretion are important for detecting a symptomatic prostatitis and ultimately preventing cystitis and epididymitis. However, prostatic massage is contraindicated in patients suffering from acute urethral discharge, acute prostatitis, acute prostatocystitis, carcinoma or those with nearly complete urinary retention.

The prostatic fluid obtained by prostatic massage, called 'resting fluid', differs in composition from 'stimulated' secretion during ejaculation since during sexual excitement, certain compounds are secreted at an accelerated rate. For example, 'resting' fluid contains a lower concentration of acid phosphatase than does stimulated secretion (Eliasson and Lindholmer 1976).

The fluid obtained by prostatic massage is a homogeneous, serous, milky fluid that is normally only slightly acid (i.e., pH 6.5) and becomes basic (i.e., pH 7.7) in men afflicted by prostatitis. Less than 1 percent of the prostatic secretion is protein; and the relative enrichment of prostatic secretion (compared to blood plasma) with free amino acids may be due to the action of proteolytic and transaminating enzymes in the prostatic epithelium (Farnsworth 1976).

In general cystic dilation of the spermatic cord is associated with hydrocele or hernia. Diffuse swelling, induration and hardness are associated with filarial funiculitis and a solid elevation may indicate a sarcoma. Fusiform enlargements of the vas may be associated with tuberculosis whereas a generalized firmness and thickening often indicates chronic infection.

Urethral stricture and prostatic obstruction often are associated with a poor urinary stream and/or tender areas of induration along the urethra. Urethral discharge, then, is examined for microorganisms, blood and pus. The viscosity and amount of the discharges provides clues to the cause(s) of the condition.

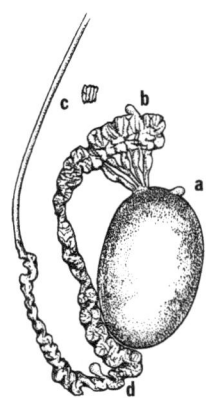

Figure 18. Congenital remnants from which a spermatocele may arise. a. Appendix testis (Müllerian origin). b. Appendix epididymis (Wollfian origin). c. Paradidymis (Wollfian origin). d. Aberrant vas deferens (Wollfian origin). From Girgis and Hafez, 1980.

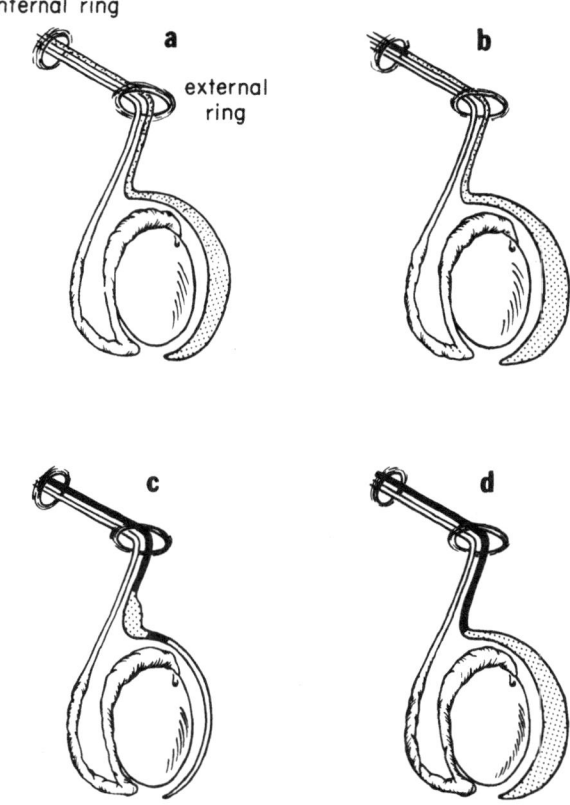

Figure 19. Various types of hydrocele. a. Congenital, b. Infantile; note closure of processus vaginalis at internal vein. c. Hydrocele of the cord. The processus vaginalis is closed at its two terminal ends whereas the middle part is patent allowing hydrocele formation. d. Vaginal hydrocele. The fluid accumulates in terminal part of processus vaginalis. From Girgis and Hafez 1980.

REFERENCES

Batra SK and Lardner TJ: Sperm transport in the vas deferens. In: Human semen and fertility regulation in men, Hafez ESE (ed), Mosby, St. Louis, 1976.

Baumgarten HG, Holstein AF and Rosengren E: Arrangement, ultrastructure and adrenergic innervation of smooth musculature of the ductuli efferentes, ductus epididymis and ductus deferens of man. Z Zellforsch Mikrosk Anat 120: 37, 1971.

Becker RF: Ph D thesis, Michigan State University, East Lansing, 1967.

Blacklock NJ: Surgical anatomy of the prostate. In: Scientific foundations of urology, Williams DI and Chisholm GD (eds), William Heinemann Medical Publ, Chicago, 1976.

Brueschke E, Burns M, Maness JH, Wingfield JR, Mayerhofer K and Zaneveld LJD: Development of a reversible vas deferens occlusive device. I. Anatomical size of the human and dog vas deferens. Fertil Steril 25: 659, 1974.

Duclos JM, Chanzy M and Alexandre JH: Contributions to the study of the prostatic vasculature. Arch Anat Path 20: 355, 1972.

Eliasson R, and Lindholmer C: Functions of male accessory genital organs. In: Human semen and fertility regulation in men, Hafez ESE (ed), Mosby, St. Louis, 1976.

Farnsworth WE: Physiology and biochemistry. In: Scientific foundations of urology, Williams DI and Chisholm GD (eds), William Heinemann Medical Publ, Chicago, 1976.

Fitzpatrick T: The corpus cavernosum intercommunicating venous drainage system. J Urol 113: 494, 1975.

Fitzpatrick TJ and Cooper JF: A cavernosogram study on the valvular competence of the human deep dorsal vein. J Urol 173: 497, 1975.

Flocks RH: The radical treatment of prostatic cancer. In: The treatment of prostatic hypertrophy and neoplasia, Castro JE (ed), University Park Press, Baltimore, 1974.

Flocks RH and Culp DA: Surgical urology. A handbook of operative surgery, third edition. Year Book Medical Publishers Inc, Chicago, 1967.

Franks LM: Biology of the prostate and its tumors. In: The treatment of prostatic hypertrophy and neoplasia, Castro JE (ed), University Park Press, Baltimore, 1974.

Girgis SM and Hafez ESE: Fundamentals of andrology in human reproduction: Conception and contraception, Hafez ESE (ed), second edition, Harper and Row, Hagerstown, Maryland, forthcoming.

Hackett RE and Waterhouse K: Vasectomy – reviewed. Am J Obstet Gynecol 116: 438, 1973.

Heidger PM and Sawatzke CL: Fine structural effects of vasectomy upon the male reproductive system. In: Male reproductive system, Yates R and Gordon M (eds), Masson Publishing Co, New York, 1977.

Holstein AF: Morphologische Studien am Nebenhoden des Menschen. In: Zwanglose Abhandlungen aus dem Gebiet der normalen und pathologischen Anatomie, Bargmann W and Doerr W (eds), Stuttgart, Georg Thieme Verlag, 1969.

Holstein AF: Structure of the human epididymis. In: Human semen and fertility regulation in men, Hafez ESE (ed), Mosby, St. Louis, 1976.

Jirasek JE: Development of the genital system and male pseudohermaphroditism. Johns Hopkins Press, Baltimore, 1971.

Jirasek JE, Sulcova J, Capkova A, Rohling S and Starka L: Histochemical and biochemical investigations of 3β-hydroxy-Δ^s steroid dehydrogenase in the chorion, adrenals and gonads of human fetuses. Endokrinologie (Dresden) 54: 173, 1969.

Mitsuya J, Asai J, Suyama K, Ushida T and Hosoe K: Application of x-ray cinematography in urology. I. Mechanism of ejaculation. J Urol 83: 86, 1960.

Newman HF, Northrup JD and Devlin J: Mechanism of human penile erection. Invest Urol 1: 350, 1964.

Pabst R: Studies on the human ductus deferens. Adv Androl 1: 135, 1970.

Pabst R and Lippert H: The vas deferens. Anat Anx 126: 543, 1970.

Price D: Concluding remarks. In: Normal and abnormal growth of the prostate, Goland M and Thomas CC (eds), Springfield, Illinois, 1975.

Schmidt SS: Anastomosis of the vas deferens: an experimental study. III. Dilatation of the vas following obstruction. J Urol 81: 206, 1959.

Schmidt SS: Megalovas: Case Report, Fertility and Steril 29: 364, 1978.

Spring-Mills E and Hafez ESE: Male accessory sexual organs. In: Human reproduction: Conception and contraception, Hafez ESE (ed), Harper and Row, Hagerstown, MD, 1980.

Wartenberg H: Human testicular development and the role of the mesonephros in the origin of a dual Sertoli cell system. Andrologia 10: 1, 1978.

Zondek T and Zondek LH: The fetal and neonatal prostate. In: Normal and abnormal growth of the prostate, Goland M and Thomas CC (eds), Springfield, Il, 1975.

II. DISORDERS OF SPERMATOGENESIS AND EJACULATION

2. ORCHIOPEXY AND THE USE OF A TESTICULAR PROSTHESIS FOR THE UNDESCENDED TESTICLE

J.N. CORRIERE, JR.

Undescended testes are comprised of two main groups: *retractile* or *truly maldescended*. Retractile testes are due to a hyperactive cremasteric reflex and will descend with maturation. Approximately 70 percent of children examined for testicular maldescent have this type of testicular abnormality which does not require surgery.

Truly maldescended testes can be further categorized as *obstructed*, *functionally dystopic* or *ectopic*. The obstructed organs, which comprise about one fourth of the truly maldescended group, usually lie in the superficial inguinal pouch or superficial to the external oblique aponeurosis. They have good cord length and are grossly normal to inspection.

Functionally dystopic testes are organs that for some unexplained reason never reach their scrotal destination but lie within the normal route of descent. They include over two thirds of the maldescended group. They can be high scrotal (49 percent), canicular or emergent i.e. in the inguinal canal (19 percent) or abdominal (9 percent). Finally, true ectopic testicles are those that lie outside the route of normal testicular descent (perineum, femoral region, pre-penile) and they represent less than one percent of all undescended testicles.

I. INCIDENCE

The true frequency of undescended testis is difficult to ascertain. The most accurate figures, when referring to a truly maldescended testis and not a retractile testis, cannot be determined until after the 3rd month of life, and spontaneous descent is unlikely to occur after one year of age, if at all. The combined incidence of obstructed, functionally dystopic and ectopic testicles, which will never descend spontaneously is approximately one percent after one year of age.

II. DIAGNOSIS

Careful examination of the relaxed, non-crying child is paramount in diagnosis. The physician's hands must be warm to avoid stimulating the cremaster reflex. After three months of age, this reflex, weak at birth, becomes strong enough to draw the testes into the superficial inguinal pouch. Extreme retraction may occur so that a normally descended testis is found in the groin and cannot be manipulated into the scrotum. The retractile testes may appear to stay in the groin on repeated examination, only to drop into its normal scrotal position as puberty approaches.

If retractile testes is suspected, the child should be observed and examined while sitting in a tub of warm water. The water may aid in relaxation and return the testicle to the scrotum. If this method fails, hormonal stimulation with human chorionic gonadotrophin (HCG) will cause retractile organs to drop to their normal position and establish the diagnosis. It should be stressed that HCG does *not* produce testicular descent; it merely overcomes the cremaster reflex and allows a proper diagnosis to be made.

III. INDICATIONS AND RATIONALE FOR SURGICAL CORRECTION

There are few comprehensive long term studies on the late results of orchiopexy. Because of this, the management, especially the timing of surgery of the undescended testicle, is controversial. There is no question that securing the testicle in the scrotum is usually a cosmetic success. However, this is not the only – or more importantly, the primary reason for surgery.

The 'problems' that frequently need to be corrected in the patient with an undescended testis are psychological, associated hernias, an increased incidence of injury, an increased incidence of malignancy and impaired fertility.

Orchiopexy should not be performed before the patient is one year of age in order to prevent operating on organs that would normally descend. Additionally, surgical anesthesia has a higher risk for children under one year of age than for the older child. However, it is preferable for psychological reasons to have the procedure performed before the child begins school, which puts the upper limit of age at five years.

Most surgeons feel that once the diagnosis is verified, a good functional result is more likely to occur if surgery is done sooner rather than later. A word of caution about predicting results: the rate of incidence of malignancy probably does not change after orchiopexy is performed, but the organ is placed in a position where it can be easily and frequently examined. Despite early orchiopexy, the majority of patients with bilateral (especially abdominal) undescended testicles have impaired fertility.

Finally, if an older child presents with an undescended testicle, particularly post-pubescent, it is wiser to remove the organ than to place it in the scrotum, because the incidence of malignancy rises proportionately to the duration the organ spends in its abnormal position. Patients with this abnormality are usually good candidates for prosthesis placement.

IV. PREOPERATIVE PREPARATION AND ANESTHESIA

No special preoperative studies are necessary. There are reports in the literature documenting an incidence of urinary tract anomalies as high as 15 percent in patients with a unilaterally undescended testis and higher in patients with bilaterally undescended testes. Many authors recommend, therefore, that a routine intravenous urogram always be performed. However, when one critically examines these series, most of the 'anomalies' are non-surgical problems (duplicated systems, ectopic or malrotated kidneys) and are of academic interest only. Certainly, if genital anomalies, especially peno-scrotal hypospadias, are present, an intersex state should be considered and appropriate studies performed.

General anesthesia, with adequate muscle-relaxation if high dissection is necessary, is advisable, and should be given with the normal precautions.

V. SURGICAL PROCEDURE

During the first part of the orchiopexy procedure, the testicle is located and mobilized. Sufficient length must be obtained on the spermatic vessels and vas deferens. The second part of the procedure involves securing the testicle in the scrotum.

A. The incision

An incision is made in the abdominal crease at the level of the internal ring and carried down to the level of the fascia of the external oblique (Figure 1). Occasionaly, the testicle is found superior to this aponeurosis or in the superficial inguinal pouch (obstructed testicle) and can be freed without a subsequent fascial incision. Electrocautery can be used on bleeding vessels or they can be ligated with 000 or 0000 absorbable suture. Scarpa's fascia can usually be incised with scissors easier than with a knife.

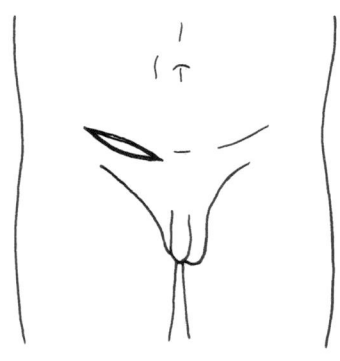

Figure 1.

B. Mobilization of the cord

In most cases it is necessary to open the fascia of the external oblique in the direction of its fibers and explore the inguinal canal to find the testicle (Figure 2). This incision should be carried through the external ring. If the testis is in the canal, the cord

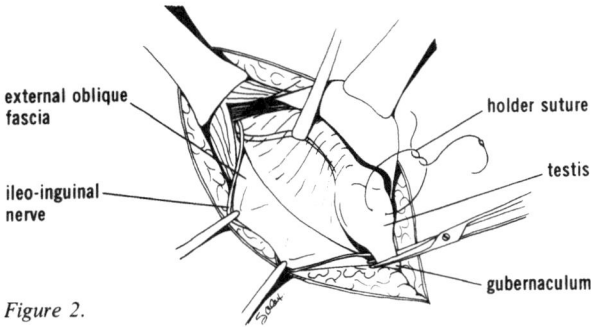

Figure 2.

structure should be mobilized by blunt dissection, and the gubernaculum isolated and transected. A 000 silk suture placed through the tunica albuginea can serve as a holder stitch. In the inguinal canal, the ileo-inguinal nerve should be identified and retracted laterally to prevent injury.

If there is concern that there will be difficulty in gaining enough length on the cord to place the organ comfortably in the scrotum, care should be taken not to disturb the tissue near the testicle. This will preserve the collateral circulation and permit division of the spermatic vessels if necessary.

C. Dissection of the sac

A hernia is commonly present medial to the cord structures. It should be isolated and dissected up toward the internal inguinal ring (Figure 3). It is often very thin and must be freed with care. Distally it should be transected as low as possible. Proximally it should be ligated with a suture ligature of

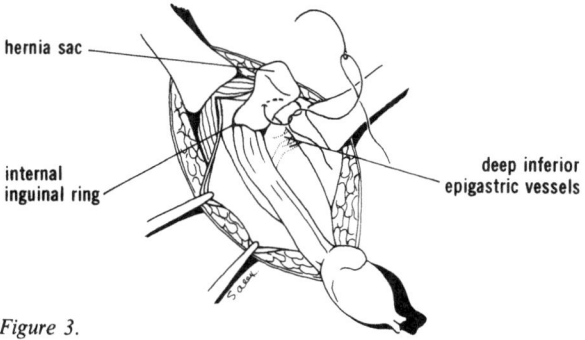

Figure 3.

000 absorbable suture as close to the internal inguinal ring as possible and the excess sac excised.

D. Transversalis Fascia Attachment – Frontal View

The vas deferens and spermatic vessels are attached to the retroperitoneal part of the transversalis fascia which is closely approximated to the posterior parietal peritoneum. This fascial attachment fans out from the spermatic vessels, especially laterally, and prevents medial displacement of these vessels if it is not divided when the vessels are separated from the peritoneum. This lateral attachment is called the lateral spermatic ligament (Figure 4).

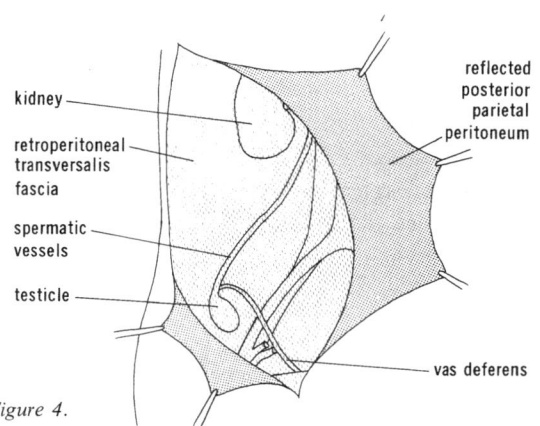

Figure 4.

E. Transversalis Fascia Attachment – Lateral View

Here can be seen the testicle and vessels attached to the transversalis fascia which overlies the peritoneum (Figure 5). Again, separation of the spermatic

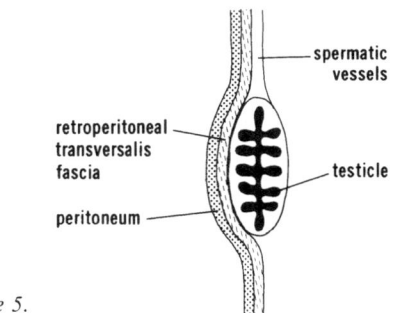

Figure 5.

vessels from the peritoneum leaves them still attached to the lateral abdominal wall by the transversalis fascia.

F. Medial Incision of the Transversalis Fascia

To gain length on the vas, an incision is made in the medial pillar of the internal ring toward the epigastric vessels (Figure 6). These vessels may be

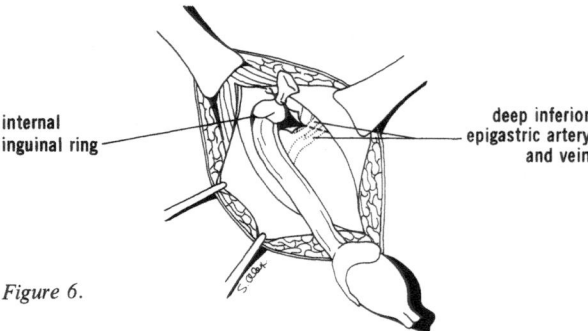

internal inguinal ring

deep inferior epigastric artery and vein

Figure 6.

cut if necessary. If the testicle is not present in the canal, it commonly can be found directly under the internal ring and is exposed by this maneuver. If it is not immediately seen, the incision in the internal ring is continued medially and, with the aid of narrow deaver retractors, the retroperitoneum explored up toward the lower pole of the kidney. If necessary, the skin incision in the external oblique may be extended superiorly to increase the exposure.

G. Incision of Lateral Spermatic Ligament

At this point, it is obvious that the only structures preventing proper placement of the testicle in the scrotum are the spermatic vessels. By drawing the testicle downward, the fibrous bands of the lateral spermatic ligament (retroperitoneal transversalis fascia) can be demonstrated. Severing these bloodless bands should allow medial displacement of the vessels to shorten their course to the scrotum and gain apparent and sufficient length to allow scrotal fixation without tension (Figure 7).

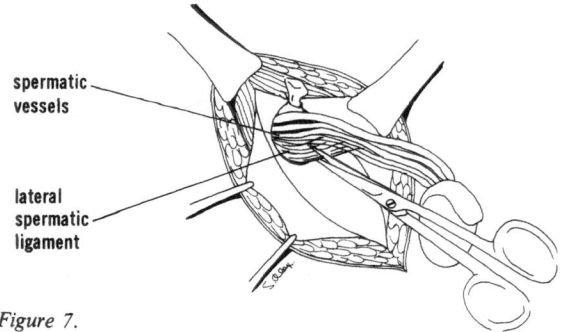

spermatic vessels

lateral spermatic ligament

Figure 7.

H. Spermatic Vessel Triangle

If the testicle still will not seat in the scrotum without spermatic vessel tension, the internal inguinal ring must be moved medially until it is directly over the scrotum and under the lateral border of the great vessels. Based on the theory that 'the shortest distance between two points is a straight line', it should be apparent that this conversion of a two-sided triangular pathway into a single straight course of the spermatic vessels to the bottom of the scrotum will gain from two to eight centimeters of length on the cord (Figure 8).

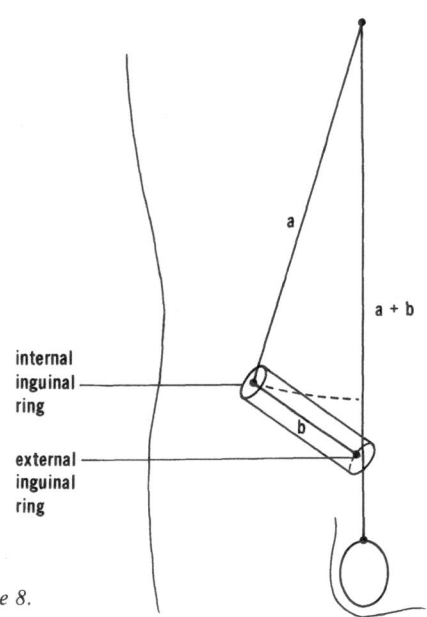

a

a + b

internal inguinal ring

external inguinal ring

b

Figure 8.

I. New Route of the Cord

After this medial displacement of the spermatic vessels, the medial incision of the internal ring is closed with 000 absorbable suture from the level of the old internal ring (which is now obliterated) to the point of exit of the vessels and vas through the 'new' ring. If the epigastric vessels were not severed during the dissection, then obviously the testicle, vas and vessels must be placed entirely medial to these structures (Figure 9).

J. Collateral Circulation of the Testicle

If the testicle is near the internal inguinal ring and has a short main vascular pedicle, a secondary vascular loop may be present from the deferential

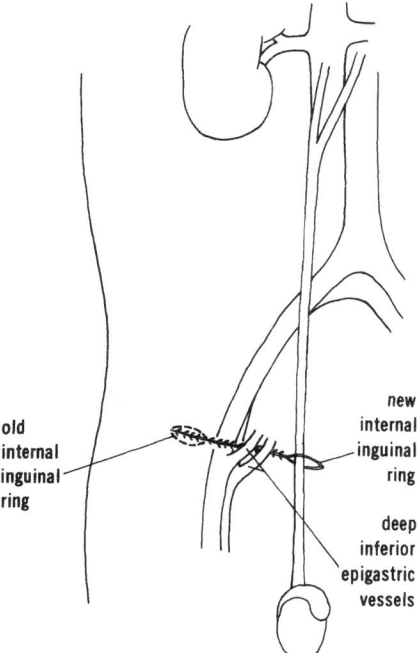

Figure 9.

artery and vein as well as the cremasteric artery and view (Figure 10). This collateral circulation arises from the *deep* epigastric vessels (the cremasterics) and the inferior vesical vessels (the deferentials); branches are also said to enter the posterior wall of the processus vaginalis from the area of the gubernaculum. This configuration allows division of the spermatic (testicular) vessels and comfortable placement of the testicle in the scrotum. Before performing this procedure, the spermatic vessels should be compressed with a vascular clamp cranial to the testicle and the tunica albuginea of the testis incised. Continued arterial bleeding from this incision indicates that adequate collateral circulation is present and that ligation of the spermatic vessels is safe.

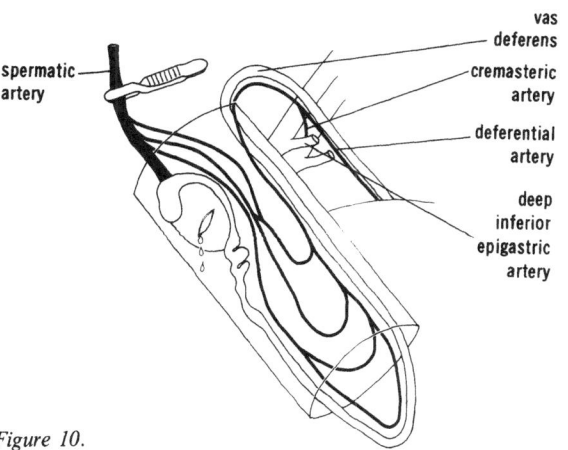

Figure 10.

K. Development of the Scrotal Canal

Once sufficient length has been obtained in the spermatic cord, attention is turned to fixing the testicle in the scrotum. A scrotal canal is prepared by pushing two fingers into the scrotum and bluntly creating a space for the organ (Figure 11).

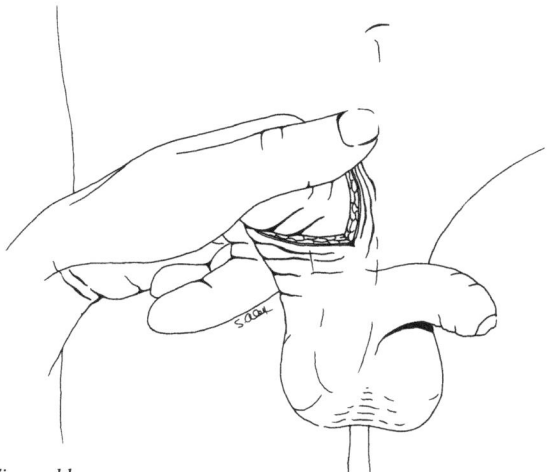

Figure 11.

L. Development of a Subcutaneous (Dartos) Pouch

A small incision is made in the scrotal skin and a pouch developed bluntly with a hemostat between the skin and the Dartos fascia. The created space must be large enough to contain both the testicle and the epididymis (Figure 12).

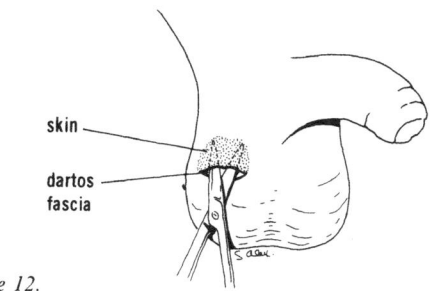

Figure 12.

M. Incising the Dartos Fascia

A buttonhole is made in.the Dartos fascia just large enough to pull the testicle through (Figure 13).

N. Placement of the Testicle

A long clamp is inserted into the buttonhole up to the abdominal incision through the newly formed scrotal canal. The holder stitch in the testicle is grasped, the clamp withdrawn, and the testicle

Figure 13.

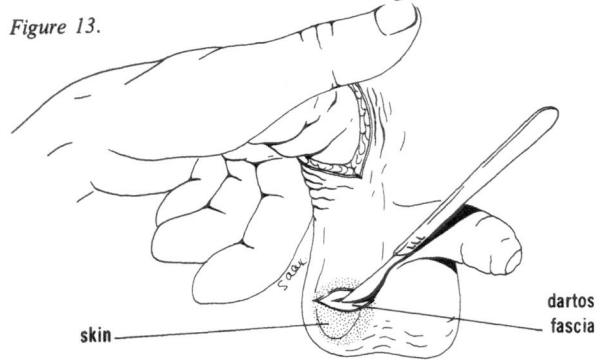

skin ———   ——— dartos
                                                           fascia

A. Incision for Prosthesis Placement

Either an inguinal incision or a high scrotal incision is acceptable (Figure 15). The incision is then carried through either Scarpa's fascia in the abdomen or Dartos fascia in the scrotum and a pouch is developed in the base of the scrotum by blunt finger dissection to accept the prosthesis. An antibiotic solution may be used to soak the prosthesis before insertion, and the pouch may be irrigated

brought through the buttonhole to its final resting place in the subcutaneous pouch. A few 000 absorbable sutures may be needed to narrow the buttonhole sufficiently to prevent retraction of the testicle into the scrotal canal. The holder stitch is removed and the scrotal skin closed with a few 0000 absorbable sutures (Figure 14). The fascia of the external oblique is closed with interrupted 000 absorbable sutures, and then the skin is closed with either subcuticular or simple skin sutures. A dry dressing is applied to the wound.

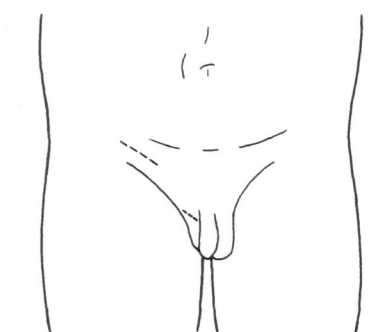

Figure 15.

with an antibiotic solution before and during placement. Many surgeons feel these patients should receive parenteral antibiotics prior to the operation and maintain them for a few days postoperatively.

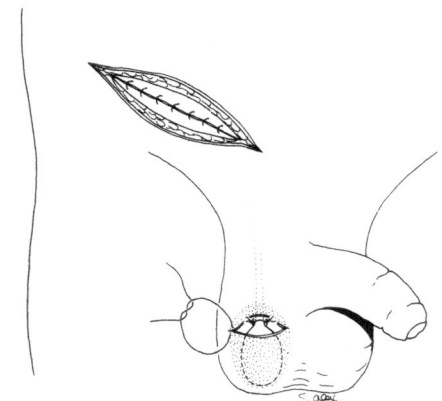

Figure 14.

VI. PLACEMENT OF A TESTICULAR PROSTHESIS

When a testicle must be removed, or if one is congenitally absent, many patients or their parents request the placement of a prosthesis for cosmetic purposes. At the present time a gel-filled silicone testicular prosthesis is available in various sizes. Because it is a foreign body, it should not be used in the presence of intrascrotal infection or if infection from a contiguous area of the body might potentially lead to contamination of the scrotal area.

B. Closing the Neck of the Pouch

A few 000 absorbable sutures should be used to close the scrotal pouch that holds the prosthesis (Figure 16). An effort should be made to separate

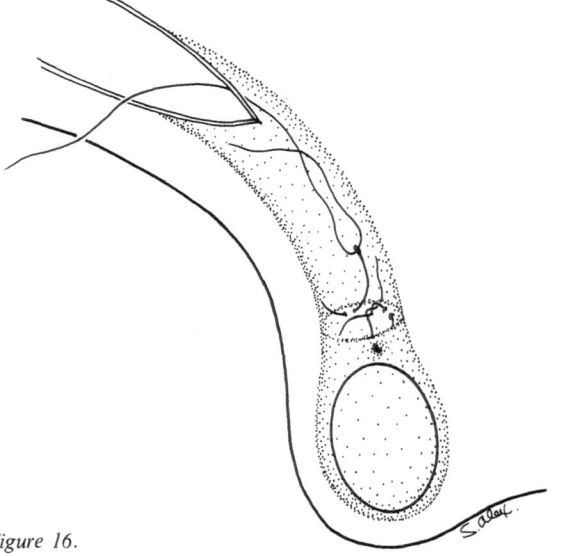

Figure 16.

the prosthesis from the skin incision with a few layers of tissue. The skin is then closed with either subcuticular or simple sutures, and a dry dressing is applied to the wound.

VII. POSTOPERATIVE CARE

Most patients may be discharged within 24 hours of the operation. However, if extensive retroperitoneal dissection has been done, a mild ileus may develop, necessitating a few days of intravenous alimentation and a delay in discharge. For the majority of patients, the dressing may be discarded after 24 hours. Ambulation is permitted immediately, and if simple nonabsorbable skin sutures have been used, they should be removed in five to seven days. An ice pack applied to the scrotum for the first eight hours postoperatively may be used to decrease scrotal edema. Salycilates should be all that are needed for analgesia. Full activity may be resumed in two to three weeks.

REFERENCES

Fowler R and Stephens FD: The role of testicular vascular anatomy in the salvage of high undescended testes. Australian and New Zealand J of Surg 29: 92, 1959.
Prentiss RJ, Weickgenant CJ, Moses JJ and Farzier DB: Undescended Testis: Surgical anatomy of spermatic vessels, spermatic surgical triangles and lateral spermatic ligament. J Urol 83: 686, 1960.
Scorer DG and Farrington GH: Congenital deformities of the testis and epididymis. New York, Appleton-Century Crofts, 1971.

3. EPIDIDYMOVASOSTOMY FOR EPIDIDYMAL OBSTRUCTION

H. FENSTER and M.G. McLOUGHLIN

The technique of epididymovasostomy dates back to the beginning of this century when Martin (1902) performed the first procedure. That operation was successful with subsequent pregnancy. Over the years the technique has been popularized by many surgeons (Hagner 1936; Humphrey and Hotchkiss 1935; Phadke 1956; Dubin and Amelar 1977). Recently the surgical procedure has become more sophisticated with the use of microsurgical techniques.

In this article we will outline some basic concepts and principles of the epididymis and then describe the macroscopic and microscopic techniques now available for epididymovasostomy.

I. ANATOMY AND EMBRYOLOGY

The epididymis is a single convoluted tube joining the testes to the vas deferens. The name is derived from epi, meaning upon, and didymus, meaning twin since the structure is found located on the twin testes (Ham 1965). The epididymis is composed of a head or caput, body or corpus and tail or cauda (Figure 1). The seminiferous tubules unite in a straight tubule, which enter the mediastinum testes to form the rete testes and the efferent ducts then exit to the caput of the epididymis. In the corpus the duct is extremely convoluted and if unwound would measure twenty feet in length. In the cauda, the convolutions straighten out until the structure becomes a mucosal lined muscular tube, the vas deferens.

The blood supply arises from the testicular, vasal and cremasteric arteries with many free anastomoses. These communications allow the surgeon to perform reconstructive surgery on this structure since it has an abundant vascular supply. The epithelial lining of the epididymis contains various forms of columnar cells with many of these cells containing cilia. Although these cilia do not allow for movement, they increase the absorptive ability of the epididymis by increasing the total surface (Jenkins 1978). Embryologically the caput of the epididymis develops from the genital ridge whereas the rest of the structure and vas deferens arises from the wolffian duct. This information is of value in exploring patients with congenital absence of the vas deferens since the upper portion of the epididymis may be present and occasionally can be utilized for reconstructive surgery.

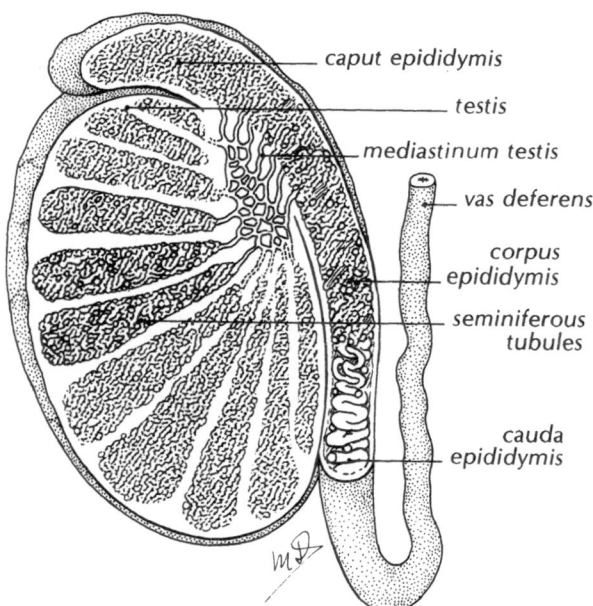

Figure 1. Anatomy of the testis, epididymis, vas.

II. PHYSIOLOGY

The functions of the epididymis are maturation, storage and transport. The ability of spermatozoa from various portions of the epididymis to fertilize the ovum has been studied and it is now known that a mammalian spermatozoon cannot successfully fertilize an ovum before passing through the cauda (Gaddum 1965). The basic problem in studies on the epididymis is that there is difficulty in separating the function of the epididymis from the inherent changes that occur in the spermatozoa as they pass through it. These changes in the spermatozoa require time and the passage through the epididymis. The question is whether the epididymis itself contributes certain factors or whether it is the spermatozoon induced activity that produces the changes observed. Presently, we believe, both factors appear to play an important role. Early studies attempting to elucidate this problem reviewed the morphological changes in the spermatozoa as they transversed the epididymis (Bedford 1975). These morphological studies documented that the middle piece cytoplasmic droplet is sloughed off as the spermatozoa reaches the distal end of the epididymis and that there is a nonnuclear loss of protein, phospholipids and cholesterol (Lavon 1970). It is possible that sperm phospholipids are changed from the head to the tail inducing some secondary permeability changes.

Studies on spermatozoa from different portions of the epididymis have shown that sperm from the restricted portions are usually mature but the majority of sperm are abnormal and pregnancy rarely occurs when these sperm are artificially inseminated (Panther 1968). This is of importance when surgically exploring the epididymis and performing reconstructive vasal anastomosis in this area since the surgery may result in a patent system whilst the sperm are not capable of fertilizing the ovum. Studies on the motility of sperm from the caput revealed that a disoriented motion was present whereas sperm from the cauda show movement similar to that of the ejaculated sperm. Investigation of human sperm also shows similar findings with the sperm from the caput showing a significant decrease in their motility when compared to sperm from the cauda (Mooney 1972). Studies on sperm motility after vasal ligation have shown that there is an increase in motility in the caput suggesting that obstruction may change the stepwise acquisition of sperm motility in the epididymis. The transport of spermatozoa in the epi-

didymis is dependent both on testicular secretion and autonomic peristaltic contractions of the epididymal wall. Both components are needed for transport of viable sperm in the ejaculate and both must be present for successful reconstructive surgery. Studies on factors important in producing fertile sperm have shown that the motility, modification of the metabolic characteristics of the sperm, structural changes in the tail organelles and the sperm nuclear chromatin, alterations in the plasma membrane, loss of the cytoplasmic droplet and acrosome modifications are changes that are needed for viable sperm to be produced. These factors plus adequate levels of circulating and tissue androgens and the correct electrolyte composition of the epididymis determine if sperm will produce fertility (Crabo 1974). The epididymis requires both androgen transport and androgen receptors to maintain the integrity of the epithelial cells. Androgen binding protein secreted from the testes transports testosterone to the epididymis where 5α reductase produces dihydrotestosterone, the active androgen metabolite. In the epididymis androgen dependent protein synthesis produces secretory products that interact with the sperm to promote maturation. These androgen dependent mechanisms are also greatly influenced by the electrolyte composition of the epididymis. It has been found that there are differences in the cellular electrolyte composition of the various portions of the epididymis. This is important in the interaction with the secretory products that affect sperm maturation (Crabo 1974).

All these factors demonstrate that the epididymis is not a passive structure but is dynamic with a major influence on the spermatozoa that traverse through it (Gaddum 1965). The epididymal influences plus the spermatozoan induced activity combine to produce fertility. Multiple factors appear to be important in sperm maturation and motility and include morphological changes in the spermatozoa, interaction of protein and electrolyte contents of the epididymis as well as the time that the sperm spend in the epididymis. It is probably a combination of all these factors plus additional unknown influences which will eventually explain the function of the epididymis and the ability of the sperm to allow for fertilization.

III. PATHOLOGY

Patients with epididymal obstruction may benefit from epididymovasostomy. The etiological factors in producing obstruction are found in Table 1. The two major categories in the pathogenesis of obstructive lesions are infection and obstruction. The

Table 1. Etiology of epididymal obstruction.

Infection	smallpox
	syphilis
	gonorrhea
	nonspecific pyrexial illness
	tuberculosis
	filiaria
	bacterial epididymitis
Obstruction	congenital
	acquired – cysts
	trauma
	surgical excisions

infective causes have been well studied in the past but are rarely seen today. The exact incidence of the congenital obstructive lesions is not well documented. In patients presenting with a primary epididymal obstruction, Hanley found 50 percent to have an obstructive congenital anomaly in the epididymis on microdissection studies. Many of these patients had multiple blocks at various sites in the epididymis. In his study, Hanley performed a primary epididymovasostomy on one side and an orchidectomy on the other so that the pathology of each patient could be studied. The most common anomaly seen was a macroscopic abnormality where the normal epididymal caput faded away into a poorly developed corpus or cauda. On the microdissection studies, multiple epididymal blocks were encountered consisting of solid growths of tissues found in the epididymal lumen. The patient who presents with epididymal obstruction secondary to a vasectomy is usually not recognized until exploration has been carried out for reversal of the vasectomy. We are now performing more epididymovasostomies in these patients and proceed early to this procedure if on exploration the cut end of the testicular side of the vas does not have any luminal dilatation, if there are no sperm found in this lumen on rush section by the pathologist and if the vasectomy involves the junction of the epididymis and the vas deferens and may have resulted

in removal of a segment of the epididymis. These patients undergo epididymal exploration with the view of finding a region in the epididymis, most preferably the tail where an adequate lumen is encountered, with viable mobile sperm seen on rush section in the operating room.

IV. DIAGNOSIS

Classically a patient with non-iatrogenic epididymal obstruction of whatever cause will present with testes of normal size, an epididymis that may be small, normal or enlarged and an ejaculate that is azoospermic. The semen fructose, serum LH, FSH and testosterone levels are all normal. The testes biopsy shows active spermatogenesis confirming a diagnosis of obstruction. Although azoospermia in the presence of normal LH, FSH and testosterone is good evidence for obstruction, one should perform a testes biopsy for confirmation. We do not perform vasograms for fear of causing obstructive injury at the site of injection from contrast media injected into the vas. The level of obstruction is defined in the operating room and if an epididymovasostomy is needed, it will be performed at the same time. Patients with congenital absence of the vas deferens may have a normal epididymal caput and therefore exploration should be carried out for possible reconstruction using the opposite vas.

Patients who have had a previous vasectomy resulting in epididymal obstruction usually have been proven fertile in the past and exploration will delineate the site of obstruction and the form of reconstructive surgery needed at that time.

V. MEDICAL MANAGEMENT

The primary therapy for epididymal obstruction is surgical with medical management being needed early in the inflammatory lesions that result in secondary obstruction since this therapy may decrease the amount of scarring and obstruction and thus facilitate reconstructive surgery. Prompt management of gonorrhea and bacterial epididymitis may decrease considerably scarring and epididymal blocks that often result. Patients with

inflammatory lesions should receive early chemotherapy and have careful follow-up so as to document and treat the onset of epididymal obstruction.

VI. SURGICAL MANAGEMENT

The treatment of most epididymal obstructions is
surgical. The surgical management can be divided
into two major categories, the macroscopic technique and the microscopic technique. In the microscopic technique, the microscope facilitates direct
mucosal anastomosis and a close approximation to
the anatomical reconstruction of the tubule. The
exploration of the scrotum is similar in both techniques and differences emerge only when the reconstruction starts.

Under general anesthetic, we explore the scrotum
to define the pathology and decide on the reconstructive technique that will be used. If the macroscopic technique is to be utilized we perform a
procedure similar to that described in the literature
(Phadke 1956; Hotchkiss 1970; Schoysman 1977;
Dubin and Amelar 1977) with modifications. The
testes, epididymis and cord structures are explored
through a horizontal scrotal incision. This incision
is generous enough so that the testes may be
delivered into the wound if needed in defining the
epididymal pathology. The vas deferens is identified
and carefully traced to its junction with the epididymis. The epididymis is exposed and examined.
If tense and turgid with tortuous tubules under the
epididymal serosa, one must suspect obstruction to
the epididymal outflow. If blue zones and/or white
sclerotic tissue are found in the epididymis, this
indicates severe long-term epididymal obstruction
(Schoysman 1977). One must take care to identify
and preserve the vessels to the vas deferens and
epididymis since injury will result in later scarring
and compromise the anastomosis. After establish-
ing the anatomy of the epididymis we mobilize the
vas deferens to provide a tension-free epididymo-
vaso-anastomosis. A 1 cm longitudinal incision is
made as distal as possible in the epididymis but
above any obvious site of obstruction (Figure 2).
The epididymal ducts are then squeezed and
opened. Often milky fluid is seen to exude from the
lumen. This material is then sent on a glass slide to
the pathologist for a rush examination to be certain

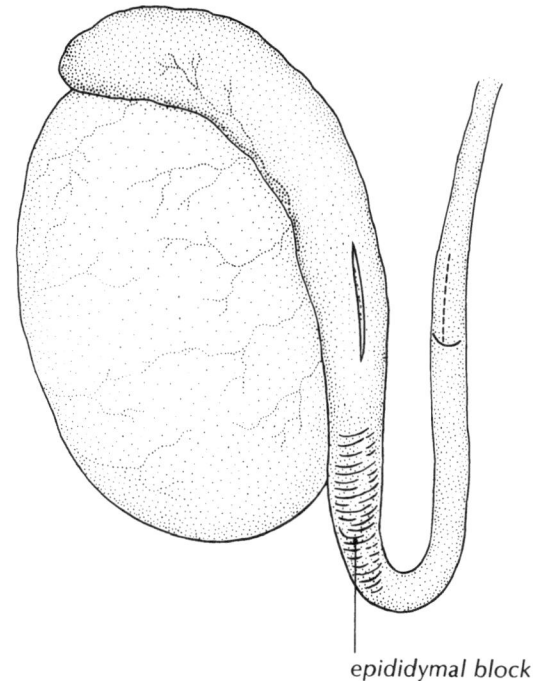

epididymal block

Figure 2. Incisions in epididymis and vas. Epididymal
block bypassed.

that live motile sperm are present. If sperm are not
seen then the epididymal incision is made higher
and closer to the caput. The initial incision in the
epididymis should be as low as possible since this
incision allows for a longer transit time of the sperm
in the epididymis and thus may provide for better
sperm maturation and fertility (Schoysman 1977).
A suitable site in the vas is then selected and the
patency checked by injecting saline proximally. We
then perform either an end of the vas deferens to the
side of the epididymis anastomosis or a side-to-side
anastomosis. In the end-to-side anastomosis, the
distal end of the vas deferens is spatulated then
anastomosed to an elliptical incision in the tail of
the epididymis (Figure 3). This anastomosis is
carried out with No. 7-0 Ethicon monofilament
suture with full thickness interrupted suture
placement. In performing the side-to-side procedure, the vas is supported by the finger and a small
transverse incision made with a No. 15 blade. A 20
gauge needle is then inserted into the lumen and a
vertical incision is made joining the previous transverse incision forming a 'T' (Figure 4). The vas is
then anastomosed to the cut end of the epididymis
with interrupted No. 6-0 or No. 7-0 Ethicon monofilament sutures. A single corner suture is placed
initially (Figure 5a) and then subsequent sutures are

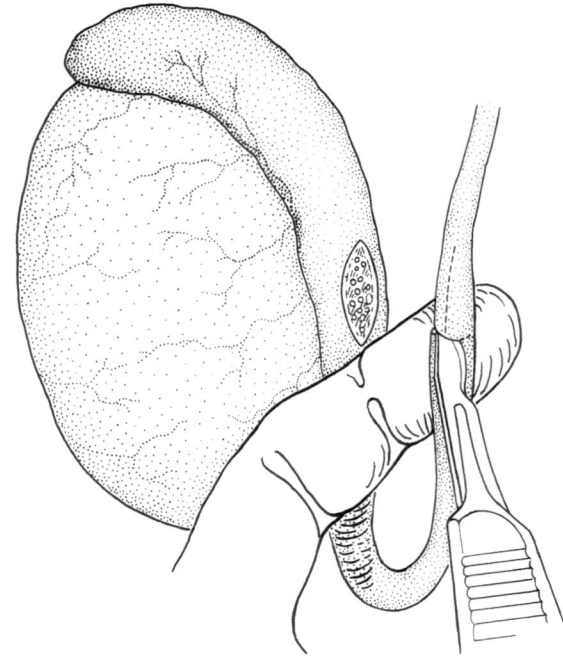

Figure 3. End-to-side anastomosis. Epididymal incision completed. Vas being cut across. Dotted line outlines spatulating incision.

placed alternately on each side (Figure 5b, c). These full thickness sutures are used to perform a sperm tight anastomosis. It usually requires approximately eight sutures to complete the anastomosis (Figure 5d). No stent is used during placement of the sutures or after the completion of the anastomosis. The end-to-side anastomosis is performed in a similar fashion (Figure 6).

The use of the microscope as an aid to vasoepididymostomy has become our mainstay in surgical reconstruction. The principles are similar with scrotal exploration and definition of the epididymal pathology and will vary with the surgeon's preference. We have found that cases of primary epididymal obstruction have better definition of the pathology with exploration of the epididymis with the microscope. In cases where a previous vasectomy has involved the vasoepididymal junction or where we have found that the luminal size of the testicular cut end of the vas deferens is small or that there are no sperm found in the cut end of the testicular vas deferens then early epididymal exploration with the microscope and epididymovasostomy is the treatment of choice. After the pathology has been defined, viable sperm identified and the epididymis and vas prepared for anasto-

mosis, the microscope is brought into the field. We do not use any approximating clamps since these are often cumbersome and hard to apply in the area of the epididymis. With proper mobilization, the structures are brought into a superficial location where they can be sutured without tension. Before starting the anastomosis, we place a colored piece of plastic material under the vas deferens and epididymis to aid in suture placement. The anastomosis is carried out with No. 9-0 monofilament nylon suture and we use a modified suction consisting of a tuberculin syringe attached to a No. 20 blunt end needle.

We perform two kinds of anastomoses, the end-to-side anastomoses and the end-to-end anastomoses. When performing an end-to-side anastomoses, we use 6-10 x's power magnification and full thickness sutures are placed in a similar manner as described in the macroscopic technique. With the microscope we are able to get better mucosal anastomoses and finer suture placement (Figure 7).

In cases where direct end-to-end anastomosis is to be performed and especially in cases where we are reversing a previous vasectomy that requires epididymal reconstruction, the end-to-end anastomosis technique has been superior. We tease out the

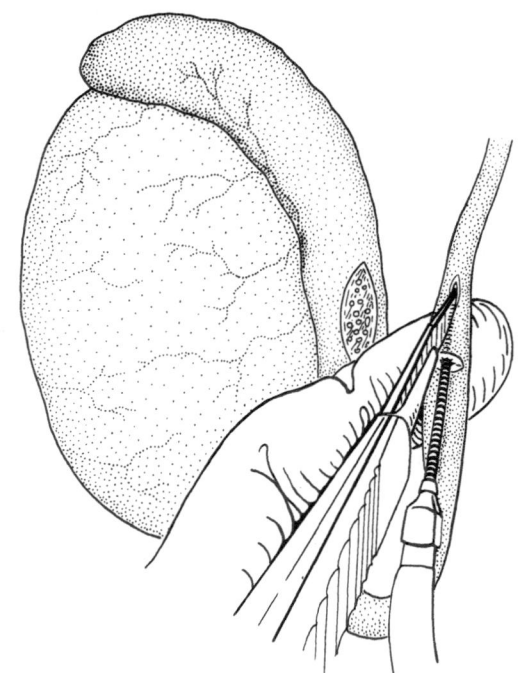

Figure 4. Side-to-side anastomosis. Epididymal incision completed. Needle in lumen of vas through horizontal incision. Vertical incision being made.

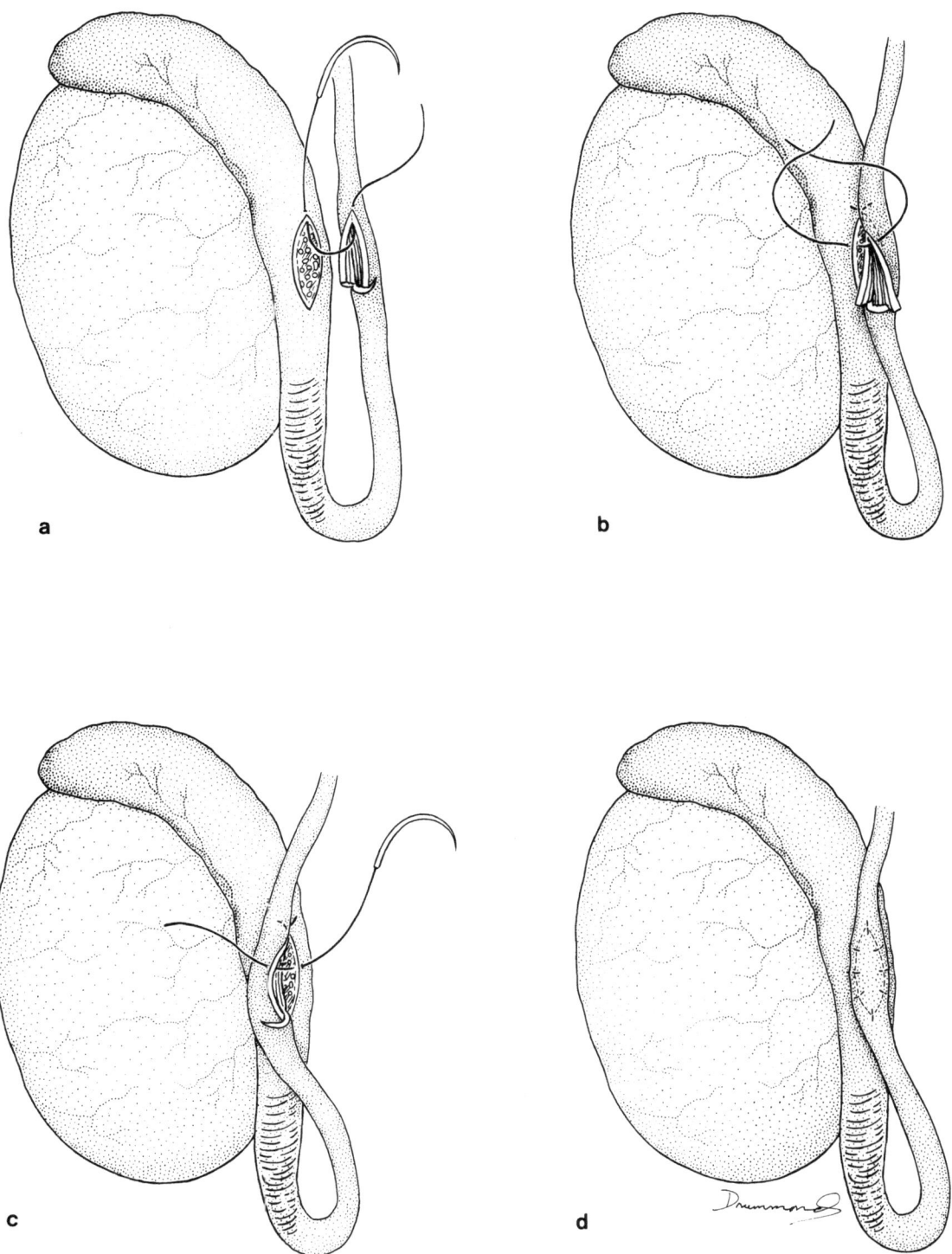

Figure 5. Side-to-side anastomosis. a. Corner suture placed. b. Anterior side suture placed. c. Posterior side sutures placed. d. Anastomosis completed.

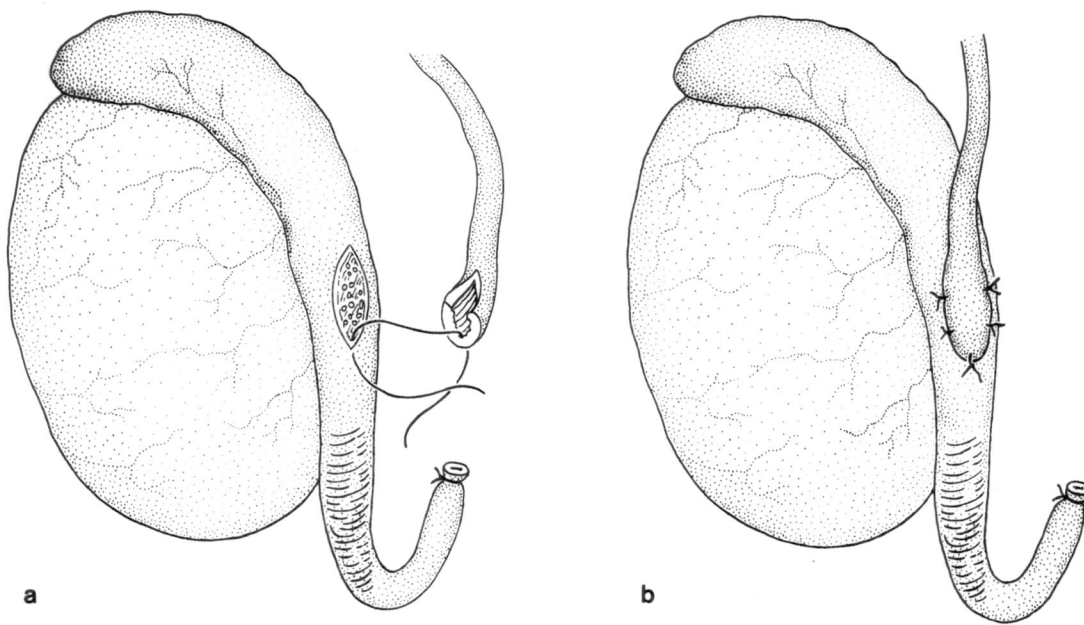

Figure 6. End-to-side anastomosis. a. Corner suture placed. b. Anastomosis completed.

epididymal duct and dilate up the lumen under microscopic control. This dilatation of the lumen is also performed on the vas deferens lumen. We then use two No. 8 Dexon sutures as corner stay sutures approximately 150 degrees apart (Figure 8a, b). These sutures are mucosal-to-mucosal with incorporation of some submucosal tissue. This material adds strength to the anastomosis and also facilitates rotation during the placement of sutures on the posterior wall. The anterior mucosal-to-mucosal sutures are then carried out with three No. 9 nylon. The corner sutures are then rotated 180 degrees and the posterior sutures are placed with No. 9 nylon. The micro instruments utilized are No. 5 Jeweler's forceps, the fine micro needle driver, and the microsurgical scissors. After completion of the mucosal sutures, a second row of serosal sutures are placed with No. 9 nylon (Figure 8c, d, e). After completion of the anastomoses, the dartos muscle is then closed with No. 3 chromic, the skin is closed with No. 4 Dexon and a pressure dressing applied for 24 hours.

The factors that seem important in the success in this type of surgery are listed in Table 2. We have found that the microscopic technique described may offer the best chance for accurate mucosal anastomosis and does provide a sperm tight conduit. For urologists inexperienced in the use of the microscope, we recommend the macroscopic technique described.

Table 2. Factors for surgical success.

1. Technique
2. Antibiotics for inflammatory lesions preoperatively
3. Site of obstruction
4. Nature of obstruction

VII. CONCLUSIONS

Certain factors are important in epididymovasostomy. Patients with blocks high in the epididymis have a very low success rate for pregnancy. This correlates with the described function of the epididymis in sperm maturation since sperm found in the head of the epididymis are not yet ready to fertilize. The nature of the obstruction is also important since the congenital obstructive lesions often have multiple blocks and are associated with a poor success rate. There are more pregnancies recorded in patients presenting with inflammatory lesions and in patients presenting with postvasectomy sterility. Finally, the surgeon must utilize a technique with which he is familiar and has experience.

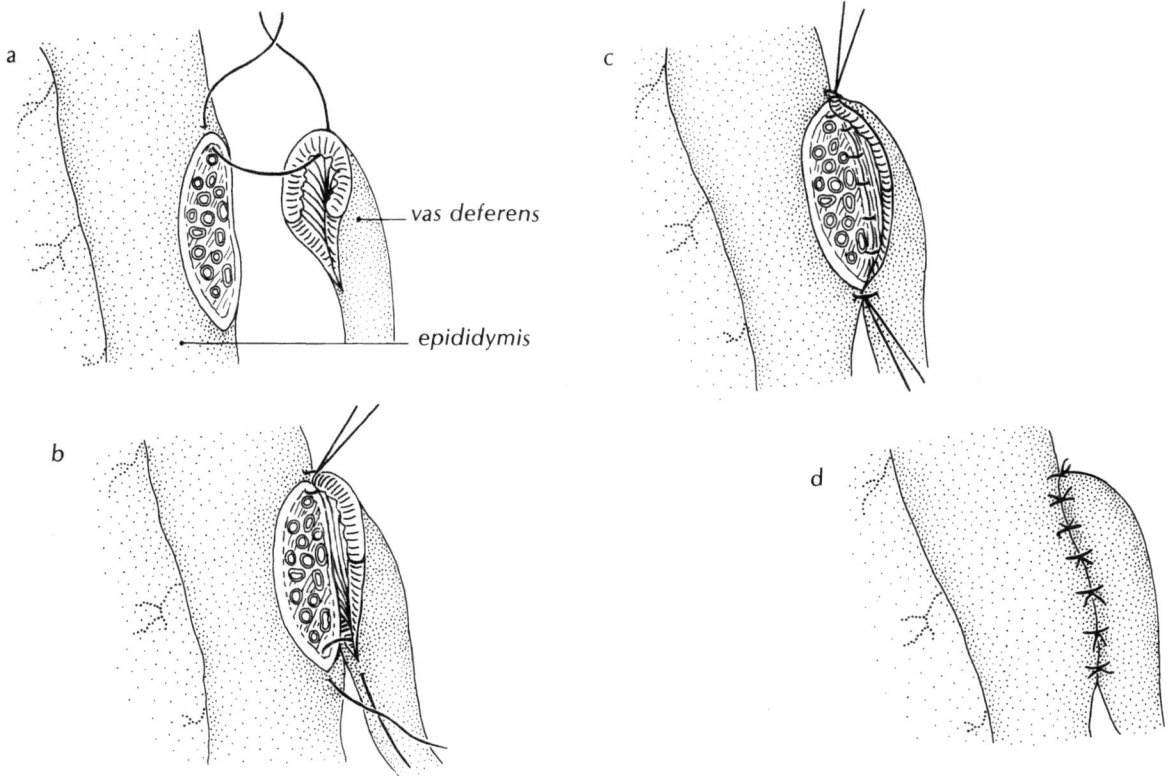

Figure 7. End-to-side anastomosis. a. Corner suture placed. b. Second corner suture placed. c. Back row completed. d. Front row completed.

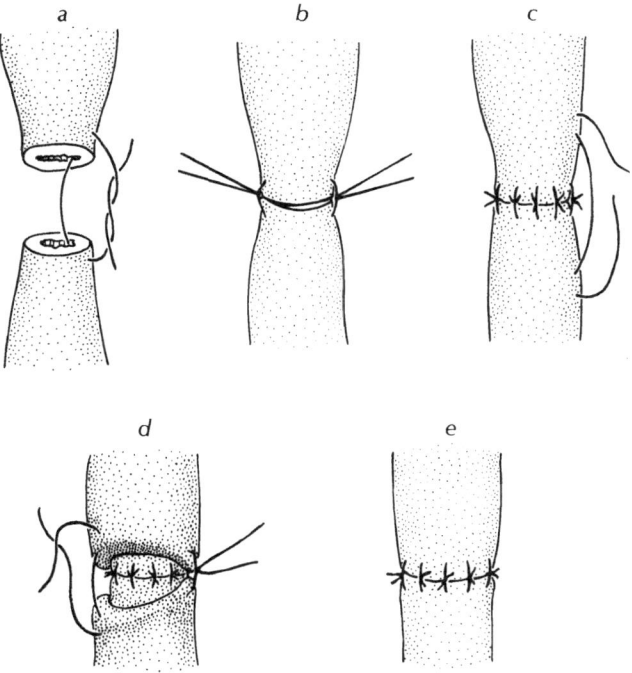

Figure 8. End-to-end anastomosis. a. Corner mucosal suture placed. b. Second corner suture placed. c. Mucosal suture line completed. First serosal suture placed. d. Serosal suture line being performed. e. Serosal suture line completed.

REFERENCES

Bedford JM: Malfunction, transport and fate of spermatozoa in the epididymis. In: Handbook of physiology, Greep RO and Astwood EB (eds), vol V, Washington DC Amer Physiol Soc 1975, p 303-317.

Crabo BG and Hunter AG: Sperm maturation and epididymal function. In Control of male infertility, Sciarra JJ et al (eds), Harper and Row, 1974, p 2-17.

Dubin L and Amelar RD: Surgery for male infertility. In: Male infertility, Amelar RD et al (eds), Philadelphia, Pa WB Saunders Co, 1977, p 222-227.

Gaddum P and Glover TD: Some reactions of rabbit spermatozoa to ligation of the epididymis. J Reprod Fert 9: 119, 1965.

Hagner FR: Operative treatment of sterility in the male. JAMA 107: 1851, 1936.

Ham AW: The male reproductive system. In: Histology, Ham AW (ed), Philadelphia, JB Lippinott Co, 1965, p 946-949.

Harley HG and Hodges RD: The epididymis in male sterility: A preliminary report of microdissection studies. J Urol 82: 508, 1950.

Hotchkiss RS: Infertility in the male. In: Urology, 3rd ed, Campbell MF and Harrison HH (eds), WB Saunders Co, 1970, p 669-673.

Humphrey G and Hotchkiss RS: Vasoepididymal anastomosis. J Urol 42: 815, 1935.

Jenkins AD, et al: Physiology of the male reproductive system. In: The Urologic Clinics of North America. Philadelphia, WB Saunders Co, 1978, p 444.

Lavon UR, et al: The proteins of bovine spermatozoa from the caput and cauda epididymis. J Reprod Fert 23: 215-222, 1970.

Martin E: Surgical treatment of sterility, Penna Med Bull 15: 2, 1902.

Mooney JK, et al: Motility of spermatozoa in the human epididymis. J Urol 108: 443, 1972.

Panther SK and Foote RH: Morphology, motility and fertility of spermatozoa recovered from different areas of ligated rabbit epididymis. J Reprod Fert 17: 125, 1968.

Phadke GM :Surgery of obstructive azoospermia. In: Proceedings of the Second World Congress on Fertility and Sterility, Tesauro G (ed), Nofles, 1956.

Schoysman R: Surgery of male genital .ract including special techniques for the correction of ductal obstruction. In: Ninth World Congress of Fertility and Sterility, Stuart BH et al (eds), 1977, p 178-185.

4. SCROTAL EXPLORATION, TESTIS BIOPSY AND VASOGRAPHY FOR TESTICULAR FAILURE

D.J. MEHAN

Testicular biopsy is a simple, safe procedure, which can frequently provide the clinician with valuable information otherwise unobtainable. Much debate has occurred relative to the merits of testicular biopsy. However, when applied with the proper indications, it is a valuable, if not indispensable diagnostic tool. Empiric testicular biopsy is to be avoided. Testicular biopsy is only a part of the entire workup of the patient, hence to achieve the fullest benefit from the procedure it must be performed in conjunction with other studies (e.g. gonadotrophins and Karyotyping) employed in the investigation of the subfertile, hypogonadic, or intersexual patient.

I. INDICATIONS FOR TESTICULAR BIOPSY

The indications for testicular biopsy are relatively simple and apply to most cases with few exceptions. In the subfertile male, we recommend biopsy in cases of azoospermia, and in most instances of severe oligospermia (counts under 10 million per cc). Exceptions to routine biopsy of the azoospermic male would be those in which the semen analysis is fructose negative, and when the Kleinfelter syndrome is suspected. Patients with fructose negative semen should be carefully examined to determine if there exists a congenital absence of the seminal vesicles or vas. If such is the case, biopsy would add little to evaluation or treatment. Should congenital absence of the vas or seminal vesicles be unproven clinically, we would consider biopsy, and probably vasography.

Any patient suspected clinically of having the Kleinfelter syndrome (azoospermia and very small gonads) should have complete gonadotrophic and chromosome studies prior to biopsy.

Once the Kleinfelter syndrome is diagnosed by laboratory studies, the need of testicular biopsy is eliminated. Without the appropriate gonadotrophic and chromosomal studies, testicular histology alone could be misleading; for example, confusing this syndrome with germinal cell aplasia or the Sertoli cell only syndrome among others.

In the severe oligospermic (sperm counts of less than 10 million per cc) testicular biopsy is recommended prior to institution of therapy. The purpose for this is to evaluate the findings to better prognosticate the effect of treatment or, in some cases, to abandon therapy. Testicular biopsy, in patients with sperm counts of greater than 10 million, although possibly demonstrating nonspecific changes in the biopsy material, will seldom provide any really useful information, and is not recommended.

Ambiguity of the external genitalia, or other findings of intersexuality, is an indication of testicular biopsy, which is often necessary for accurate diagnosis and sexing of the patient.

II. TECHNIQUE OF TESTIS BIOPSY AND SCROTAL EXPLORATION

Testicular biopsy is performed in the hospital under general anesthesia. This is done simultaneously with the assessment of gonadotrophins and karyotype, and, if appropriate, is deferred until these studies have been completed. Open biopsy is preferred over a blind needle biopsy since a significant value of the biopsy is to visualize the epididymis and vas to ascertain if there is any abnormality of these structures. General anesthesia is used to assure patient comfort, especially if a thorough examination of the vas and epididymis is contemplated. Normally only one testicle is biopsied. However, if a bilateral procedure is desired, this can easily be accomplished by making the incision in the midline of the scrotum and alternately delivering each testicle. After incising the scrotum and subcutaneous fascia, the tunica vaginalis is opened, and the testicle is delivered from the scrotum. Accurate assessment of size and consistency is made, and the epididymis and vas is carefully examined to determine any anatomic abnormality or obstruction. If desired, a vasogram can be done quite readily. The tunica albuginea is then incised with a No. 11 blade and the color and texture of the seminiferous tubules noted. Frequently the testicular material will spontaneously extrude from the testicle, and this can be sectioned with a sharp knife, being careful not to squeeze or manipulate the tissue. The normal testicular tissue is a golden brown and tends to string when teased with a fine tissue forceps. In instances of severe testicular dysfunction, the color may be a dark brown and the tissue tends to compact and will not string. The biopsied material must not be handled and should be cleanly incised from the bulk of the testicle and placed immediately in a proper fixative. Either Bouin's, Clelland's or Zenker's solution will do an adequate job of fixing the material, preventing disruption of the testicular histology. Under no circumstances should Formalin be used as a fixative, since this will disrupt the normal histology and make reading of the stages of development of the spermatocytes difficult.

After satisfactory tissue is obtained, the tunica albuginea is closed with 4-0 chromic sutures, either running or interrupted. The testicle is then replaced in the scrotum, and a two layer closure of the fascia and skin of the scrotum is made with 4-0 chromic catgut. Drains are not necessary.

An ice bag is applied to the scrotum and the patient is usually discharged the same day with a scrotal support and mild analgesics. Customarily we stain biopsy material only with Hematoxylin for the best visualization of the cells, although special stains such as Trichrome may be desired in specific situations. Separate biopsy specimens can be taken for culture, karyotyping or meiotic preparations at the time of the original surgery.

III. RESULTS

In general, the results of testicular biopsy can be classified into two categories, those which absolutely preclude pregnancy, and those which do not.

The lesions which preclude pregnancy would include the following: (1) the Kleinfelter syndrome, (2) the Sertoli Cell Only syndrome, (3) hyalinization (e.g., mumps), (4) germinal cell aplasia (e.g., cryptorchid testicle), and (5) idiopathic atrophy. All of these lesions demonstrate a degree of overlap insofar as the histologic picture is concerned. Again the need for thorough evaluation of the patient is apparent.

The Kleinfelter syndrome is usually characterized by tubules void of germ cells, frequently hyalinized, with peritubular fibrosis and often a relative increase in the interstitial cells (Leydig cell hyperplasia) (Figure 1).

The Sertoli Cell Only syndrome may produce a similar picture relative to the seminiferous tubules, although there is seldom the degree of hyalinization or Leydig cell hyperplasia (Figure 2). Certain inflammatory lesions can produce enormous hyalinization of which mumps is indeed the classic example (Figure 3). A cryptorchid testicle may demonstrate changes which are difficult to distinguish histologically from the preceding, with no germ cells present in the tubules and a mild degree of peritubular fibrosis. Lesions producing atrophy with absent germinal epithelium of an unknown etiology are often seen and will preclude pregnancy (Figures 4, 5, 6). In general, the lesions which preclude pregnancy are those which show a degree of hyalinization, marked peritubular fibrosis, absent germinal cells and significant Leydig cell hyperplasia.

The lesions, though not precluding pregnancy, that may well prove refractory to treatment are many and varied. These include all the various stages of spermatocytic arrest, disorganization and sloughing of cells to varying intensity. Slight increases in the interstitial cells and minimal peritubular fibrosis need not in themselves be a contradiction to therapy. Some authors do quantitative studies of the ratios of the various cellular components in the biopsy, and while we believe this to be a useful research tool, we do not believe it worthwhile for the practicing clinician. Varying stages of arrest and

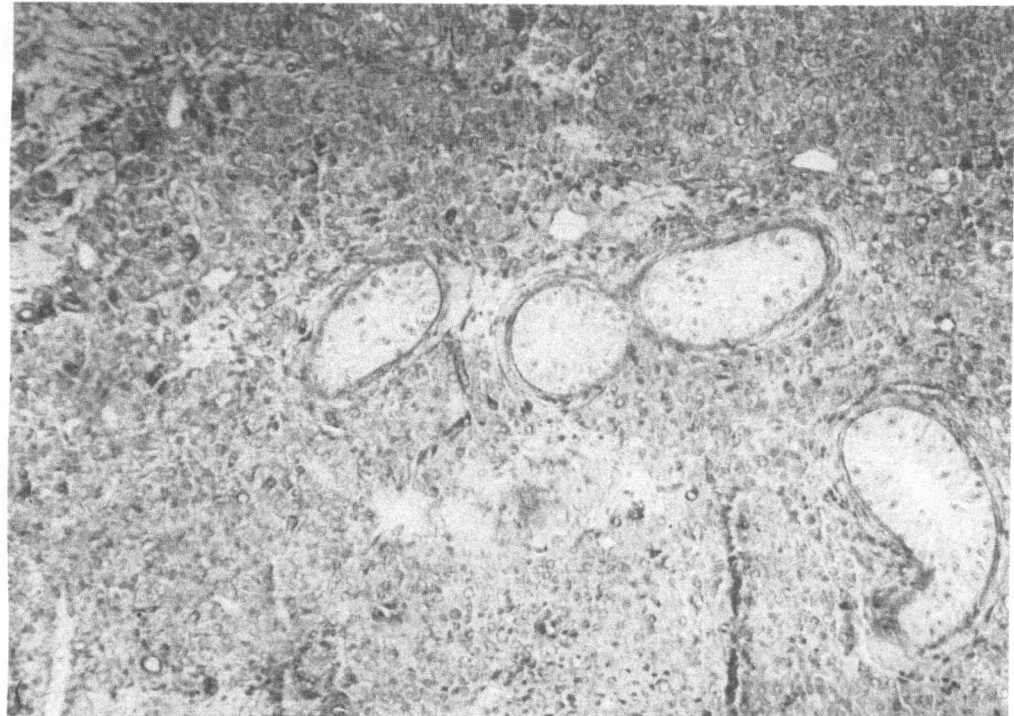

Figure 1. The Kleinfelter syndrome in this instance showing enormous Leydig cell hyperplasia. Seminal tubules void of any spermatogenic elements with a modest amount of peritubular fibrosis. Conspicuous by its absence is the lack of tubular hyalinization in this specimen.

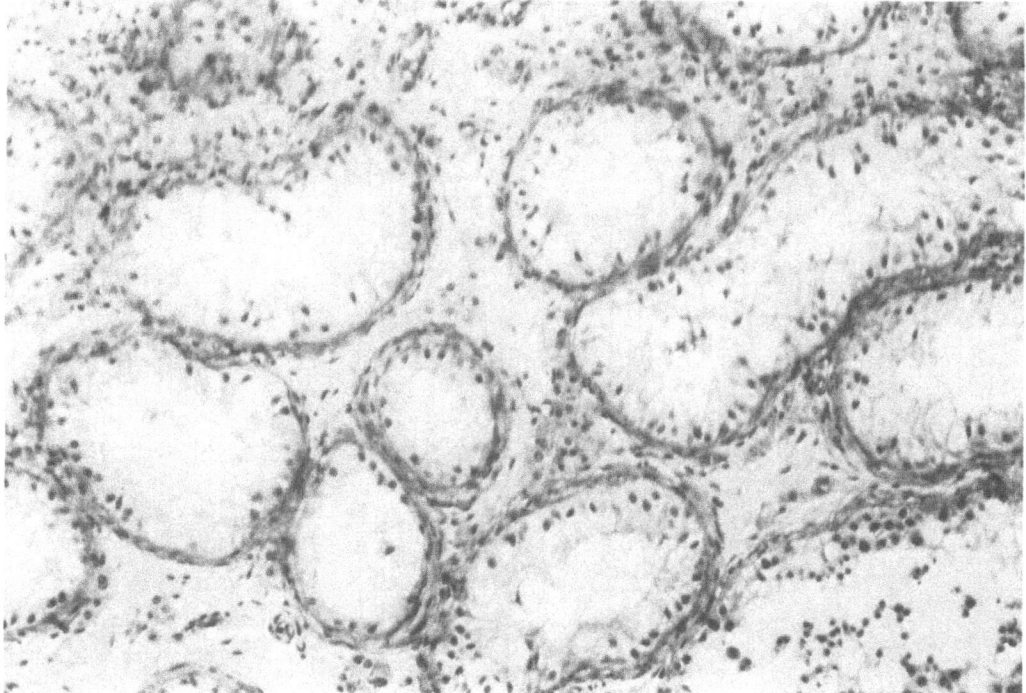

Figure 2. An example of the Sertoli Cell Only syndrome showing Sertoli Cells only within the seminiferous tubules. No evidence of hyalinization, minimal peritubular fibrosis, and no apparent Leydig cell hyperplasia.

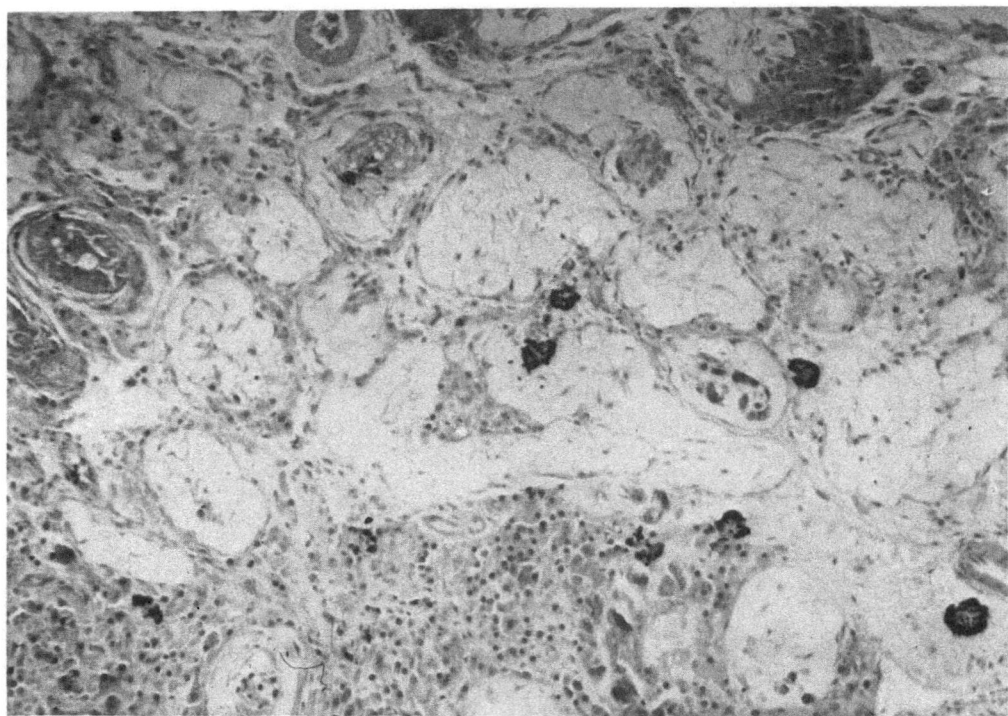

Figure 3. Inflammatory reaction producing enormous hyalinization and apparent Leydig cell hyperplasia, as seen in a post-mumps testicular biopsy.

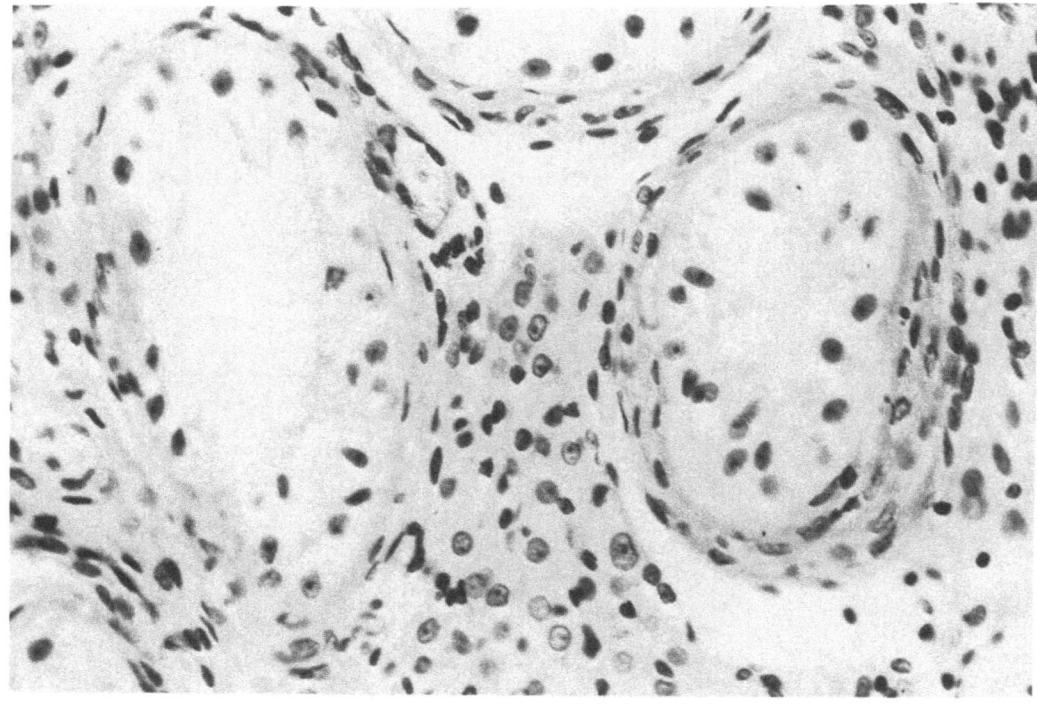

Figure 4. Unexplained germinal cell aplasia with modest peritubular fibrosis and no Leydig cell hyperplasia or hyalinization.

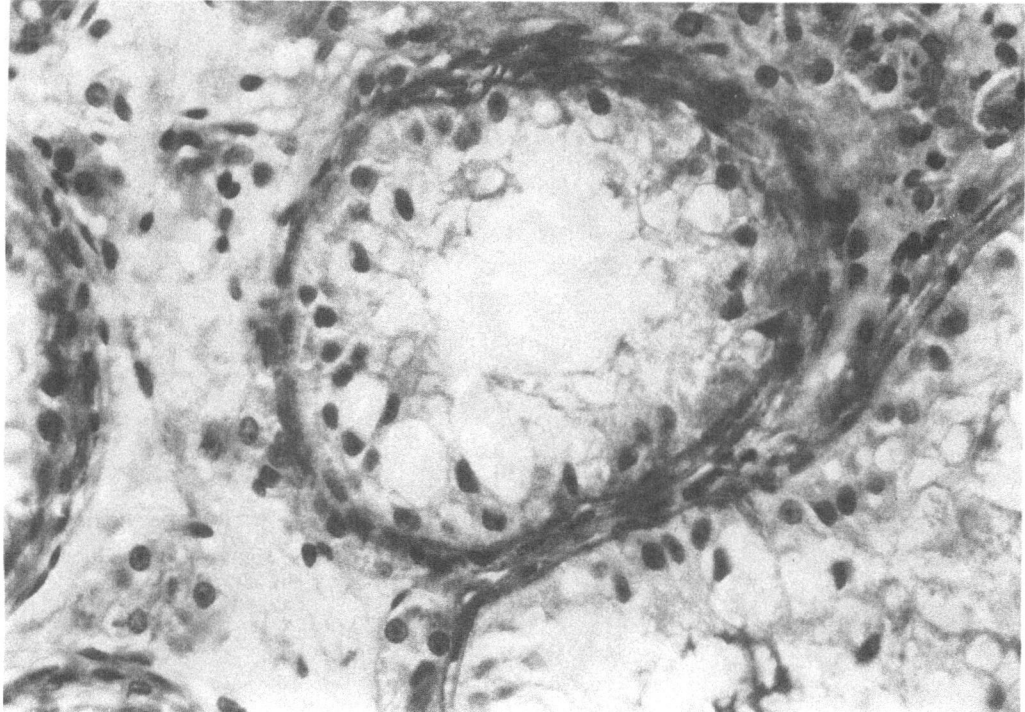

Figure 5. Another example of germinal cell aplasia without fibrosis, hyalinization or Leydig cell hyperplasia, possibly related to a Kleinfelter mosaic, though not proven.

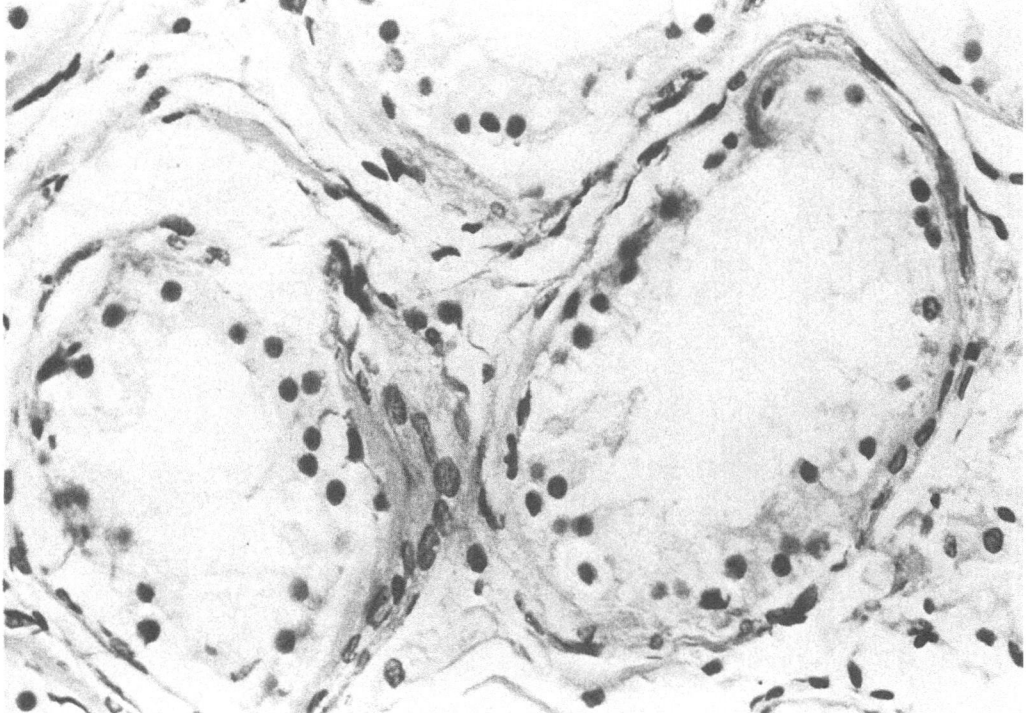

Figure 6. Tubules void of germinal cells without hyalinization. In this instance the result of an undescended testicle operated on at age 20.

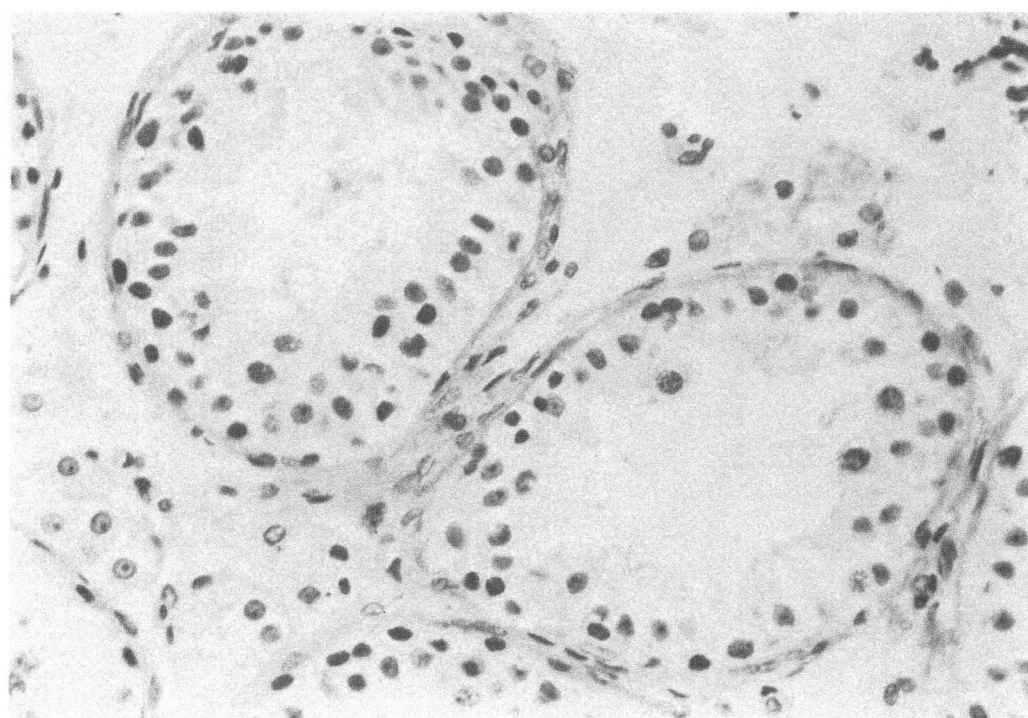

Figure 7. Marked spermatogenic arrest, the tubules showing only occasional primary spermatocytes or pachytene cells, but without hyalinization, peritubular fibrosis or Leydig cell hyperplasia. Pregnancy resulted in this patient following varicocele ligation and treatment with human chorionic gonadotropins.

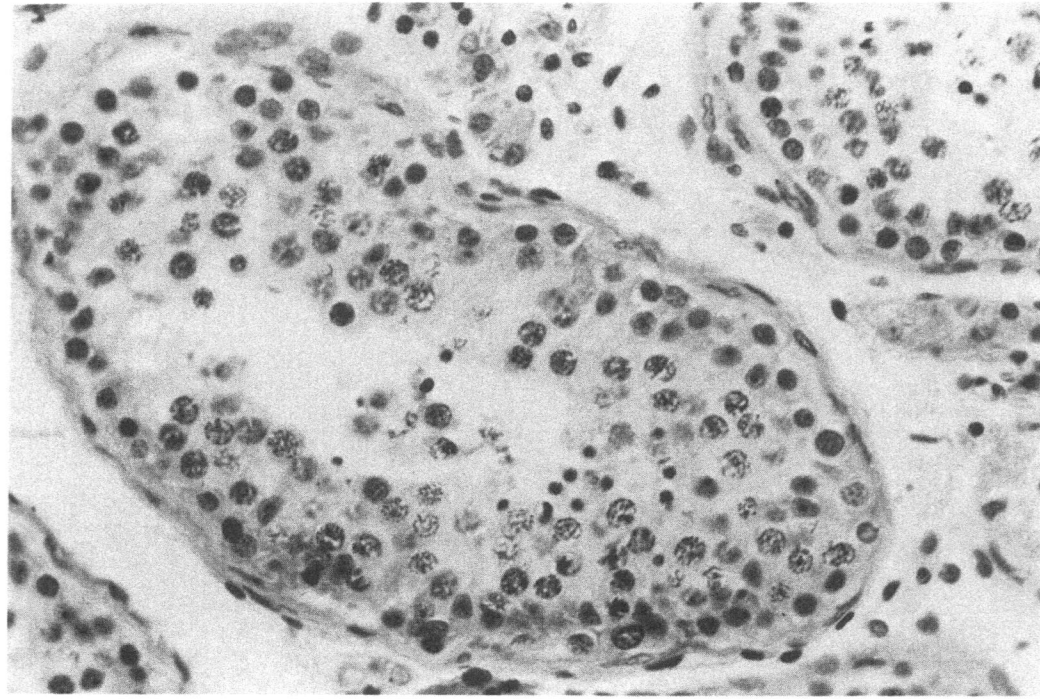

Figure 8. Spermatogenic arrest at a higher level than seen in the previous figure with good profuse demonstration of pachytene cells and various stages of meiosis in the testicular biopsy. Some spermatids are noted.

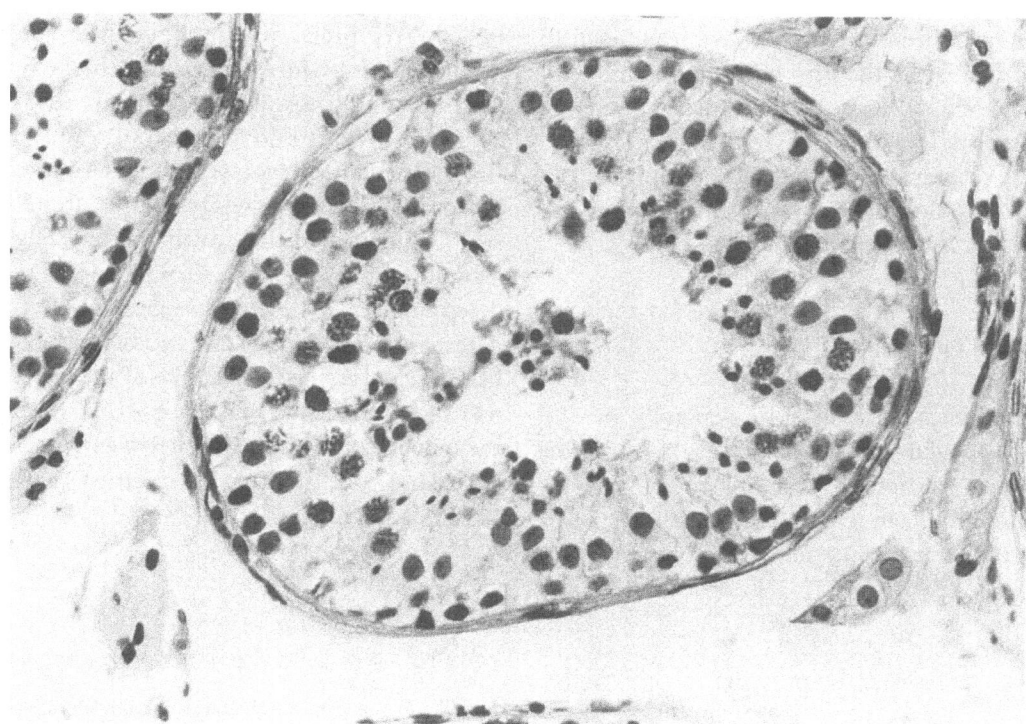

Figure 9. Good progression noted in this biopsy in a severely oligospermic male without great numbers of spermatids seen, and some evidence of premature sloughing of the germinal epithelium. Pregnancy in this case did result following varicocele ligation and chorionic gonadotropins.

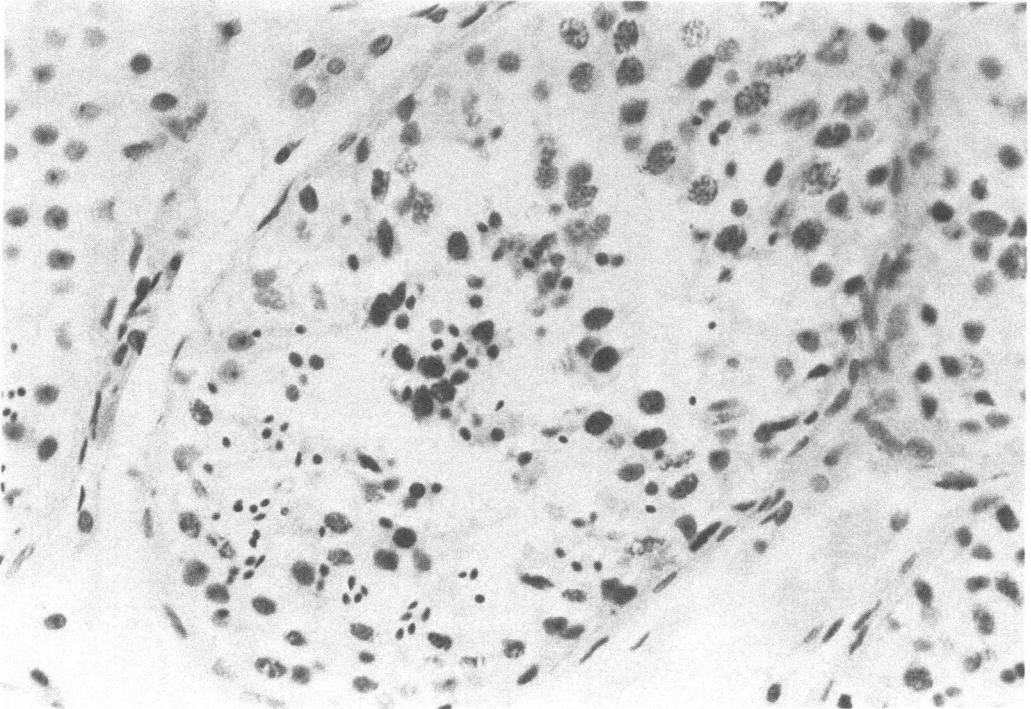

Figure 10. Severe disorganization and sloughing of germinal epithelium in a testicular biopsy which otherwise contains all the elements normally seen. The key factor in this biopsy is the lack of organization and the intense sloughing of the material.

sloughing have been noted and have responded to surgical or medical therapy or a combination of the two (Figures 7, 8, 9, 10). As long as there are primary spermatocytes (pachytene cells) present in the biopsy, a reasonable chance for improvement does exist. We do not feel that primary spermatocytic arrest is a contraindication to surgery.

IV. VASOGRAPHY

The indications for vasography generally parallel those for testicular biopsy. When vasal obstruction is suspected, vasography should be done. Frequently we do it in conjunction with testicular biopsy in the azoospermic (fructose positive)

patient. We prefer to use a small 25 gauge scalp needle, carefully inserting it into the lumen of the vas, directing it toward the seminal vesicles. Some clinicians prefer to do a vasostomy, and then close this with microsurgical techniques. Although this is a more complex procedure than is usually necessary, it does have the advantage of being able to aspirate fluid from the testicular side of the vas to determine if any sperm are present in the fluid. Alternate placement of the needle may be done to better visualize the testicle side of the vas if needed, and methylene blue may be injected to determine the patency of the vas, although we find this seldom necessary. One to 3 cc of contrast material will usually suffice.

REFERENCES

Garduno A and Mehan Donald J: Testicular biopsy findings in patients with impaired fertility. J Urol 104: 871, 1970.

McFadden Micheal R and Mehan Donald J: Testicular biopsies in 101 cases of varicocele. J Urol 119: 372, 1978.

Mehan Donald J, Chehval Micheal J and Wolk Sr Leo rita: Meiotic indices in the oligospermic male. Fert and Steril 28: 952, 1977.

Ting-Wa Wong, Straus FH, Jones TM and Warner NE: Pathologic aspects of the infertile testis. Surg Clin N Am 5: 503, 1978.

Weiss DB, Rodriguez-Rigau LJ, Smith KD and Steinberger E: Leydig cell function in oligospermic men with varicocele. J Urol 120: 427, 1978.

5. INTERNAL SPERMATIC VEIN LIGATION FOR VARICOCELE

L. DUBIN and R.D. AMELAR

Varicocele was mentioned as a cause of male infertility as early as the 1880s by a British surgeon named Barfield (Zorgniotti 1975). In 1929, Macomber and Sanders reported restoration of fertility in men following bilateral varicocele surgery. However, it was not until Tulloch's report in 1952 of restored spermatogenesis in an azoospermic man with a varicocele that real notice was taken of the problem; unfortunately, in general, therapeutic results in azoospermic men since that time have been poor (Dubin and Hotchkiss 1969; Mehan 1976; Stewart 1974). Since Tulloch's work in the 1950s, numerous reports of success following varicocele ligation have appeared in the literature. The major reports are listed in Table 1.

The incidence of varicocele in the general population has been reported by Clarke to be as low as

7 percent, but most surveys have found the incidence to be between 15 and 20 percent (Lewis 1950; Lipshultz and Corriere 1977; Oster 1971; Scott 1962; Uehling 1968).

The incidence of varicocele in a subfertile male population is much higher. Of 1,294 consecutive cases of male infertility seen from 1965 to 1970, we found 39 percent to be caused by varicocele (Dubin and Amelar 1971). Although our figure may be somewhat high because of the pre-selected patient population that we see, other authors have confirmed that the incidence is significant and deserves attention in the diagnosis and therapy of male subfertility (Greenberg 1977; Hamen 1944; Hendry 1973; Russell 1954; Stewart 1973).

The deleterious effect of varicocele on fertility was well established by Johnson et al. in 1970. They found in routine physical examinations for military induction performed on 1,592 young males that 9.5 percent (151 men) had asymptomatic varicocele. Ninety-three agreed to have a semen analysis performed, and 63 of these had significant abnormalities.

In 1977, Lipshultz and Corriere noted a significant loss of testicular mass in a small group of young men with incidentally diagnosed varicocele, as compared with age-matched controls. However, abnormal semen quality was not consistently demonstrated.

The seminal status encountered in subfertile men with varicocele was described in 1965 by MacLeod. Oligospermia of varying degrees was noted, but of more importance were the signs of a marked impairment of the motility of the sperm and a definite increase of immature and tapering sperm forms in the ejaculum. Indeed, although the sperm count frequently improves following ligation of the varicocele, the response is often limited to an

Table 1. General results of varicocele ligation.

Investigator	No. patients	Semen improvement	Pregnancy
Tulloch 1955	30	66%	not reported
Charny 1962	36	64%	30%
Scott and Young 1962	166	70%	not reported
Hanley and Harrison 1962	60	70%	30%
Brown et al. 1968	185	55-60%	43%
Charny and Baum 1968	104	61%	24%
Dubin and Amelar 1970	111	81%	48%
Stewart 1974	20	85%	55%
Dubin and Amelar 1975	504	71%	55%
Brown 1976	295	58%	41%
Glezerman et al. 1976	52	60%	25%
Greenberg et al. 1977	68	65%	not reported
Dubin and Amelar 1977	986	70%	53%

improvement in motility and a decrease in immature sperm forms.

Dubin and Hotchkiss in 1969 studied testicular biopsies from subfertile men with varicocele and found germinal cell hypoplasia and a premature sloughing of immature sperm forms within the lumina of the seminiferous tubules. These cells were similar to those seen in the ejaculum and included tapering forms and spermatids in a stage between Clermont Sb-1 and Sb-2 (Heller and Clermont 1964). The testicular histology in patients with unilateral varicoceles was similar on both sides. Those patients who did not improve showed no specific histologic pattern. It is significant that an increase in interstitial tissue was noted on the biopsies of these men, but one could not be sure whether this represented hyperplasia or hypertrophy of Leydig cells. However, it may be that the mode of action of varicocele is related to abnormal Leydig cell function.

I. ETIOLOGY OF INFERTILITY

The reason that varicocele causes male infertility has not been completely elucidated. One suggestion is that the effect is secondary to increased heat in the scrotum caused by stasis of blood (Hanley 1955; Hanley and Harrison 1962). This, however, has been disputed (Tessler and Krahn 1966).

Zorgniotti and MacLeod (1973) reported that the intrascrotal temperature in 50 oligospermic men with varicocele was an average of 0.6° C higher than that in a control group of 35 medical students with normal semen. Some oligospermic men without palpable varicocele had abnormal intrascrotal temperatures similar to those in men with varicocele. There is a possibility that this was caused by clinically undetectable retrograde blood flow in the left internal spermatic vein. More recently, Comhaire et al. (1976) found abnormal thermograms in 37 of 39 oligospermic men with varicocele. Among 36 men suspected of having subclinical varicocele, 19 had abnormal thermograms, and 16 of these showed reflux in the left internal spermatic vein on venography. Kay and Alexander (1977) have also recently reported increased scrotal temperature in Rhesus monkeys with experimental creation of varicocele by partial occlusion of the left renal vein.

Swerdloff and Walsh (1975) studied 13 subfertile men with clinical varicocele. The levels of luteinizing hormone (LH), follicle-stimulating hormone (FSH), testosterone, and estradiol in the peripheral veins were obtained, as were the levels of testosterone and estradiol in the internal spermatic vein. Secretion of both gonadal steroids and pituitary gonadotropins was normal. It appears likely that mechanisms other than abnormal reproductive hormonal factors are responsible for the poor quality of the semen in these patients.

Another theory became more acceptable when the rich anastomoses of the veins of the pampiniform plexus between the venous drainage of the left and right testicles were demonstrated (El-Sadr 1950). Because of venous valvular incompetence, the blood flows in a retrograde manner down the left internal spermatic vein in patients with varicocele (Brown et al. 1967). It has been shown radiographically, using radiopaque contrast media injected into the internal spermatic vein, that the blood on the left side in the man with varicocele mixes with that on the right side, allowing for an adverse effect on the two sides (Brown, Dubin, Becker and Hotchkiss 1967).

By injecting radiopaque dye directly into the left renal vein via a catheter, it has also been demonstrated that the blood from the left renal vein can flow in a retrograde manner along the left internal spermatic vein in patients with varicocele (Ahlberg et al. 1965). It is hypothesized that blood from the left adrenal and left renal veins, carrying a relatively high concentration of toxic metabolic substances such as steroids, which are potential spermatogenic inhibitors, can enter the left internal spermatic vein directly and in an undetoxified state. These 'toxins' can reach both testicles and affect sperm production. Comhaire and Vermeulen (1974) have suggested that chronic testicular exposure to catecholamine-rich blood might explain the disturbance in spermatogenesis found in the patients.

Varicocele usually occurs on the left side, due to the insertion of the left internal spermatic vein into the renal vein at a right angle; the right internal spermatic vein usually enters the inferior vena cava at an oblique angle. Man's erect posture may contribute to the increased pressure in the venous system. In addition, the superior mesenteric artery and aorta may squeeze the left renal vein while beating in synchrony, causing increased pressure on the valves at the junction of the internal spermatic and left renal veins.

If this causal theory of blood toxins and retrograde venous flow is correct, then the solution to the problem of male infertility is ligation of the left internal spermatic vein at a point above the cross-over anastomosis with the venous drainage from the right testicle. If this is done surgically at or above the level of the internal inguinal ring, the venous drainage from the left testicle will take the routes of the uninterrupted external spermatic and deferential veins. This theory implies that varicocele itself is a result of retrograde venous blood flow in the internal spermatic veins, rather than a cause of male infertility. This concept has been corroborated by recent studies showing that the size of varicocele preoperatively has no effect on the results of ligation of the internal spermatic vein (Dubin and Amelar 1970). The effects on semen quality and fertility are similar, regardless of whether the varicocele has been judged preoperatively to be large, moderate, or small.

II. FERTILITY RESULTS WITH SPERMATIC VEIN LIGATION

A. Semen Analysis

In 1977 we published the largest reported series of varicocelectomies for male infertility (Dubin and Amelar 1977).

Nine hundred and eighty-six patients were studied. All patients were evaluated preoperatively and had normal thyroid, adrenocortical, and pituitary gonadotropin function. At least two semen specimens from each patient were examined prior to surgery; all specimens showed varying amounts of oligospermia, severely impaired motility of sperm, and an increase in immature and tapering forms in the ejaculate. Azoospermic patients were eliminated from the study. All patients had tried unsuccessfully to produce a pregnancy for at least one year prior to evaluation, and many had received previous therapy with medications elsewhere. Of these, 838 had unilateral varicocele

and 148 had bilateral varicocele (15 percent). Six patients had right-sided varicocelectomy; one had situs inversus; three had undergone previous orchiectomy; and two had had previous left varicocelectomy. Improvement in semen quality was demonstrated in 690 (70 percent), while 296 (30 percent) did not improve. There were 523 pregnancies (53 percent).

Of 416 men who had preoperative sperm counts of over 10 million per ml, 354 (85 percent) had improved semen quality with 292 (70 percent) resultant pregnancies.

Of the 570 men who had preoperative sperm counts of less than 10 million per ml, 143 received no additional therapy; 50 (35 percent) of these had improved semen quality with 39 (27 percent) resultant pregnancies.

In our effort to improve on these results, 427 of the patients who had preoperative sperm counts below 10 million per ml were treated with varicocelectomy and postoperative human chorionic gonadotropin, 400 units twice weekly for 10 weeks. Improved semen quality was shown in 235 men (55 percent) and 192 pregnancies (45 percent) resulted.

The supplemental HCG therapy causes Leydig cell stimulation, which increases androgen production in these severely oligospermic patients and appears to have a definite beneficial effect on quality of the semen.

Of the 690 men who demonstrated improvement of semen quality, all had improvement in sperm motility. Improvement in sperm count levels was noted in 501 men (73 percent) and 435 (63 percent) had improvement in sperm morphology.

B. Pregnancies

The 523 pregnancies occurred at a mean of 4.4 months and a median of 5.3 months after varicocelectomy.

Five hundred and twenty-three patients' wives delivered 637 babies; 322 were female and 315 were male. There were four sets of twins. Thirty-one miscarriages and five ectopic pregnancies occurred.

Many of the patients fathered more than one child after varicocelectomy. Two patients underwent subsequent bilateral vasectomy after each fathered three children. Five men had improved semen quality and were able to produce pregnancies with an unexplained semen deterioration three years later.

It is noteworthy that pregnancy occurred following varicocelectomy in the wives of seven patients who failed to demonstrate improved semen quality.

III. SURGICAL PROCEDURES

The major problem in varicocele seems to be retrograde blood flow from the renal vein into the scrotal circulation secondary to incompetent valves

in the internal spermatic venous system. The problem can be corrected by interrupting the course of the internal spermatic vein to prevent retrograde flow, rather than by removing the dilated scrotal veins. Three approaches are available.

A. High inguinal procedure

In this procedure (our modification of Ivanissevich's technique) an inguinal incision is made over the area of the internal inguinal ring (Figure 1). The external oblique muscle is incised through the external ring, and a self-retaining retractor is

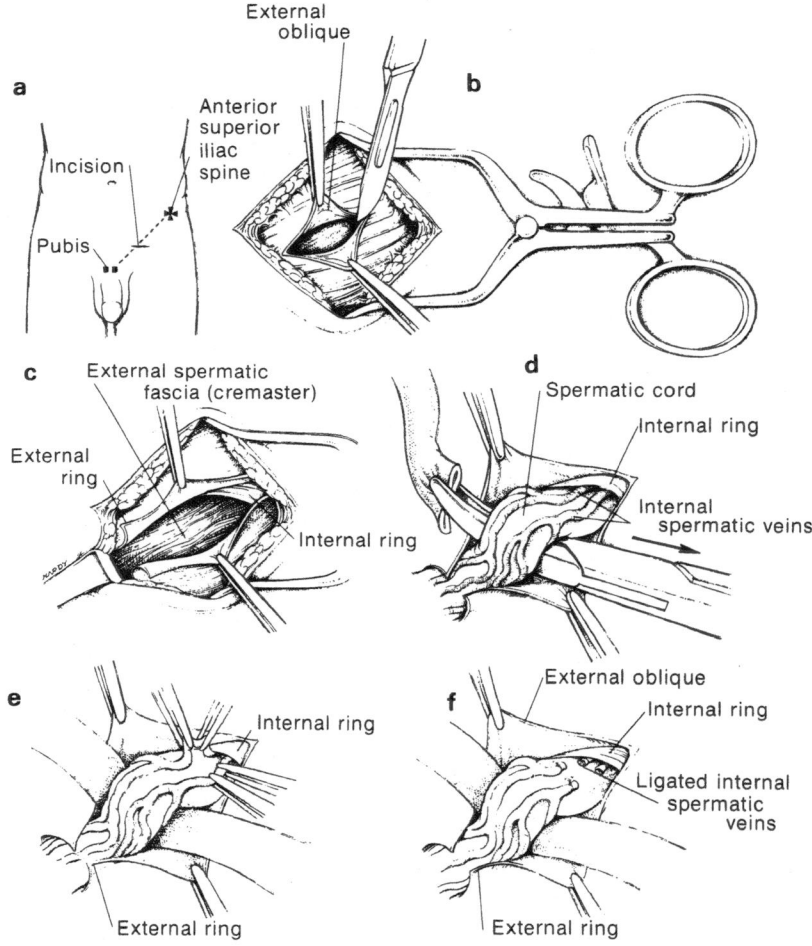

Figure 1. Varicocelectomy (high inguinal procedure modified by Amelar and Dubin) (from Amelar et al. 1977). a. An inguinal incision is made over the area of the internal inguinal ring. b. and c. An incision is made in the external oblique muscle extending through the external inguinal ring, and a self-retaining retractor is placed in the wound. d. The spermatic cord is dissected free. A Penrose drain is then placed under the spermatic cord. e. and f. The internal spermatic veins are then dissected while attempting to preserve all lymphatic channels. The veins are then interrupted, ligated and partially excised at the internal inguinal ring.

placed in the wound. The spermatic cord is dissected free. A Penrose drain is then placed under the spermatic cord and the cord is lifted out of the incision by the drain, which is then clamped on each end to the drapes. The external spermatic fascia is incised, and the veins are dissected free, while trying to preserve all lymphatic channels. The internal spermatic veins are then ligated and partially excised at the internal inguinal ring. Usually two or three branches of the internal spermatic vein are located in this area. The spermatic cord is returned to its position and the external oblique fascia is closed with 2-0 chromic catgut. The skin is closed with interrupted silk or nylon sutures. No drains are used. The patient is ambulatory two hours after the procedure and is discharged from the hospital one or two days after the operation (Ivanissevich 1960).

B. Retroperitoneal procedure

In this procedure an inguinal incision similar to that used in the Ivanissevich procedure but slightly higher and extended through the external oblique fascia in the direction of the muscle fibers, approximately 2 inches above the internal ring is used (Palomo 1949). The internal oblique fascia is spread apart, and retroperitoneal dissection is performed; this usually exposes two branches of the internal spermatic vein, which are ligated and incised. The internal spermatic artery is not intentionally ligated as was described by Palomo in his original article. The internal oblique fascia is then closed with 2-0 chromic catgut, and the remainder of the closure proceeds as described previously.

C. Scrotal approach

The transcrotal approach, which utilizes multiple clamping and ligation of the numerous vessels of the pampiniform plexus, is not recommended because many veins may be missed and end-artery damage at this level is a danger. Scrotal swelling and hematoma may also lead to delayed recovery of fertility.

D. Postoperative complications

The relatively few postoperative complications attest to the benign nature of the surgery (Table 2).

Recurrence on the varicocele occurred in one

Table 2. Postoperative complications from varicocelectomy in 986 men.

Complication	Number
Hydrocele not requiring surgery	25
Hydrocele requiring hydrocelectomy	5
Wound infection	7
Inguinal hematoma	10
Epididymitis	2
Atelectasis	2
Varicocele recurrence	1
Bladder hernia injury	1

patient. This patient and his wife had been attempting a pregnancy for four years. The patient's initial sperm count was over 10 million per ml, but semen quality was poor. A left varicocelectomy was performed on February 10, 1966; semen quality improved, and pregnancy occurred 12 months after surgery. A son was born November 9, 1967. Difficulty in achieving a second pregnancy and poor semen quality were noted again three years after surgery. Examination revealed that the varicocele had recurred. Reflux of blood was again noted during scrotal palpation using the Valsalva maneuver. The patient was operated on again and a large internal spermatic vein was ligated. Postoperatively, a marked improvement in semen quality was noted and pregnancy occurred three months after surgery. A daughter was born on August 10, 1970. A third pregnancy then occurred and a son was born on January 6, 1972.

Thirty (3 percent) patients had hydrocele formation postoperatively. The exact etiology of this is unknown, but the low incidence is probably related to care in only ligating the veins, while trying to preserve all lymphatic channels. Five patients required operative hydrocelectomy.

We also reported on five other patients who had previously had varicocelectomy performed by other physicians. Three of the five had improvement in semen quality and pregnancy resulted. These cases were not included in this reported series.

IV. CONCLUSIONS

The effectiveness of varicocelectomy in the therapy of male infertility has been well demonstrated.

We favor a high inguinal ligation procedure. It is simple and can be done well by most surgeons, and results have been excellent.

Surgery is indicated by poor sperm motility and immaturity. The presence of a varicocele in the absence of this combination of semen defects is not a sufficient indication for surgery.

Patients with initial sperm counts less than 10 million per ml did not yield spectacular results.

The empirical administration of gonadotropin therapy, however, almost doubled the pregnancy rates in a similar group of patients.

All of the actual effects of varicocele on fertility are still unknown. Many men with varicocele have normal semen qualities and adequate fertility. The study of varicocelectomy failures does not reveal any preoperative differences between this group and the group that showed improvement. Nevertheless, the good results in improvement of semen and pregnancy rate continue to make this form of therapy one of the most effective in the treatment of male infertility.

REFERENCES

Ahlberg NE, Bartley O and Chidekel N: Retrograde contrast filling of the left gonadal vein: a roentgenologic and anatomical study. Acta Radiol (Diag) 3: 385, 1965.

Amelar RD and Dubin L: Male infertility, current diagnosis and treatment. Urology 1: 1, 1973.

Amelar RD and Dubin L: Basic and practical aspects of the etiology and management of male infertility. Urol Digest 14: 19, 1975.

Amelar RD, Dubin L and Walsh P: The varicocele and infertility. In: Male infertility, WB Saunders Co, June 1977, p 57-68.

Brown JS: Varicocelectomy in the subfertile male: A 10 year experience with 295 cases. Fertil Steril 27: 1046, 1976.

Brown JS, Dubin L, Becker M and Hotchkiss RS: Venography in the subfertile man with varicocele. J Urol 98: 388, 1967.

Brown JS, Dubin L and Hotchkiss RS: Varicocele as related to fertility. Fertil Steril 18: 46, 1967.

Brown JS, MacLeod and Hotchkiss RS: Results of varicocelectomy in subfertile men. Exhibit at American Fertility Society, Miami, Florida, 1968.

Charny CW: Effect of varicocele on fertility. Fertil Steril 13: 47, 1962.

Charny CW, Baum S: Varicocele and infertility. JAMA 204: 1165, 1968.

Clarke BG: Incidence of varicocele in normal men and among men of different ages. JAMA 198: 1121, 1966.

Comhaire F, Monteyner R and Kunnen M: The value of scrotal thermography as compared with selective retrograde venography of the internal spermatic vein for the diagnosis of subclinical varicocele. Fertil Steril 27: 694, 1976.

Comhaire F and Vermeulen A: Varicocele sterility; cortisol and catecholamines. Fertil Steril 25: 88, 1974.

Dubin L and Amelar RD: Varicocele size and results of varicocelectomy in selected subfertile men with varicocele. Fertil Steril 21: 606, 1970.

Dubin L and Amelar RD: Etiologic factors in 1294 consecutive cases of male infertility. Fertil Steril 22: 469, 1971.

Dubin L and Amelar RD: Varicocelectomy as therapy in male infertility: A study of 504 cases. Fertil Steril 26: 217, 1975.

Dubin L and Amelar RD: Varicocelectomy as therapy in male infertility. J Urol 113: 640, 1975.

Dubin L and Amelar RD: 986 cases of varicocelectomy: A 12 year study. Urology 10: 446, 1977.

Dubin L and Hotchkiss RS: Testis biopsy in subfertile men with varicocele. Fertil Steril 20: 50, 1969.

El-Sadr Ar and Mina E: Anatomical and surgical aspects in operative management of varicocele. Urol Cutan Rev 54: 257, 1950.

Glezerman M, Rakowszczyk M, Lunenfeld B, Beer R and Goldman B: Varicocele in oligospermic patients: pathophysiology and results after ligation and division of the internal spermatic vein. J Urol 115: 562, 1976.

Greenberg SH, Stanley H: Varicocele and male fertility. Fertil Steril 28: 699, 1977.

Greenberg SH, Lipshultz LI, Wein AJ: Experience with 425 subfertile male patients. J Urol 119: 507, 1978.

Hamen R: Studies on impaired fertility in men with special reference to the male. London, Oxford University Press, 1944, p 22, 108.

Hanley HG: The surgery of male sub-fertility. Ann R Coll Surg Eng 17: 159, 1955.

Hanley HG and Harrison RG: Nature and surgical correction of varicocele. Br J Surg 50: 64, 1962.

Heller CG and Clermont Y: Kinetics of the germinal epithelium in man. Prog Horm Res 20: 545, 1964.

Hendry WF, Sommerville IF, Hall RR and Pugh RLB: Investigation and treatment of the subfertile male. Br J Urol 45: 684, 1973.

Ivanissevich O: Left varicocele due to reflux, experience with 4470 operative cases in 42 years. J Int Coll Surg 24: 742, 1960.

Johnson D, Pohl D and Rivera-Correa H: Varicocele: an innocuous condition? South Med J 63: 34, 1970.

Kay RM and Alexander NJ: Experimental creation of varicocele in Rhesus monkeys. Abstract Fertil Steril 28: 339, 1977.

Lewis EL: The Ivanissevich operation. J Urol 63: 165, 1950.

Lipshultz LI, Corriere JN: Progressive testicular atrophy in the varicocele patient. J Urol 117: 175, 1977.

MacLeod J: Seminal cytology in the presence of varicocele. Fertil Steril 16: 735, 1965.

Macomber D and Sanders MD: The spermatozoa count. N Engl J Med 200: 981, 1929.

Mehan DJ: Results of ligation of internal spermatic vein in the treatment of infertility in azoospermic patients. Fertil Steril 27: 110, 1976.

Oster J: Varicocele in children and adolescents. Scand J Urol Nephrol 5: 27, 1971.

Palomo A: Radical cure of varicocele by a new technique. J Urol 61: 604, 1949.

Russell JK: Varicocele in groups of fertile and subfertile men. Br Med J 1: 1231, 1954.

Scott LS and Young D: Varicocele. Fertil Steril 13: 325, 1962.

Steeno O, Knops J, Declerck L, Adimoelja A and Van De Voorde H: Prevention of fertility disorders by detection and treatment of varicocele at school and college age. Andrologia 8: 47, 1976.

Stewart N: Varicocele in infertility: incidence and results of surgical therapy. J Urol 112: 222, 1974.

Stewart B and Montie J: Male infertility. an optimistic report. J Urol 110: 216, 1973.

Swerdloff RS and Walsh P: Pituitary gonadal hormones in patients with varicocele. Fertil Steril 26: 1006, 1975.

Tessler AN and Krahn HP: Varicocele and testicular temperature. Fertil Steril 17: 201, 1966.

Tulloch WS: Consideration of sterility, subfertility in the male. Edinburgh Med J 59: 29, 1952.

Tulloch WS: Varicocele in subfertility: results of treatment. Br Med J 2: 356, 1955.

Uehling DT: Fertility in men with varicocele. Int J Fertil 13: 58, 1968.

Zorgniotti AW: The spermatozoa count, a short history. Urology 5: 672, 1975.

Zorgniotti AW and MacLeod J: Studies in temparature, human semen quality and varicocele. Fertil Steril 24: 854, 1973.

6. BLADDER NECK RECONSTRUCTION FOR RETROGRADE EJACULATION

A.D. JENKINS and S.S. HOWARDS

I. PHYSIOLOGY OF EJACULATION

The ejaculatory process may be divided into two phases, the pre-ejaculatory or emission phase and the ejaculatory phase. During emission, secretions from the periurethral glands, the seminal vesicles, and the prostate are deposited in the posterior urethra. In addition, spermatozoa from the ampulla of the vas deferens, the vas itself, and the cauda epididymidis are propelled by peristalsis into the posterior urethra. The emission process is primarily mediated through the sympathetic nervous system. At the time of ejaculation, the bladder neck, or so-called internal sphincter, closes. Both emission and closure of the bladder neck can be prevented by alpha-adrenergic blocking agents (Shishito and Kimura 1973).

The exact neurophysiology of emission and ejaculation is not known. Afferent sensory stimuli are thought to be relayed from the genitalia to the cerebral cortex via the pudendal nerve. The efferent fibers travel in the spinal cord to the thoracolumbar sympathetic outflow (Kedia and Markland 1975).

During the final phase of ejaculation, the external urethral sphincter relaxes and the striated bulbocavernosus and ischiocavernosus muscles contract, expelling the ejaculate from the posterior urethra and through the urethral meatus. This phase is thought to be triggered by the presence of seminal fluid in the posterior urethra and to be mediated through the parasympathetic sacral outflow (Kedia and Markland 1975).

II. EVALUATION

Retrograde ejaculation is the propulsion of seminal fluid from the posterior urethra into the bladder. Emission is intact and seminal fluid reaches the posterior urethra, but retrograde flow occurs because the bladder neck does not completely close. If emission does not occur, seminal fluid is not deposited in the posterior urethra during the first phase of the ejaculatory process (Rieser 1961). Any man who states that he has an erection, comes to a climax, but sees scant semen, should be suspected of having retrograde ejaculation. This diagnosis can be confirmed by demonstrating reduced semen volumes and the presence of fructose and numerous spermatozoa in a post-ejaculatory urine specimen. Patients with retrograde ejaculation may have no outward or antegrade component during ejaculation or they may have an ejaculate of low volume. In the latter case, there is antegrade ejaculation of the initial sperm-free portion of ejaculate and retrograde ejaculation of the sperm-rich fraction which also contains fructose from the seminal vesicles (Keiserman et al. 1974).

If there is failure of emission, there will be no sperm or fructose in a post-ejaculatory urine specimen or in any ejaculate that might be present.

III. ETIOLOGY

Any process which interferes with the anatomic integrity or sympathetic innervation of the bladder neck can alter bladder neck contractility and result in retrograde ejaculation. Interruption of sympathetic innervation can also cause failure of emission.

Retrograde ejaculation may follow transurethral or open resection of the bladder neck or prostate (Ochsner et al. 1970), bilateral sympathectomy (Whitelaw and Smithwick 1951), extensive pelvic surgery, especially colectomy and proctectomy, abdominal aortic aneurysmectomy (Weinstein and

Machleder 1975), and unilateral or bilateral retroperitoneal lymphadenectomy. However, in one series of patients undergoing high retroperitoneal lymphadenectomy for testicular tumors, 35 of the 36 patients studied had no evidence of ejaculation, either antegrade or retrograde (Kedia et al. 1975). During the dissection, all of the sympathetic ganglia and some of the preganglionic fibers involved with emission were necessarily removed with the lymphatics, thus leading to failure of emission.

A functional sympathectomy may result from diabetic visceral neuropathy (Greene and Kelalis 1968). Drugs such as guanethidine, which interfere with the release of norepinephrine at terminals of the sympathetic nervous system, may also result in a temporary chemical sympathectomy (Goodman and Gilman 1975).

IV. TREATMENT

A. Surgical

The only paper describing a surgical procedure for the correction of retrograde ejaculation is a report concerning two patients who developed retrograde ejaculation following Y-V plasties for bladder neck obstruction (Abrahams et al. 1975). Preoperative cystograms showed contrast material in the posterior urethra and panendoscopy confirmed the presence of a wide open bladder neck in both patients.

With the patient in the supine position, a 16 Fr Foley catheter is passed per urethra. The old scar is excised and the bladder is entered through an anterior cystotomy. An inverted U incision is made in the mucosa surrounding the bladder neck (Figure 1a). The mucosa is elevated for a distance of approximately 1 cm into the prostatic urethra and is excised. The bladder neck muscle is exposed by sharply dissecting and removing any scar tissue. The repair is performed by joining the two limbs of the inverted U anterior to the Foley catheter using four sutures of 0 chromic catgut (Figure 1b, c). The bladder is closed in a routine fashion and the perivesical space is drained. The Foley catheter is removed three weeks postoperatively. In this series, both patients reported antegrade ejaculation by the fourth postoperative week and one patient subsequently fathered a child.

The authors emphasize the importance of exposing the bladder neck muscle by excising any scar tissue that might have resulted from a previous operation. No separate attempt was made to close the mucosa.

No other reconstructive procedures of the bladder neck have been described specifically for the correction of retrograde ejaculation. However, several procedures have been described for the correction of urinary incontinence (Young 1975). One technique that may be useful to correct retrograde ejaculation is the transvesical bipennation and keeling operation of Stephens (Stephens 1970). A midline, full thickness, longitudinal incision is made in the trigone. This is carried from the verumontanum, to and through the interureteric ridge. The resultant lateral wings of trigonal muscle are then plicated. The deep muscle is closed with a running suture of 4-0 chromic catgut and the more superficial muscle is closed with interrupted 4-0 chromic catgut sutures. This forms a thick keel-like bundle in addition to narrowing the bladder neck.

The implantable urinary sphincter prosthesis of Scott is also potentially applicable for the correction of retrograde ejaculation (Scott et al. 1973).

B. Artificial Insemination

When retrograde ejaculation occurs, spermatozoa can be recovered from the bladder following ejaculation and used as an inseminate. In the past, this has been the standard treatment for retrograde ejaculation. The original technique of semen recovery was described by Hotchkiss (Hotchkiss et al. 1955). In this method, the bladder is first washed with Ringer's solution after the patient has had a period of fluid restriction. The bladder is emptied and 2 ml of the same solution are instilled into the bladder. Following ejaculation, the contents are recovered by voiding or catheterization and are used for artificial insemination. Other physicians have alkalinized the urine or washed and concentrated the spermatozoa gently during their processing from the urine (Glezerman et al. 1976).

Pregnancies will result when care is taken to time the insemination precisely with ovulation and to use specimens which contain motile spermatozoa. There is even a case report of a conception which

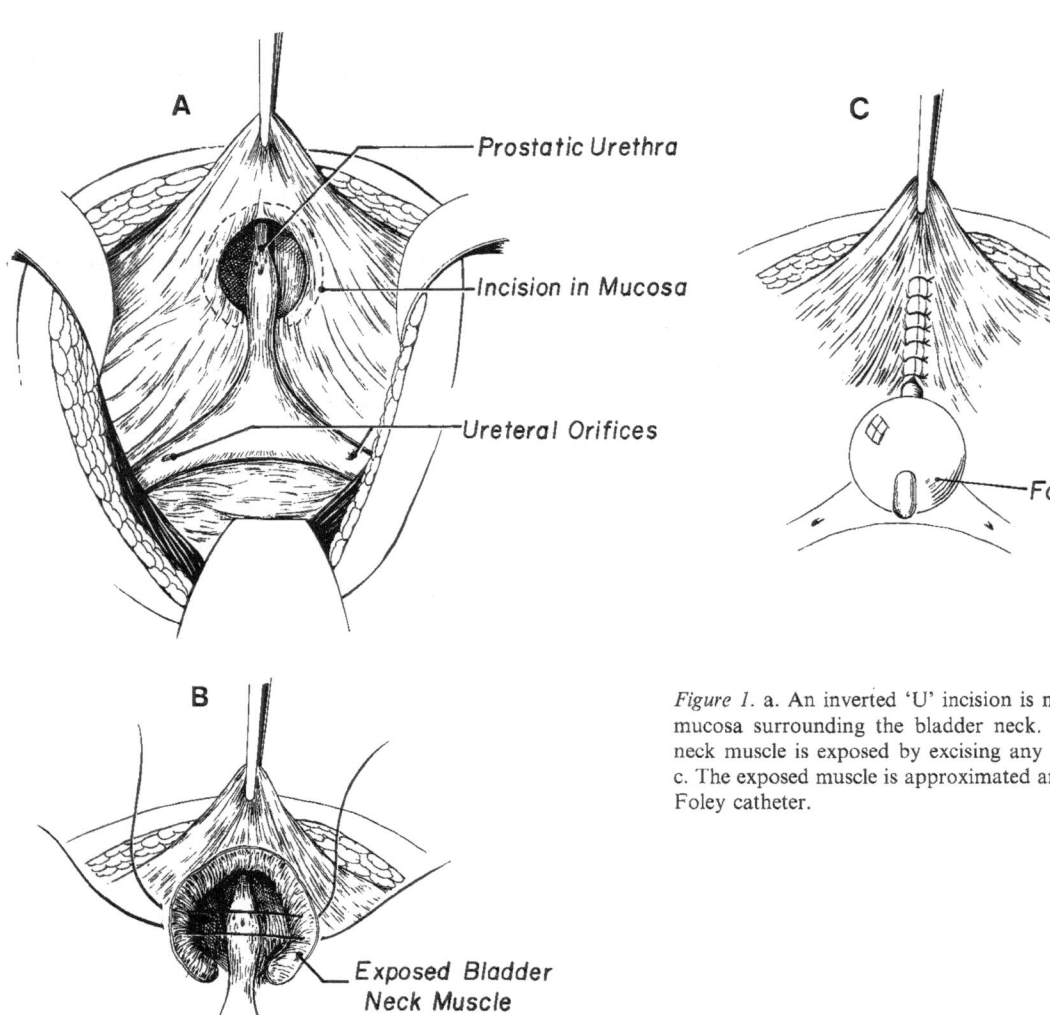

Figure 1. a. An inverted 'U' incision is made in the mucosa surrounding the bladder neck. b. Bladder neck muscle is exposed by excising any scar tissue. c. The exposed muscle is approximated anterior to a Foley catheter.

occurred following the voiding of a postejaculate specimen directly into the vagina (Schram 1976).

C. Medical

There are a few case reports suggesting that sympathomimetic drugs and certain antihistamines may be effective in diabetic and postsurgical retrograde ejaculation. Phenoxybenzamine (an alpha-blocking agent) has been used to improve bladder emptying in patients with abnormally high bladder neck resistance due to hyperactivity of smooth muscle in this area (Krane and Olsson 1973), while ephedrine (alpha and beta receptor activity) has been used to restore continence in patients with stress in-

continence (Stewart and Bergant 1974). Intravenous synephrine (almost exclusive alpha agonist activity) has been administered to patients who have previously undergone retroperitoneal lymphadenectomy for testicular tumors (Stockamp et al. 1974). In that study, only one of six patients had a high sperm count in a postejaculation urine specimen and this patient achieved antegrade ejaculation following the injection of synephrine. Oral ephedrine (50 mg, 1 to 2 hours prior to intercourse) has also been used to treat retrograde ejaculation (Stewart and Bergant 1974); however, ephedrine is often ineffective. This is not surprising since the drug works, at least in part, by releasing local norepinephrine.

Bethanechol (a parasympathomimetic drug) has been shown to open the bladder neck, while epinephrine will reverse this effect (Kleeman 1970). Consequently, some investigators have postulated that stimulation of the sympathetic nervous system causes closure of the bladder neck, while stimulation of the parasympathetic nervous system causes the bladder neck to open (Kleeman 1970). Brompheniramine maleate (Dimetane-Robins) is an antihistamine with anticholinergic side effects. It has been reported to reverse retrograde ejaculation in a patient with juvenile onset diabetes mellitus (Andaloro and Dube 1975).

Ornade (Smith, Kline, and French Laboratories) has also been reported to correct documented retrograde ejaculation in a diabetic patient (Stewart and Bergant 1974). Ornade contains three drugs: chlorpheniramine (an antihistamine), phenylpropanolamine (a sympathomimetic agent), and isopropamide (a synthetic anticholinergic agent). Therefore, it can theoretically close the bladder neck both through stimulation of the sympathetic innervation and antagonism of the parasympathetic innervation of the bladder neck. Recently, two successful conceptions have been reported following the augmentation of antegrade ejaculation with Ornade and artificial insemination using the resultant ejaculate (Thiagarajah et al. 1978).

At the present time, the treatment of retrograde ejaculation with artificial insemination or pharmacologic agents is preferable to surgical reconstruction of the bladder neck.

REFERENCES

Abrahams JI, Solish GI, Boorjian P and Waterhouse RK: The surgical correction of retrograde ejaculation. J Urol 114: 888, 1975.

Andaloro VA Jr and Dube A: Treatment of retrograde ejaculation with brompheniramine. Urology 5: 520, 1975.

Glezerman M, Lunenfeld B, Potashnik G, Oelsner G and Beer R: Retrograde ejaculation: Pathophysiologic aspects and report of two successfully treated cases. Fertil Steril 27: 796, 1976.

Goodman LS and Gilman A (eds): The pharmacological basis of therapeutics, 5 ed, New York, MacMillan, 1975.

Greene LF and Kelalis PP: Retrograde ejaculation of semen due to diabetic neuropathy. J Urol 98: 693, 1968.

Hotchkiss RS, Pinto AB and Kleegman S: Artificial insemination with semen recovered from the bladder. Fertil Steril 6: 37, 1955.

Kedia KR, Markland C and Fraley EE: Sexual function following high retroperitoneal lymphadenectomy. J Urol 114: 237, 1975.

Kedia K and Markland C: The effect of pharmacological agents on ejaculation. J Urol 114: 509, 1975.

Keiserman WM, Dubin L and Amelar RD: A new type of retrograde ejaculation: report of three cases. Fertil Steril 25: 1071, 1974.

Kleeman FJ: Physiology of the internal urinary sphincter. J Urol 104: 549, 1970.

Krane RJ and Olsson CA: Phenoxybenzamine in neurogenic bladder dysfunction, II. Clinical considerations. J Urol 110: 653, 1973.

Ochsner MG, Burns E and Henry HH II: Incidence of retrograde ejaculation following bladder neck revision as a child. J Urol 104: 596, 1970.

Rieser C: The etiology of retrograde ejaculation and a method for insemination. Fertil Steril 12: 488, 1961.

Schram JD: Retrograde ejaculation: A new approach to therapy. Fertil Steril 27: 1216, 1976.

Scott FB, Bradley WE and Timm GW: Treatment of urinary incontinence by an implantable prosthetic urinary sphincter. Urology 1: 252, 1973.

Shishito S and Kimura Y: Peripheral nerves controlling ejaculation and receptor mechanism. Urology Digest, p 9, August 1973.

Stephens FD: A form of stress incontinence in children: Another method of bladder neck repair. Aust N Z J Surg 40: 124, 1970.

Stewart B and Bergant JA: Correction of retrograde ejaculation by sympathomimetic medication: preliminary report. Fertil Steril 25: 1073, 1974.

Stockamp K, Schreiter F and Altwein JE: α-Adrenergic drugs in retrograde ejaculation. Fertil Steril 25: 817, 1974.

Thiagarajah S, Vaughan ED Jr and Kitchin JD III: Retrograde ejaculation: successful pregnancy following combined sympathomimetic medication and insemination. Fertil Steril 30: 96, 1978.

Weinstein MH and Machleder HI: Sexual function after aorto-iliac surgery. Ann Surg 181: 787, 1975.

Whitelaw GP and Smithwick RH: Some secondary effects of sympathectomy. N Engl J Med 245: 121, 1951.

Young BW: The vesical neck. In: Urologic surgery, 2 ed, Glenn JF (ed), Hagerstown, MD, Harper and Row, 1975.

III. DISORDERS OF ERECTION, EMISSION AND VAGINAL PENETRATION

7. URETHROPLASTY FOR HYPOSPADIAS

J.N. CORRIERE, JR.

Hypospadias is a developmental anomaly of the penis and urethra in which the uretral meatus is situated on the ventral aspect of the penis at any point from the glans to the perineum. Meatal stenosis is also commonly present. In most cases, the corpus spongiosum distal to the meatus, along with the dartos and Buck's fascia, is replaced by a tough fibrous band which bends the penis ventrally. The curvature is called chordee. During erection, the chordee becomes more severe, making sexual intercourse difficult or impossible. The prepuce is also deficient ventrally and forms a dorsal hood over the glans. Incontinence is never a problem.

These anomalous arrangements prevent the patient from accomplishing the two acts the penis and pendulous urethra are designed to perform – allowing the patient to direct his urinary stream while in the standing position and vaginal penetration during coitus with deposition of semen at the female's cervical os.

I. INCIDENCE, ETIOLOGY AND ASSOCIATED ANOMALIES

The incidence of hypospadias has been reported in ranges of 1:160 to 1:1800 births; it is probably somewhere between 1:300 and 1:500 live births. During recent years, an increased occurrence of three percent per year has been reported in the United States. An increased incidence has also been reported in England, Wales and Norway.

Partial explanation of this increase is unquestionably due to improved recognition and reporting of cases, but there is some evidence that exposure of the fetus to exogenous maternal progestins during the first trimester of pregnancy, either as hormonal pregnancy tests or to prevent abortion, may be an etiologic factor (Aarskog 1979).

Studies of families in which one individual has hypospadias have also revealed that this congenital defect is not necessarily a sporadic event but has a familial occurrence tendency. Although the mode of inheritance has not been completely verified, it seems to be multifactorial with multiple gene factors combining under appropriate intrauterine environmental influences to produce the anatomic defect (Bauer et al. 1979).

The incidence of a second family member having hypospadias is about 25 percent. A brother will be affected 14 percent of the time, the father nine percent of the time and uncles and cousins less than five percent of the time. If both the father and index child are affected, a second male sibling has a 27 percent chance of having the anomaly. Finally, the more severe the anomaly, the greater the chance of another family member being affected.

Associated anomalies are present in up to 27 percent of affected children (Table 1). Most authors feel that the incidence of other malformations increases with the severity of the hypospadias (Bauer et al. 1979; Fallon et al. 1976; Lutzker et al. 1977; McArdle and Lebowitz 1975). Most of the associated anomalies are present in the genitourinary tract, but the documented literature is unclear as to whether radiographic or endoscopic studies are productive. If there are no clinical indications

Table 1. Anomalies associated with hypospadias.

Congenital inguinal hernia
Cryptorchidism
Ambiguous genitalia
Ureteropelvic junction obstruction
Vesicoureteral reflux
Renal rotation and ascent anomalies
Heart disease
Orthopedic defects

of urinary tract disease, further investigation is probably not necessary. However, the presence of bilateral cryptorchidism or other ambiguous genitalia (bifid scrotum, micropenis) mandate a search for an intersex state.

II. DEVELOPMENTAL ANATOMY AND CLASSIFICATION

A. Embryology

The genital tubercle develops cranial to the cloacal membrane. A midline groove persists in the tubercle for its entire length to its tip where an epithelial tag is formed. With male differentiation, the genital tubercle grows and assumes a more cylindrical shape. The midline urethral groove deepens and the urethral folds become prominent. By 16 weeks, the urethral folds have fused proximal to distal forming a tube – the urethra. The fused edges remain as the median raphe. During fusion, mesenchyme coalesces around the deepening groove forming the corpus spongiosum and covering fascia.

As the urethral folds meet distally, the glans enlarges and the urethral groove deepens. The glans closes over the groove, but its edges do not fuse, leaving a deep epithelial-lined tract. A roll of skin then arises on either side of the urethral opening and encircles the penis. This skin grows out to form the prepuce. As the prepuce grows, the edges of the glans seal over the glanular urethra until the urethral meatus reaches its ultimate location at the site of the epithelial tag. The deep epithelial tract forms the fossa navicularis. This segment of the urethra forms from the terminal plate or epithelial tag and is not part of the epithelial groove.

If this distal event does not occur, glanular hypospadias and a hooded prepuce result. If the terminal urethra closes without meeting the penile urethra, a blind-ending glanular canal forms, the urethral meatus is hypospadiac, and the prepuce is hooded. The mesenchyme around the unfused urethral groove becomes a fibrous band instead of corpus spongiosum, dartos and Buck's fascia.

B. Types of Anomalies

1. Chordee without hypospadias. In as many as ten

percent of some reported patients series, the urethra is normally formed but the penis has a chordee. In this anomaly, the skin overlying the urethra is inelastic because it is attached to the urethra. The curvature usually only appears to involve the glans but it may be more severe. Treatment involves appropriate correction of the chordee.

2. Glanular or Balanic. This is the most common type of anomaly, being present in 40 to 80 percent of the reported studies. The urethra opens at the site of the frenulum, which is rudimentary or absent. The meatus may be slit-like or pocket-like with downward chordee and commonly is stenotic. If no chordee is present, meatotomy may be the only treatment needed. Chordee correction with or without meatal advancement should be performed in more severe cases.

3. Penile. Ten to 30 percent of the time the urethra opens somewhere between the penoscrotal junction and glans. Various severities of chordee may be present. The chordee should be corrected and the meatus advanced to the tip of the penis.

4. Penoscrotal, Scrotal or Perineal. This severest group of deformities occurs in three to 15 percent of the cases. The urethra opens anywhere from the penoscrotal junction back to the perineum. The chordee is usually quite marked and the meatus stenotic. A cleft or bifid scrotum is common. In severe cases, intersex evaluation is indicated. Treatment consists of chordee correction, meatal advancement and possibly scrotal reconstruction.

III. PREOPERATIVE EVALUATION AND COUNSELING

These children should be seen by a urologist during the neonatal period. The severity of the anomaly as well as other clinical findings may dictate that an excretory urogram or renal scan be performed. More importantly, if there is a question of an intersex state, a retrograde urethrogram ('vaginogram'), chromosomal, chemical and hormonal evaluation and subsequent determination of the patient's sex rearing must be done as quickly as possible for both medical and psychological reasons.

If the meatus is stenotic, meatotomy should be performed immediately. Circumcision is contra-indicated because the preputial skin may be needed at the time of surgical repair. The parents should then be counseled concerning the familial aspects of the problem and be assured that in most cases, surgical correction can produce a cosmetically acceptable and functional organ. It should be emphasized that hypospadias surgery is commonly a 'multi-staged procedure' even for those patients for whom one-staged operations are attempted. The child should be re-examined at no less than yearly intervals to ensure that meatal stenosis does not develop and this also allows the parents to ask any questions they may have concerning the upcoming hospitalizations and repair.

The most hazardous time psychologically for elective surgery on the genitalia is between the ages of six months and three years. The most optimum time, both psychologically and medically, is during the fourth or fifth year of life. Beyond the age of six, although the adverse effects of hospitalization and separation diminish, anxiety about the impending surgery may increase.

However, since the degree of deformity and thus the complexity and number of procedures varies from case to case, it is difficult to make strict guidelines. Correction should not be started before the patient is age one and if possible, it should be deferred until after the third birthday. Repair should be completed by the fifth birthday so the child may enter school without the stigma of a genital anomaly.

Aside from adequate psychological counseling and a detailed explanation of the entire preoperative, operative and postoperative procedures, no special preparation or studies are necessary. A complete history and physical examination, blood count, urinalysis, urine culture and chest roentgenogram are performed in keeping with good preoperative surgical practice. Any abnormalities that are found are then investigated further. As with all pediatric surgery, the operation should be scheduled as early in the day as possible. All oral intake should be forbidden for at least six hours before the operative procedure.

IV. SURGICAL PROCEDURES

The goals for surgical repair are complete straightening of the penis and bringing the urethral meatus as close to the tip of the glans as possible. It is also hoped that the patient will have a controlled full urinary stream without spraying, plus a normal penile appearance. The deformity present, as well as the experience of the surgeon, dictates which procedure to utilize. Herein are detailed some of the more popular approaches, all of which have advocates and all of which will lead, if properly chosen and performed, to a satisfactory result. No attempt has been made to catalogue the multitude of procedures that have been described over the years.

A few technical points that are applicable to all forms of reconstructive surgery should be reviewed. First, it must be remembered that the edges of raised skin flaps will become functional tubes and covering layers. They should be handled with skin hooks or holding sutures when at all possible and never crushed with forceps. Second, minor bleeding can be controlled with epinephrine-soaked sponges. Large vessels may be ligated with fine absorbable suture or lightly electrocoagulated. Use of the ophthalmologic battery powered cautery is usually satisfactory. Third, chromic sutures are probably the best material to use on a neourethra. The synthetic absorbable sutures can be used but they are absorbed at an unpredictable rate and may act as wicks encouraging fistula formation. Either chromic or the synthetic material can be used for skin closure. Many surgeons prefer a running subcuticular nonabsorbable suture closure which is removed about 14 days postoperatively.

A. Chordee without Hypospadias (Allen-Spence Procedure)

When the patient has a curvature of the penis but the urethral meatus is on the glans, the pathology appears to be abnormal development of the distal corpus spongiosum and attachment of the urethra directly to the overlying skin of the shaft. If the skin is dissected free from the urethra, this 'skin-chordee' is released, the penis straightens, and then merely needs dorsal prepuce transposition to cover the ventrally denuded penis (Allen and Spence 1968).

A circumcising incision is made proximal to the meatus and the attachments of the skin to the underlying urethra and corpora are dissected free (Figure 1a). The urethra directly under the distal and ventral skin is paper-thin and can be inadvertently entered if care is not taken during dissection. Should this occur, the rent may be closed with interrupted 6-0 chromic sutures. When all the skin attachments are lysed, the ventral skin will drop quite a ways down the shaft. The hooded prepuce is then unrolled and divided by the Byers' incision technique (Figure 1b). An alternate method is to employ the Nesbit button-hole for closure (Figure 6a, b). Finally, the flaps are wrapped around the shaft to cover the ventral defect and sutured in place with interrupted 5-0 chromic or polyglycolic sutures (Figure 1c). A compression dressing and urethral catheter drainage are employed for three to five days.

B. The Flip-Flap (Mustarde Procedure)

If the meatus is near the glans, a minor meatal advancement procedure combined with correction of chordee is indicated (Mustarde 1965). A flap of skin on the ventral shaft of the penis, proximal to the meatus, is elevated to act as the ventral surface of the neourethra, and the glans is triangularized to allow appropriate removal of all underlying fibrous bands creating the chordee (Figure 2). The apex of the middle glanular flap is then sutured back to the distal rim of the old meatus and the shaft flap to the edges of this middle glanular flap to bring the urethra to the tip of the glans (Figure 2b, c). The prepuce must be unrolled and incised for use in ventral closure (Figure 2b, c). During tube construction, interrupted 6-0 chromic suture is employed. Closure is then performed by wrapping the lateral glanular flaps and preputial skin flaps around the ventral side of the denuded penis (Figure 2d), using interrupted 5-0 chromic or polyglycolic sutures. Urethral or proximal diversion are used for five days or longer. A compression dressing is applied for about five days.

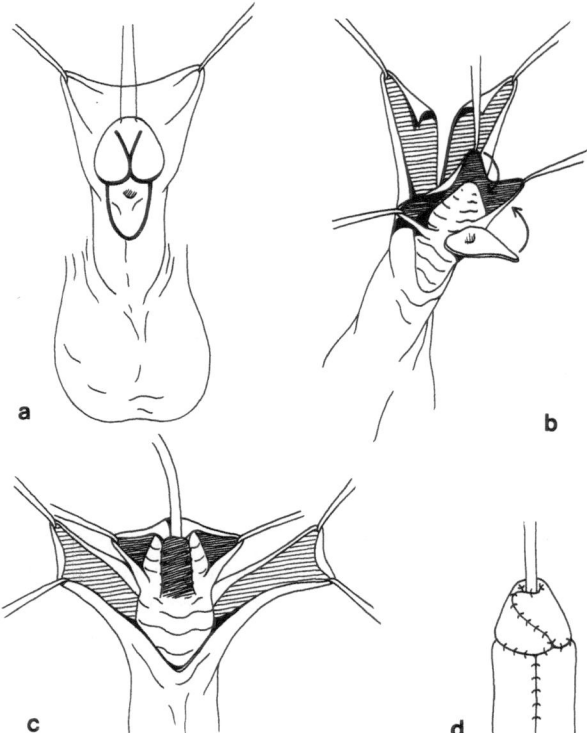

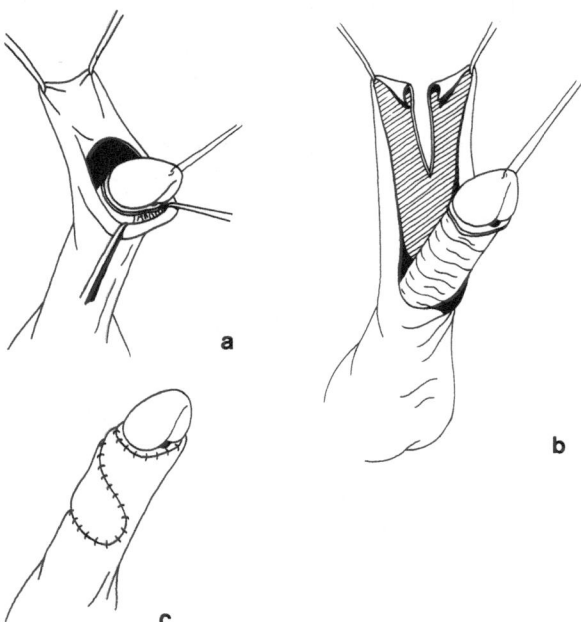

Figure 1. a. Circumcising incision made proximal to the meatus. Note attachment of urethra by fibrous bands directly to skin near incision and use of skin hooks on flaps. b. Skin completely dissected off penis. Prepuce unrolled and midline incision performed. Note holder stitch in glans. c. Skin flaps brought ventrally to cover defect. Excess skin discarded.

Figure 2. a. Incisions for ventral flap and triangularizing of glans are outlined. b. Skin flaps are elevated by skin hooks. All fibrous bands are removed. Middle glanular flap is now sutured to the edge of the old meatus. Ventral flap is then sutured to edges of this glanular flap. Prepuce is unrolled and incised. c. Flap suturing completed. Neourethra constructed with the neo-meatus at the tip of the glans. Note urethral catheter in place. d. Lateral glanular flaps cover neourethra. Preputial flaps cover the shaft defect. Excess skin discarded. Urethral catheter in place.

C. Rolled Penile Skin Tube (King Procedure)

When there is a more proximal meatus and the chordee is cutaneous or absent, a neourethra can be created by rolling a skin tube from the ventral penile skin (King 1970). The skin tube incision should be wide enough to create a urethra of at least a 12 French diameter. The incision should extend into the glans and a circumcising incision should be used to free the prepuce (Figure 3a). The skin tube is not extensively freed from the underlying penis in order to preserve its blood supply. Interrupted 5-0 or 6-0 chromic sutures are used to create the neourethra (Figure 3b). The lateral glanular flaps and penile skin must be widely freed. When the tube is complete, the prepuce is unrolled and divided (Figure 3c). The prepuce is now used to cover the ventral defect. A compression dressing is employed for about four days and proximal urinary diversion for at least one week. A urethral stent may be used for a few days.

D. One-Stage Pedicle Graft (Hodgson II Procedure)

In the early 1970s Hodgson described three ways to use the skin of the prepuce as a pedicle graft to create a neourethra (Hodgson 1970). In his Type I procedure, the mucosal side of the prepuce is rolled into a tube and in Type III, the dorsal side is rolled into a tube. The Type II procedure is useful when a minimal defect and minimal chordee are present in which the pedicle graft is taken from the dorsal side of the prepuce and becomes the ventral side of the neourethra, while the ventral penile shaft skin becomes dorsal neourethra.

The dorsal side of the neourethra is outlined on the penile shaft and a circumcising incision performed (Figure 4a). On the dorsal surface of the prepuce the corresponding ventral side of the neourethra is outlined (Figure 4b). Care is taken not to dissect this delicate strip of skin from the ventral

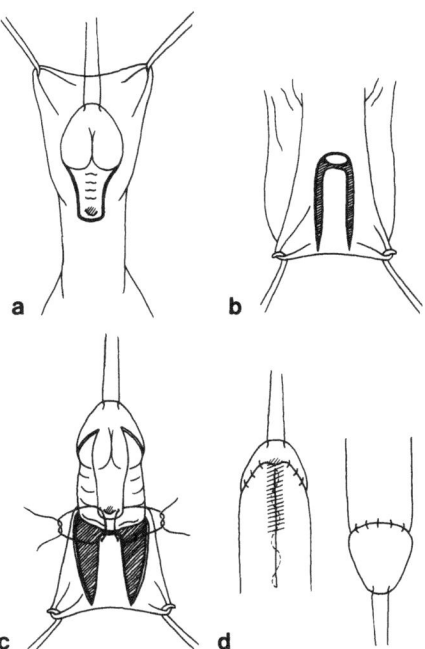

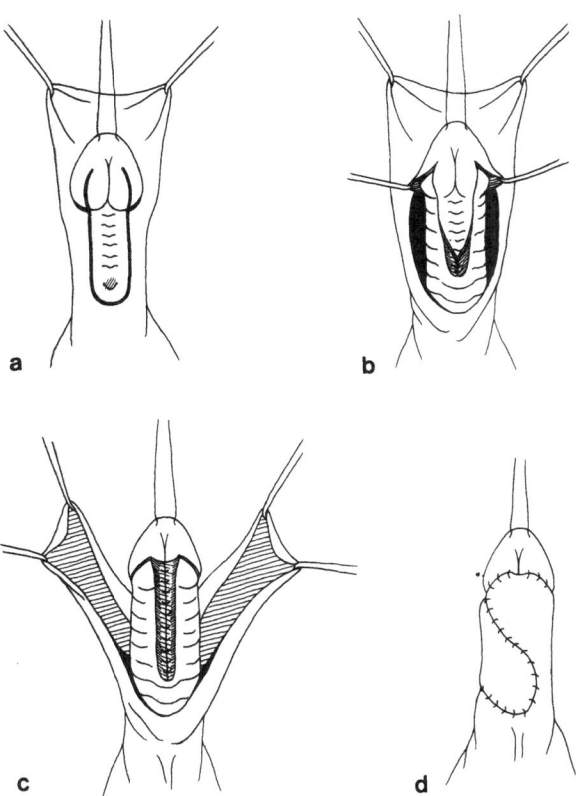

Figure 3. a. Skin incision outlined for tube and circumcision. Holder stitch in glans. b. Skin hooks elevate lateral flaps. Tube being rolled with interrupted sutures. c. Neourethra completed. Prepuce unrolled and divided. d. Preputial flaps cover the ventral shaft defect. Excess skin discarded.

Figure 4. a. The dorsal side of the neourethra on the ventral side of the penis and circumcising incisions are outlined. A holder stitch is in the glans. b. The dorsal preputial pedicle graft has been incised and a buttonhole made in the ventral prepuce at its base. c. The penis has been brought through the buttonhole. The two halves of the neourethra are being sutured. d. The neourethra has been completed (shaded area) and a running suture (dotted line) is shown closing the ventral opening which used to be the circumcising incision. Excess skin discarded. Note there is no suture line on the dorsal side of the penis.

prepuce to preserve its blood supply. A buttonhole is made in the ventral pepuce at the level of the proximal end of the skin flap (Figure 4b). The penile shaft is brought through the buttonhole and the two layers of the neourethra are joined by interrupted 5-0 or 6-0 chromic sutures (Figure 4c). Adequate dissection must be performed laterally on the penile shaft, but the ventral skin graft should not be lifted from the penis so that its blood supply will be preserved. Excess skin is trimmed from the ventral skin incision (which is the old circumcising incision) and closed with either interrupted or continuous suture (Figure 4d). A stent is left in the urethra for three to seven days and a compression dressing is utilized for four days. Urethral or proximal diversion is used for at least seven days.

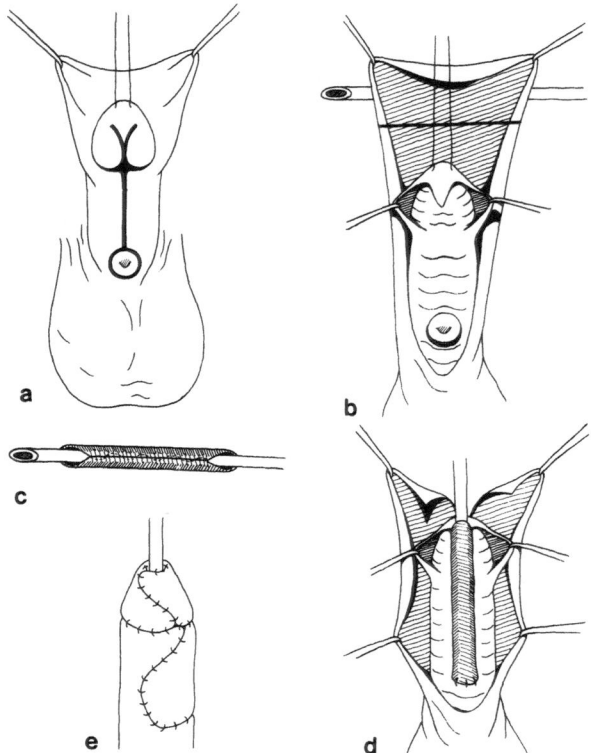

Figure 5. a. Incisions are made around the meatus, in the ventral midline from the meatus to the glans and around the glans in a circumferential manner. The glans is also triangularized. b. The lateral glanular flaps and ventral skin of the penis are widely dissected. They are shown here retracted with skin hooks. All chordee is removed. A holder stitch is in the glans. The prepuce is unrolled and measured with a 12 French catheter for a free graft. C. The subcutaneous tissue has been removed from the free graft which is now sutured, skin side down, over the catheter. Note spatulated ends of the tube. d. The proximal end of the tube is sutured to the old meatus and the distal end to the medial glanular flap. The remaining prepuce has been divided. e. The glanular flaps and preputial flaps are brought ventrally to cover the denuded shaft and skin graft. Excess skin discarded.

E. One-Stage Free Graft (Devine-Horton Procedure)

When chordee is extensive, dissection must be done from the level of the glans to and around the normally formed urethra. This leaves an extensive denuded area on the ventral surface. An alternative to a pedicle tube graft is a free preputial graft (Devine and Horton 1961). In this procedure, an incision is made around the meatus, up the middle of the ventral shaft to the glans and around the glans (Figure 5a). The glans is also triangularized. When all of the chordee is freed, the prepuce is unrolled and the distal end measured for a free skin graft (Figure 5b). The subcutaneous tissue is removed from the graft which is sutured, skin side down. over a 12 French urethral catheter with interrupted 5-0 chromic (Figure 5c). The tube is sutured proximally to the old meatus and distally to the medial glanular flap with chromic sutures (Figure 5d). The remaining prepuce is divided and the lateral glanular flaps and prepuce are used to close the ventral defect (Figure 5e). Either chromic or polyglycolic sutures are used for this closure. A compression dressing is left in place for three to seven days, the stent for seven days and proximal diversion for at least ten days.

F. Two-Stage Technique (Belt-Fuqua Procedure)

Many times extensive dissection is necessary to remove the chordee or the surgeon may feel uneasy about completing such an operation in one stage. In these instances, a two-stage procedure is useful (Fuqua 1971). In the first stage, the chordee is corrected, the penis straightened and the dorsal hooded prepuce transferred to the ventral side of the shaft for use in subsequent repair. In the second stage, a neourethra is formed.

In the first stage, a midline incision from the meatus to the glans as well as a circumcising incision are performed. All fibrous bands are excised and the foreskin is unrolled (Figure 6a). A buttonhole is created in the foreskin (Figure 6a), the penis is brought through this buttonhole, and all suture lines are closed with interrupted 5-0 chromic or polyglycolic suture (Figure 6b). A urethral catheter and compression dressing are used for about five days.

About six months later, when healing has been completed and all the tissues are soft and pliable, the second stage of the operation is performed. A tube of skin that becomes the neourethra is freed from the old meatus in length sufficient distally on the redundant ventral skin to reach the base of the glans penis (Figure 6c). The neourethra is closed with interrupted 5-0 or 6-0 chromic and an opening is made at the base of the glans for the neomeatus (Figure 6c). The meatus is sutured to this area with interrupted 5-0 chromic and after trimming excessive skin, the ventral incision is also closed (Figure 6d). If a more cosmetically pleasing result is desired, glanular triangularization may be performed. A urethral stent and compression dressing are employed for three to five days and proximal diversion for at least ten days.

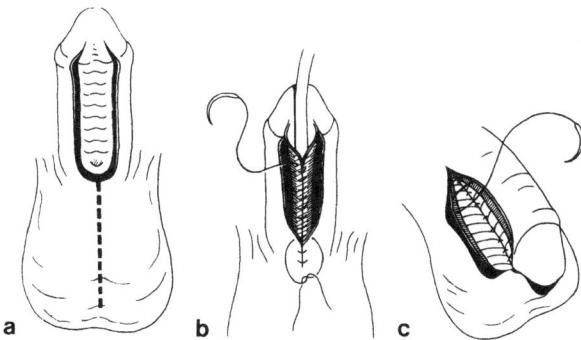

Figure 7. a. Incisions made for neourethra. If Cecil-Culp procedure is to be used, scrotum must be opened in the midline for the same length as the neourethra (dotted line). b. Neourethra being closed. Catheter in urethra. If Byars procedure is used, note closure of skin overlying neourethra in same direction. c. If Cecil-Culp procedure is to be used, the edges of the opened skin are sutured to the edges of the opened scrotum. Here can be seen a fascial layer being closed. The skin will then be approximated.

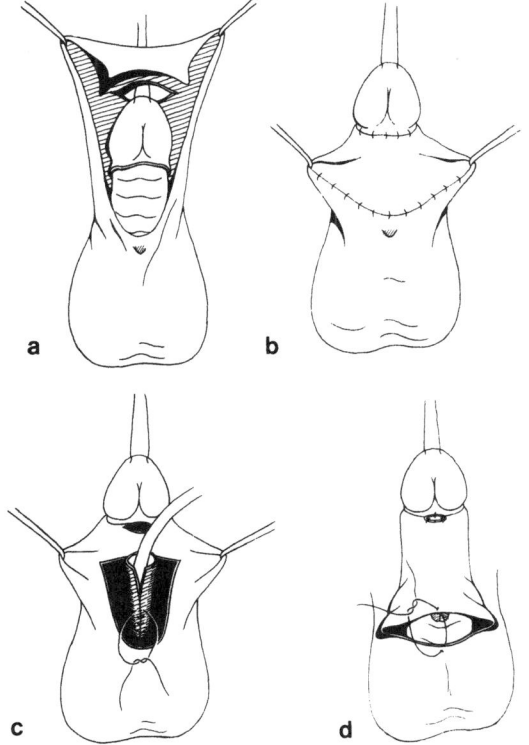

Figure 6. a. Midline incision from meatus to base of glans and circumcising incision performed. All fibrous bands dissected free. Prepuce unrolled, buttonhole made. Holder stitch in glans. b. Penis brought through buttonhole, skin closed. No skin is excised. c. Neourethra outlined and closure beginning. Neourethral opening made at base of glans. d. Urethra sutured to neomeatus. Excess skin excised and ventral incision closed horizontally.

G. Other Second Stage Techniques (Byars Procedure; Cecil-Culp Procedure)

If there is insufficient skin to perform the second stage of the Belt-Fuqua procedure, a neourethra may be created from the meatus to the glans as shown in Figure 7. If the skin can then be closed over the top of this layer the procedure may be completed (Byars 1955). If there is insufficient skin, the penis may be sutured to the scrotum and released at a later date when healing has taken place (Culp 1966).

In both procedures, the neourethra is rolled from the ventral skin of the penis, large enough to accept a 12 French catheter from the old meatus into the glans (Figure 7a). If a Cecil-Culp procedure is to be performed, the scrotum must be opened in the midline for an equal distance (Figure 7a, dotted line). The neourethra is closed with interrupted 5-0 or 6-0 chromic sutures (Figure 7b). If possible, the overlying skin is closed with either interrupted 5-0 absorbable sutures or a running pullout non-absorbable nylon suture (Figure 7b). If there is tension on this suture line, a dorsal linear relaxing incision may be performed. This defect may be grafted or allowed to heal on its own. A stent and compression dressing are left in place for three days and proximal diversion for at least ten days. If a subcuticular pullout suture is placed, it should be removed at about ten days.

If there is insufficient skin to close over the neourethra, the scrotum should be opened as described above and the edges of the penile wound sutured to the edges of the scrotal wound with interrupted absorbable sutures (Figure 7c). As many fascia layers as possible should be closed between the neourethra and the skin. A stent is left in place for three days and proximal diversion is employed for at least ten days. Four to six months later, when healing has been completed, a third procedure is necessary to release the penis from the scrotum and close the penile and scrotal wounds created. No diversion is usually needed. Compression dressings may be used for a few days if desired.

V. URINARY DIVERSION

As mentioned in the previous section, the patient with a neourethra should be put at rest for a period of five days to two weeks to allow healing to occur. To this end, tube diversion of the urine is accomplished by one of the following procedures:

A. Urethral Catheter

Many surgeons, especially those performing one-stage procedures, utilize an indwelling urethral catheter to both stent the anastomosis and divert the urinary stream. A silastic catheter is preferred and is usually taped up to the abdomen to prevent kinking the urethra at the peno-scrotal junction. In a small child, the balloon of a Foley catheter sitting on the trigone may induce bladder spasms. Thus, some authors advocate the use of a straight catheter sewn to the glans penis for this form of diversion.

One advantage of the urethral catheter is that it can be replaced if it inadvertently is removed, or if at the time of planned removal a fistula mandates further diversion. A disadvantage is the presence of a foreign body (the catheter) across the most important suture line in the repair (the urethral tube) which may lead to suppuration and necrosis.

B. Perineal Urethrostomy

For many surgeons, the most popular form of diversion is the placement of a Foley catheter through a urethrotomy proximal to the repair. To perform this procedure, the patient is placed in the dorsal lithotomy position, a sound or catheter introduced into the bladder and a midline incision made through the perineum into bulbous urethra. The edges of the urethra are tagged with 4-0 chromic suture and the sound removed. A Foley catheter is then placed into the perineal urethrotomy and advanced into the bladder. No sutures or dressings are necessary. At the time of catheter removal, the urethrotomy promptly heals without further surgical manipulation.

The advantages of this form of diversion are that it prevents having a catheter across a suture line and the wound is in an inconspicuous position. The disadvantages are the need for repositioning the patient after diversion for the repair, increased expenditure of surgical time, the fact that once the catheter is removed, it cannot be replaced, and the recent evidence that urethral diverticulae develop at the site of the urethrostomy in some patients.

C. Suprapubic Cystostomy

In the child, the bladder is an abdominal organ which is quite accessible for suprapubic diversion. Formal cystostomy can be performed through a three centimeter transverse skin incision. The fascia can be opened vertically, the recti separated, the bladder identified and opened in its dome. A mushroom catheter can be placed in the opening and the bladder, fascia and skin closed around the tube. In the last few years, the development and use of percutaneous suprapubic cystostomy tubes has become popular and has even outmoded the formal cystostomy. Early models drained poorly because of the inadequate size of the catheter lumen and drainage ports and induced bladder spasms by contacting the trigone. Newer models of larger sizes and drainage ports which can be affixed to the dome of the bladder have been developed and are quite satisfactory.

The major disadvantage, the presence of an abdominal scar, is more imagined than real, for when pubic hair grows, the wound is well hidden. The increased surgical time for the formal cystostomy can be reduced to a minimum by employing one of the percutaneous procedures.

However, this procedure does not require a foreign body across a suture line; it can be clamped to test voiding and, if need be, unclamped for further drainage; and trigonal irritation and bladder spasms are reduced to a minimum. The advantages of this procedure greatly outweigh the disadvantages, thus making it an attractive form of diversion.

D. Catheter Care

Closed drainage should be employed but antibiotics are unnecessary until the catheter is removed. High fluid intake should be encouraged to prevent clogging of the tube with debris. Intake of dairy products, popular with children, especially milk and ice cream, should be severely restricted as the resulting phosphaturia and alkaline urine will increase crystaluria and the chances of catheter obstruction. If bladder spasms occur, first the catheter should be irrigated to rule out obstruction, and then an anticholinergic such as probanthine in doses of 7.5 to 15 mg should be prescribed at six-hour intervals.

VI. POSTOPERATIVE CARE AND FOLLOW-UP

A. Immediate Care

Aside from the customary problems with urinary diversions, most postoperative difficulties occur from wound disruption and flap necrosis. Devascularized tissue cannot be saved, but the use of an ice pack for the first 12 to 24 hours will keep wound edema and hematoma formation to a minimum.

Most surgeons prefer to keep a compression dressing on the patient's penis for three to five days. When it is removed, some swelling is inevitable. After dressing removal, warm soaks three or four times a day will keep the wound clean and help decrease edema. These soaks should be continued for at least two weeks postoperatively. Any eschar or devitalized tissue should be debrided to allow secretions under these tissues to drain rather than burrow deeper into the wound.

Finally, if a urethral tube, stent or diversion is used, the possibility of urethritis and poorly drained urethral secretions is likely. Some authors advocate a fenestrated catheter to give these secretions egress, while others apply antibiotic ointments to the urethral meatus, attempting to prevent their formation. There is serious doubt as to whether they can be prevented, and there is some thought that ointments at the meatus may in fact provide further jeopardy by gluing the tube to the neourethra and, in effect, preventing natural drainage. If a fenestrated catheter is used, the holes in the tube must be carefully positioned to lie only in the urethra, for if they lie outside the meatus, urine will constantly leak onto the genitalia and macerate the skin.

Moderate urethral secretions are commonly seen after urethral surgery and must be allowed to exit at the meatus. The presence of a urethral catheter or stent increases the amount of these secretions and probably prevents adequate drainage. For this reason, urethral tubes should be removed at the earliest possible time.

If diversion is to be used for only a few days, the patient is kept in the hospital until the tube is removed, the wounds are well on their way to healing and the patient can void without difficulty. Many surgeons fill the bladder with contrast material and perform a voiding urethrogram when the catheter is withdrawn to check for fistulae. If one is present, diversion may be continued for a longer period of time. It is doubtful that a fistula which is present for over four weeks, even with diversion, will ever close without a second surgical procedure.

If diversion is to be used for over a week, the patient and his parent or guardian should be instructed in the use of a leg bag and the child sent home with instructions to continue his soaks. Obviously both the family and patient should be confident that they can handle home care, and the surgeon should be sure that the patient's wound does not need frequent expert attention. The child can then return as an outpatient for catheter removal and voiding evaluation.

B. Longterm Follow-up

Because of the indwelling catheter, a urine culture should be done once the patient is voiding well and has discontinued all antibiotics in order to confirm that the urine is sterile. The penis should be observed in the erect state to insure that chordee has been eliminated; the child should be observed while voiding to be sure he has a full straight stream that he can direct without spraying and that there is no fistula formation. If there is any question about the urinary stream, a voiding flow rate or urethrogram may be diagnostically helpful. A few urethral dilatations may correct minor stream deviation.

The parents should be warned that strictures may not become evident for years, so continued observation is warranted. Occasional flow rates have been suggested as a noninvasive way to follow these patients until maturity is reached.

VII. RESULTS AND COMPLICATIONS

The problems that are evident in the immediate postoperative period, namely bleeding with hematoma formation, edema, devitalized flaps and infections have all been discussed in previous sections. Strict attention to detail, proper wound care and increased experience of the surgeon are necessary to keep these problems to a minimum. Certainly they should occur infrequently under the care of a competent surgeon who does frequent hypospadias repairs.

The complications of failure to release the chordee, urethral diverticulae, stricture formation and meatal stenosis are most likely errors in technique which can be improved with surgical experience. If scrotal skin is used for the urethral tube, hair may grow in the neourethra at puberty and act as a nidus for calculi formation. Endoscopy may be necessary to remove these concretions.

Urinary fistulae may be related to technique; nevertheless, they are the most common complication in hypospadias surgery. The incidence varies according to the technique employed, and usually occurs less commonly with the planned multiple-staged procedures. The Cecil-Culp three-staged procedure has the lowest incidence (six percent), the two-staged repairs from six to 14 percent and one-staged procedures from eight to 25 percent. Again, the surgeon's experience with these repairs seems to be the key to success. Recently, Smith (1973) described a de-epithelialized overlay flap technique which lowered his fistula rate in two-staged repairs to less than one percent.

Because this anomaly presents with varying complexity, no one technique is applicable in all cases. Similarly, the complication rate, or rather the 'unplanned re-operation' rate in many surgical series approaches 50 percent. Many of these 're-operations' are only meatotomies or removal of excess skin tags, but they are operations nevertheless. The measures of success in hypospadias repairs are the demonstrated results of a cosmetically pleasing, straight penis with the urethral meatus as close to the tip as possible and the ability of the patient to void with a full straight stream that he can direct while standing, not speed or limited intraoperative time.

REFERENCES

Aarskog D: Maternal progestins as a possible cause of hypospadias. N Engl J Med 300: 75, 1979.

Allen TD and Spence HM: The surgical treatment of coronal hypospadias and related problems. J Urol 100: 504, 1968.

Bauer SD, Bull MJ and Retik AB: Hypospadias: A familial study. J Urol 121: 474, 1979.

Byars LT: A technique for consistently satisfactory repair of hypospadias. Surg Gynecol Obstet 100: 184, 1955.

Culp OS: Struggles and triumphs with hypospadias and associated anomalies: Review of 400 cases. J Urol 96: 339, 1966.

Devine CJ and Horton CE: One-stage hypospadias repair. J Urol 85: 166, 1961.

Fallon B, Devine CJ and Horton CE: Congenital anomalies associated with hypospadias. J Urol 116: 585, 1976.

Fuqua F: Renaissance of urethroplasty: The Belt technique of hypospadias repair. J Urol 106: 782, 1971.

Hodgson NB: A one-stage hypospadias repair. J Urol 104: 281, 1970.

King LR: Hypospadias – A one-stage repair without skin graft based on a new principle: Chordee is sometimes produced by the skin alone. J Urol 103: 660, 1970.

Lutzker LG, Kogan SJ and Levitt SF: Is routine intravenous urography indicated in patients with hypospadias? Pediatrics 59: 630, 1977.

McArdle R and Lebowitz R: Uncomplicated hypospadias and anomalies of upper urinary tract. Need for screening? Urology 5: 712, 1975.

Mustarde JC: One-stage correction of distal hypospadias: and other people's fistula. Br J Plast Surg 18: 413, 1965.

Smith D: A de-epithelialised overlap flap technique in the repair of hypospadias. Br J Plast Surg 26: 106, 1973.

8. GENITAL RECONSTRUCTION OF ANOMALIES OF THE GENITALIA OTHER THAN HYPOSPADIAS

W.J. CROMIE and J.W. DUCKETT JR.

I. CLINICAL EMBRYOLOGY

The penis and scrotum develop well toward the end of the third trimester and are dependent on hormonal factors, separate from urinary tract development. This hormonal stimulus involves high local androgen production by the fetal testes with conversion of testosterone to dihydrotestosterone by five alpha reductase in the genital skin. This specific biochemical step is critical in genital differentiation and any combination of factors affecting this series of events probably accounts for many of the genital anomalies in males (Raifer and Walsh 1978).

The penis itself is developed from paired genitourinary tubercles that fuse to form a mound of tissue between the allantois and cloacal membrane. Not until the eighth week of life does actual sexual development occur and not until the third month does the penis become recognizable (Arey 1965). Abnormalities in the formation of the urethral groove, or cessation of urethral development, results in hypospadias which will be the topic of a subsequent article (Aarskog 1970).

In addition, improper differentiation and development of the genital tubercle can result in a spectrum of defects from penoscrotal transposition to absent penis (Kernahan 1973).

Correspondent with genital development, other associated defects can occur such as abnormalities in the cloacal membrane resulting in varying degrees of the exstrophy-epispadias complex (Marshall and Muecke 1962).

Thus it appears that abnormalities of the genitalia in the male result from mechanical or hormonal derangements and in some cases, a combination of both.

II. PHIMOSIS AND PARAPHIMOSIS

The prepuce forms initially as a roll of epithelium at the coronal sulcus which is incomplete ventrally. In the normal penis the frenulum is the hallmark of this defect. It is of interest that the development of the ventral aspect of the foreskin is dependent upon normal urethral formation. Thus, in patients with hypospadias, failure of urethral advancement restricts the ventral development of the foreskin. Conversely, in patients with epispadias, dorsal foreskin development is lacking (Belman 1978).

Although the prepuce is formed distinctly separate from the glans, the two opposing epithelial surfaces fuse but later separate gradually as desquamated cells build up between the two layers. Bearing this in mind, only four percent of males have retractable foreskins at birth. Phimosis, on the other hand, is the inability to retract the foreskin because of circumferential inflammatory tissue that is actually too small to admit the glans. This condition occurs secondary to inflammation. A point of confusion exists in terminology when one lumps the nonretractable foreskin and true phimosis into the same category. Oster, in a series from Denmark, noted that one third of boys of ages six through sixteen still had failure of complete separation of the foreskin, while only four percent had true phimosis. In those boys aged six through seven years, 63 percent had residual preputial adherence, whereas those aged sixteen through seventeen years had persistence of these adhesions in only three percent.

Paraphimosis is the same basic pathological condition as phimosis, however, the inflammatory ring has been brought above the corona and cannot be readily returned to the normal position because of edema. Manual reduction of paraphimosis can be accomplished in essentially all cases if persistent pressure is applied to the glans. With phimosis or paraphimosis, a dorsal slit interrupting the circumferential band may be required to reduce the obstruction or to provide adequate drainage and recovery of infection where balanoposthitis occurs. In either circumstance, elective circumcision is carried out when the inflammation has resolved (Belman 1978).

III. CIRCUMCISION

The ritual of circumcision predates biblical history with the underlying idea probably that of sanctification of an organ of reproduction to a deity. This, of course, can be extrapolated to a tribal mark, a step toward marriage, or a sign of manhood antedating sexual activity (Hastings 1911). Circumcision today is carried out for a large number of reasons, probably unrelated to the historical origins. The medical indications are based on hygiene with the subsequent influence of carcinoma on the penis, as previously noted in uncircumcised patients. However, in view of the low incidence of penile carcinoma in western Europe where newborn circumcision is not the rule, the current thinking toward making a circumcision an elective procedure has resulted (Preston 1970). Positive aspects of neonatal circumcision assure the patient of complete freedom from the hazard of penile cancer in later years, as well as the relative freedom from inflammatory disorders of the glans, reduced problems of condyloma and virtually no possibility of phimosis or paraphimosis. On the negative side, serious complications requiring surgical repair do occur. The most common, and often most disconcerting, complication is the penis with the glans covered by the skin of the shaft with adherence to the glans. This is the result of excessive shaft skin adhering to the raw surface of the glans resulting in dense scar tissue, in some cases requiring sharp dissection for removal resulting in a pocked-appearing glans (Belman 1978). Less severe degrees of this obviously occur. A more difficult complication is a urethral fistula secondary to removal of excessive ventral tissue. Usually this occurs at the level of the coronal sulcus and unfortunately there is less flexible tissue in this area necessitating a rather

formidable hypospadias repair. With proper attention to detail, the overall incidence of complications is approximately 0.2 percent (Gee and Answell 1976; Shulman et al. 1964).

The basic techniques for circumcision by the freehand circumcision or the dorsal slit technique are well known to most surgeons. Less familiar may be mechanical devices such as the Gomco clamp or plastibell set. To use either device, a dorsal slit is first made to allow the foreskin to be retracted and adhesions between the foreskin and underlying tissue of the glans broken down. The bell of either clamp is placed over the glans, the foreskin drawn over the bell and clamped or tied depending on the type of device used. It is most important to select the proper size of bell, particularly in the case of plastibell circumcisions, as too large a bell can slip behind the corona of the glans and present a potential strangulation situation. The excess skin is removed and with nothing more than routine care, the penile skin recovers quickly. In the case of the plastibell, the distal portion of the plastic ring often sloughs within four to five days with primary healing over the glandular shaft skin. If the child is beyond six weeks of age, a specific indication is required as general anesthesia is necessary. In our experience, older children can have the procedure done, usually by freehand technique, with local anesthesia as a day surgical procedure.

IV. MEATAL STENOSIS

The normal urethral meatus, as noted previously, develops as an inversion of an epithelial tag meeting the anterior urethra at the fossa navicularis. In the uncircumcised male, the glans and meatus are protected by the foreskin from diaper irritation, thus the irritation produces posthitis, while the circumcised male has direct irritation of the glans and meatus. A lip of tissue often forms secondarily under the ventral portion of the meatus deflecting the urinary stream upward (Allen et al. 1972). Allen et al., calibrated the urethral meatuses of one hundred newborn boys and found the majority to have openings of 6, 7 or 8 french. It was the conclusion that a 4 french meatus could be considered to have meatal stenosis. Actually the diagnosis of meatal stenosis is established more accurately by a method that defines the physiologic impairment produced by narrowing. An example of this is the technique of Gleason et al. (1972), describing energy loss during voiding on the basis of pressure flow relationship. Practically speaking, it is a rare occurrence indeed, as the most severe degrees of meatal stenosis are seen in the hypospadiac patient and they rarely have any proximal abnormalities related to the small meatus. Thus, the relationship of a tight meatus to vesicoureteric reflux, enuresis and urinary infection, is seriously in doubt. The American Academy of Pediatrics has suggested guidelines for meatotomy which include: bulging of the penile meatus with voiding indicating obstruction, significant deflection of the urinary stream with voiding, and a history or clinical findings of significant meatitis (Belman et al. in press). Should these occur, a simple meatotomy can be carried out in the office using local xylocaine or ethyl chloride spray on the inferior portion of the meatus, followed by application of a small mosquito hemostat across the intervening tissue and a ventral cut with tenotomy scissors. It is important for the parents to

pull the edges apart once or twice daily for the ensuing four to five days to prevent reapproximation of the raw skin edges. For more severe degrees of meatal stenosis or for recurrences, the technique depicted in Figure 1 can be carried out.

V. DIPHALLUS

Duplication of all or portion of the penis is a rare urologic occurrence resulting from a failure or incomplete fusion of the lateral plate mesoderm of the genital tubercles. It thus follows that the development of the penis from bilateral analogs can result in any degree of division of the penis (Remzi 1973). The condition of diphallus may range from a mere fissure or split of the glans to two well developed penes placed widely apart. In Figure 2, a classification of diphallus is presented.

Numerous variations in the anatomy of the genitalia have been described in association with diphallus (Wilson 1973). The penis may be symmetrical or asymmetrical with an equal or unequal

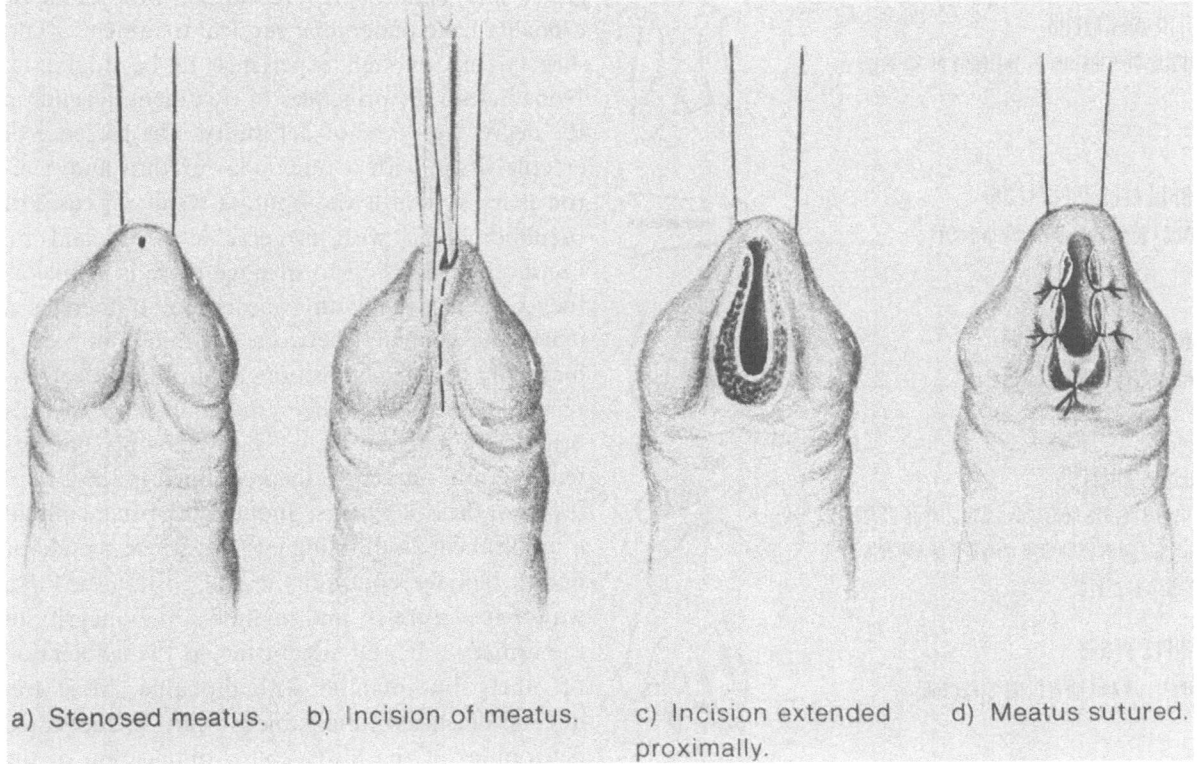

a) Stenosed meatus. b) Incision of meatus. c) Incision extended proximally. d) Meatus sutured.

Figure 1. Technique of meatotomy (from Eckstein et al. 1977 p. 418).

variation in size. They may lie side by side or one above the other. Occasionally they may be ectopic and based in the thigh or perineum. The penes usually have a prepuce, the glans may be perforate or imperforate, reflecting an absent or present urethra. If the urethra is duplicated, it commonly drains a septate or double bladder; rarely, the double urethras will unite and enter a single bladder.

The scrotal sac is often duplicated, but it may be normal, bifid, found in the usual scrotal position or in fact in an ectopic position. When a double scrotum is present it usually contains a single testis which may be normal, atrophic, descended or undescended, depending on the location of the scrotum.

For purposes of clarification, diphallus falls into two clinical categories, first *bifid penis*, and secondly true *diphallia*. A bifid penis is characterized by a vertical longitudinal cleft that divides the penis into two halves. The duplication may involve only the glans or it may involve the entire penile shaft in which case each half contains only one corporal body. The urethral opening is usually in the depth of the cleft between the two corpora (Alleem 1972). It would appear that these patients can be approached much like hypospadias. If two corporal bodies exist, then reconstruction can be undertaken by suturing them together. As a rule, the urethral meatus is in the cleft between the corpora and at a subsequent stage, a urethral tube can be rolled and advanced to the fused glans.

True diphallia differs from bifid penis in that two fully formed penes are found each with its own urethra. The innumerable variations in position, location and configuration have been previously discussed. In each case a thorough urologic evaluation is essential, including intravenous pyelography, retrograde urethrography, voiding cystogram, and endoscopic evaluation. Few cases of diphallia have undergone surgical treatment, so no surgeon has enough experience to be dogmatic. Nonetheless, the principles of treatment depend on the degree and type of deformity. The presence of erectile tissue with a functional urethra and genitourinary system is the optimal result. In cases of pseudodiphallia with no erectile tissue and no urethra, the decision to manage these is simple as they can be dealt with by excision. If there is a marked asymmetry between the bifid unit or a markedly abnormal position, again excision of this unit is preferable. Where there are two distinct organs, investigation usually reveals only one patent urethra. Surgery is then confined to the amputation of the other penis. Should both penes contain a urethral canal, draining either a single septate or double bladder, continuity must be established in a way that is simplest and maintains the integrity of the urinary tract. Of significance is the association of other abnormalities with diphallia. Most frequent is diastasis of the pubic symphysis, duplicated deformities of the lower spine, duplication of the bowel, and occasionally anomalies of the upper

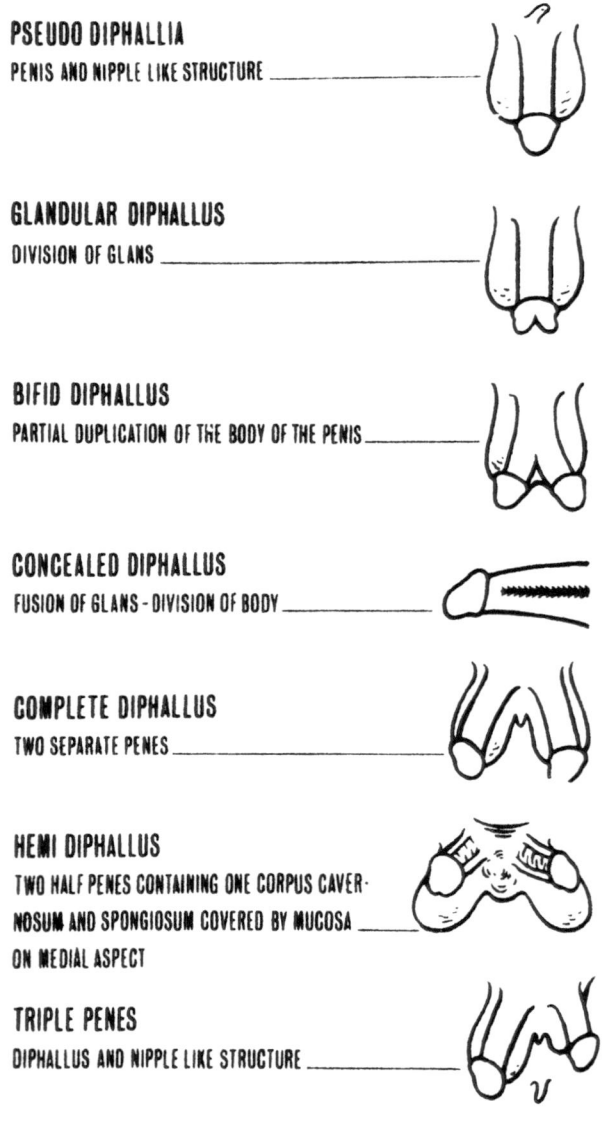

PSEUDO DIPHALLIA
PENIS AND NIPPLE LIKE STRUCTURE _____

GLANDULAR DIPHALLUS
DIVISION OF GLANS _____

BIFID DIPHALLUS
PARTIAL DUPLICATION OF THE BODY OF THE PENIS _____

CONCEALED DIPHALLUS
FUSION OF GLANS - DIVISION OF BODY _____

COMPLETE DIPHALLUS
TWO SEPARATE PENES _____

HEMI DIPHALLUS
TWO HALF PENES CONTAINING ONE CORPUS CAVERNOSUM AND SPONGIOSUM COVERED BY MUCOSA _____
ON MEDIAL ASPECT

TRIPLE PENES
DIPHALLUS AND NIPPLE LIKE STRUCTURE _____

Figure 2. Classification of diphallia (from Horton 1973 p. 165).

urinary tract (Kossow and Morales 1973). Considering all of these factors, the ultimate goal essentially is preservation of the urinary tract with a functional and cosmetically acceptable appearance of the penis.

A. Diphallia in Cloacal Exstrophy

The most severe degrees of diphallia are associated with cloacal exstrophy in the male. In these cases there are very small hemipenes with no continuity to the urinary tract as the ureters go to separate hemibladders flanking a hindgut eventration and often an omphalocele. In all but the most minimal degrees of this deformity, it is unreasonable to attempt phallic reconstruction in these children and it is our recommendation that they be reassigned to the female gender.

VI. MICROPENIS

Microphallus is a congenital disorder in which the penis, although diminutive, is anatomically normal with the urethral meatus at the tip of the glans. For purposes of this discussion, a true micropenis measures approximately one cm in length at birth as compared to 3.75 cm for the average male neonate (Hinman Jr. 1972). Although the etiology of microphallus is unknown, several lines of evidence suggest that it may be caused by a defect in androgen secretion in the third trimester of pregnancy. It is during these last two trimesters that the normal penis increases in size about tenfold, reaching a length of approximately 3.5 cm at birth. The major stimulus for this growth is androgen secretion and action on the target cells of the genitalia. At the clinical level, two categories of microphallus can be outlined. First, an association with a wide assortment of disorders that affect the hypothalamic pituitary axis, such as anencephaly, Fanconi's anemia, Meckel's syndrome, and Prader-Willi syndrome. It is also seen and associated with syndromes affecting the testes such as Borjeson and Robinows syndromes (Allen 1976). In these disorders, the diagnosis is usually apparent from the overall clinical picture. In other instances, microphallus occurs as an isolated disorder unassociated with other major abnormalities. Walsh et

al. (1978), in a study of eight patients with microphallus, found these two distinct categories to hold true. In five patients the disorder appeared to be familial with low gonadotrophin levels that responded to stimulation with chorionic gonadotrophin. It appeared that three and possibly five of these patients clearly had hypogonadotropic hypogonadism and he concluded that this probably is the major cause of the syndrome of microphallus. In the other group, the cases are sporadic with elevated serum luteinizing hormone and follicle stimulating hormone levels. Plasma testosterone failed to increase after short-term treatment with chorionic gonadotrophin. In these patients, a primary testicular disorder appeared to be responsible.

Clinically, in both types of these patients, bilateral cryptorchidism is usually present or the testes are small and poorly developed. The phallus may enlarge somewhat at puberty, but it remains diminutive relative to the overall body size.

Treatment of secondary hypogenitalism is directed at diagnosis of the primary defect. A logical step would be to treat the patients with H.C.G.; however, as a practical matter testosterone has usually been preferred because it is less expensive, widely available, and in the last analysis is the final common pathway of all the therapeutic agents (Allen 1976). Wilson et al. (1974), discovered a familial type of hypogenitalism where androgen production is normal, but there is a genetic resistance to the action of androgen at the cellular level. In these patients, as in patients with idiopathic microphallus, it becomes essential in the newborn period to determine that a boy can respond to testosterone and that some penile growth can be anticipated. Topical testosterone cream, 2.5-5 percent, can be applied, but the absorption is less controlled than depo-testosterone which has a more controlled uptake (Guthrie et al. 1973). Penile enlargement is sometimes seen, but often there is an increase in bone age as well. Following cessation of therapy, the bone growth returns to the normal range, but there likewise is some recession of penile growth. The question remains whether prepubertal treatment borrows from further potential growth and although it is highly desirable psychologically that the penis be more normal size in childhood, its ultimate size probably will be less than normal as an adult (Belman 1978). If the child presents after the neonatal period and is firmly fixed in his gender, it is important to make the maximum therapeutic attempts at obtaining the best penile length. In patients with severe hypospadias, a chordee release can be helpful, and the penile lengthening procedure described by Johnston et al. (1977) (Figure 3) can be used in very selected cases of micropenis. In the neonatal period, the presence or absence of significant corporal tissue is important. In the absence of corporal tissue, a sexual reassignment is the only reasonable approach. In the remainder of

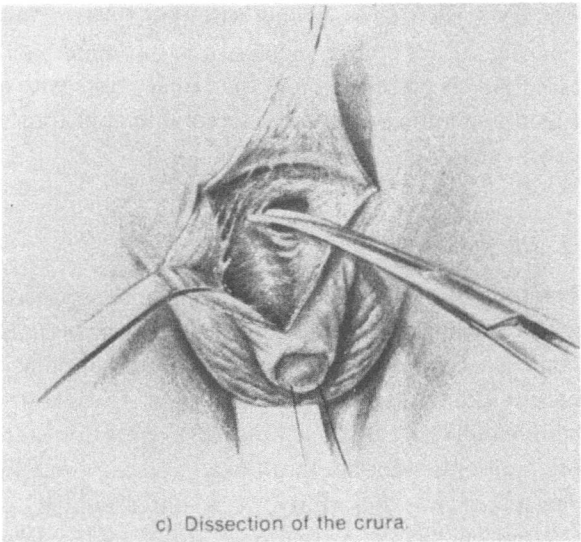

c) Dissection of the crura.

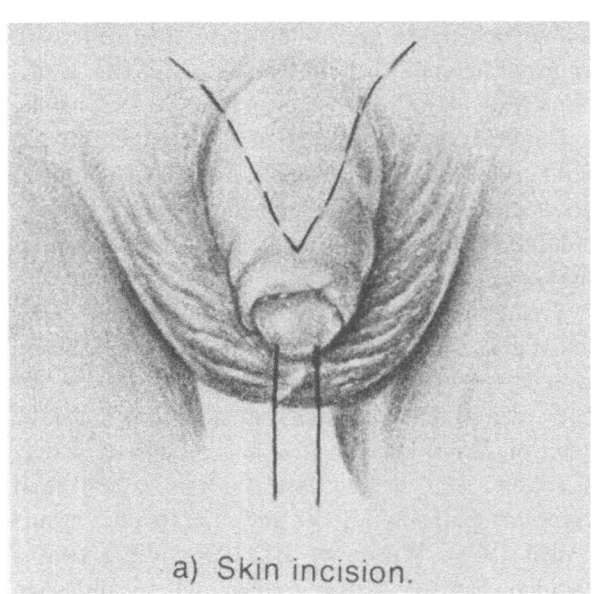

a) Skin incision.

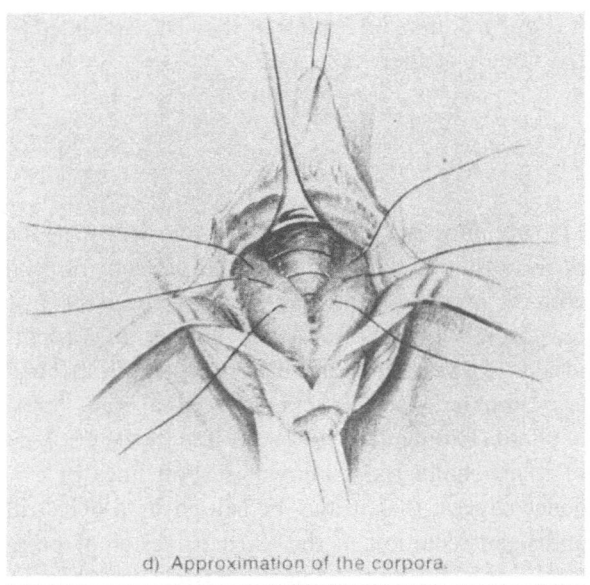

d) Approximation of the corpora.

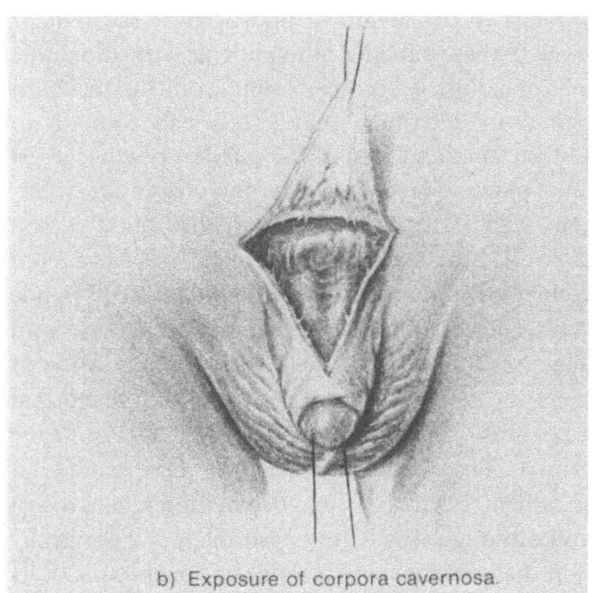

b) Exposure of corpora cavernosa.

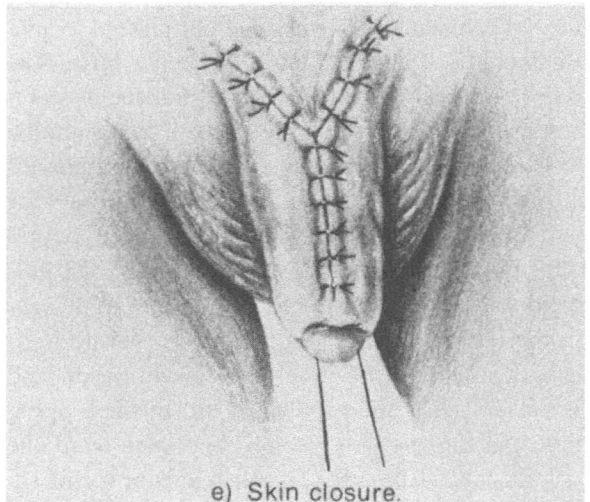

e) Skin closure.

Figure 3. Penile lengthening procedure (from Eckstein et al. 1977 p. 412).

cases, the patients with penile stretchlength less than 2.5 cm that do not respond to topical or depo-testosterone also represent another indication for sexual reassignment.

VII. ABSENT PENIS

Complete absence of the penis is an extremely rare abnormality due to failure of the development of the genital tubercle. With rare exceptions, the physical findings on examination are quite similar, the urethral opening is located just inside or anterior to the anal opening, in association with a small tag of skin. The scrotum is usually well formed, but hydroceles, hernias or cryptorchid testes do occur (Lisa et al. 1973).

Various anorectal abnormalities are found in association with penile agenesis such as congenital rectal stricture, imperforate anus and rectovesical fistula. Renal dysplasia and agenesis are often encountered and account for one third of the deaths in infancy with these children. The remainder are healthy otherwise (Richart and Benirschke 1960).

A recent report by Johnston et al. (1977), stressed the importance of early sexual conversion to the female role, with plans for formation of the appropriate sexual structures later. This is much easier said than done as in most cases the proximity of the urethra to the anus precludes any simple solution to the formation of a vagina. If a tag of penile tissue remains between the area of the rectum and the urethra, it might be important to save it for conversion of this skin to a neovagina in much the same manner as with transsexual surgery.

VIII. WEBBED PENIS

This is a term applied to the condition when scrotal skin is attached to the undersurface of the penis throughout its length (Kenawi 1973). This is in distinction to the chordee and deficiency of ventral penile skin seen in patients with intersex and perineal hypospadias. Treatment consists of resection and Z-plasty of the web, or incising the skin transversly and closing it longitudinally as described by Perlmutter and Chamberlain (1972) (Figure 4).

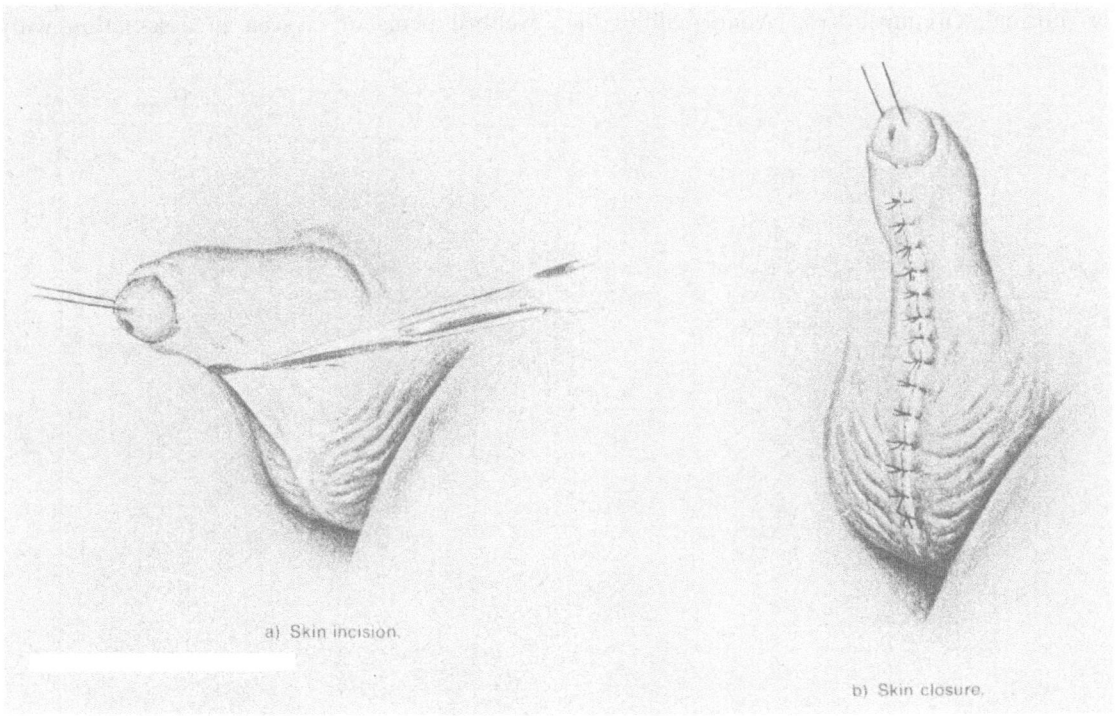

a) Skin incision.

b) Skin closure.

Figure 4. Repair of webbed penis (from Eckstein et al. 1977 p. 411).

IX. PENILE TORSION

Clockwise or counterclockwise torsion of the penis can occur independent of the hypospadias complex. It is evident by the off-center location of the midline raphe and is usually associated with incomplete development of the ventral foreskin. Surgical correction is usually requested for a misdirected urinary stream. Johnston (1974), has proposed a detorsion circumcision at the base of the shaft of the penis (Figure 5). We feel that this can be more easily accomplished by an encircling incision at the subcoronal level, denuding the penis of skin to the base, and then re-approximating the skin in the normal relationship. In some cases overcorrection is necessary so that the penis will lie in a normal configuration.

X. SCROTUM

The scrotum is the structure found only in mammalian species and serves as a temperature regulating mechanism for the testes. It is formed from the genital swellings and arises lateral to the genital tubercle. These swellings undergo migration caudally, fusing in the midline beneath the phallus under normal circumstances. Abnormalities in

scrotal positioning can occur primarily or in association with intersex disorders (Allen 1976).

A. Transposition of the Scrotum

This rare abnormality is also referred to as pre-penile scrotum and is often associated with other congenital defects incompatible with life. The clinical appearance (Figure 6) is that of a penis developed to a greater or lesser degree, lying behind an essentially well formed scrotum. The majority of the cases have associated abnormalities, the most frequent being hypospadias. Improvement in the appearance of the genitalia may be brought about by a variety of procedures designed to restore the normal relationship of the penis to the scrotum. The most recent technique has been described by Glenn and Anderson (1973), in which the lateral scrotal folds are transposed to the ventral position on the shaft of the penis. If, however, the surgeon is faced with the situation where a functional repair would result in inadequate corpora for erections or insufficient penile length coupled with severe hypospadias, a consideration of sexual reassignment must be made.

Milder forms of peno-scrotal transposition often fall into the category of the previously discussed webbed penis or is seen in association with the

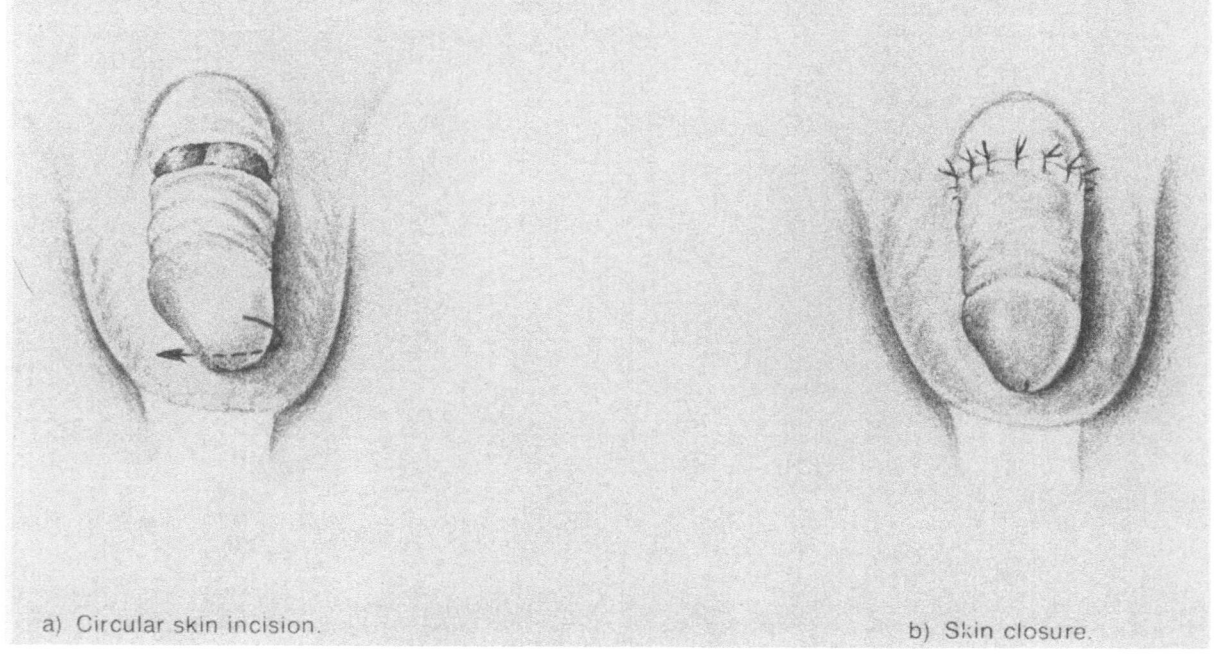

a) Circular skin incision.   b) Skin closure.

Figure 5. Penile detorsion procedure (from Eckstein et al. 1977 p. 413).

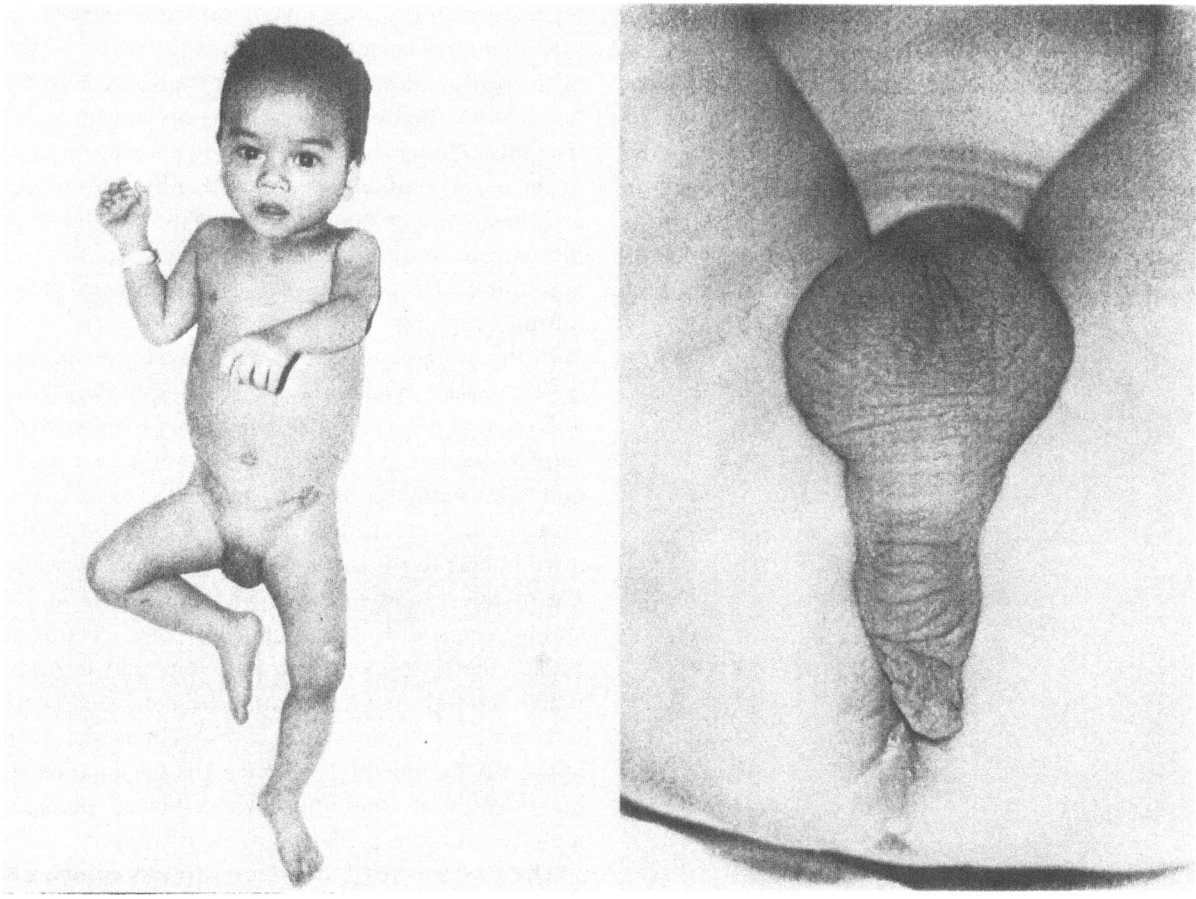

Figure 6. Picture of severe penoscrotal transposition (from Horton 1973 p. 177).

rather severe degrees of peno-scrotal hypospadias. The freeing of this band between the penis and scrotum with release of the chordee is part of the overall repair and actual scrotal repositioning is not required.

B. Ectopic Scrotum

Complete dislocation of the scrotal tissue from its normal location is a rare anomaly (Figure 7), usually associated with advanced forms of exstrophy, diphallia or the popliteal pterygium syndrome (Mininberg and Richman 1972). There have been three reported cases of isolated unilateral scrotal ectopia with two of them having associated absence of the kidney on that side (Milroy 1969). Other common locations for ectopic tissue include the groin, external inguinal ring, inner thigh, and abdominal wall.

Basically, treatment is the moving of the affected skin tag back to its normal position by rotating skin flaps and subsequently relocating the testicle. If the ectopic tissue is at a very distant site, often the testicular tissue is atrophic and excision of both is probably the procedure of choice.

XI. EXSTROPHY-EPISPADIAS COMPLEX

This complex of abnormalities is a rare congenital defect resulting from the persistence of the large cloacal membrane that serves as a wedge between the developing mesodermal structures of the lower abdominal wall (Muecke 1964). Muecke was able to create this abnormality in the chick embryo by placing a tantillum wedge on the cloacal membrane causing the same obstructive effect. It thus appears that a mechanical event can produce this abnormality, most likely accounting for the broad variation in presentation of the exstrophy-epispadias complex, from simple balanitic epispadias to the massive defect of cloacal exstrophy. The incidence of epispadias is approximately one in every 100,000 males with a five to one male to female ratio. Exstrophy of the bladder associated with epispadias, however, is one in 30,000 with a 3:1 male preponderance, making the more severe exstrophy complex ten times more common than epispadias alone (Duckett Jr. 1978).

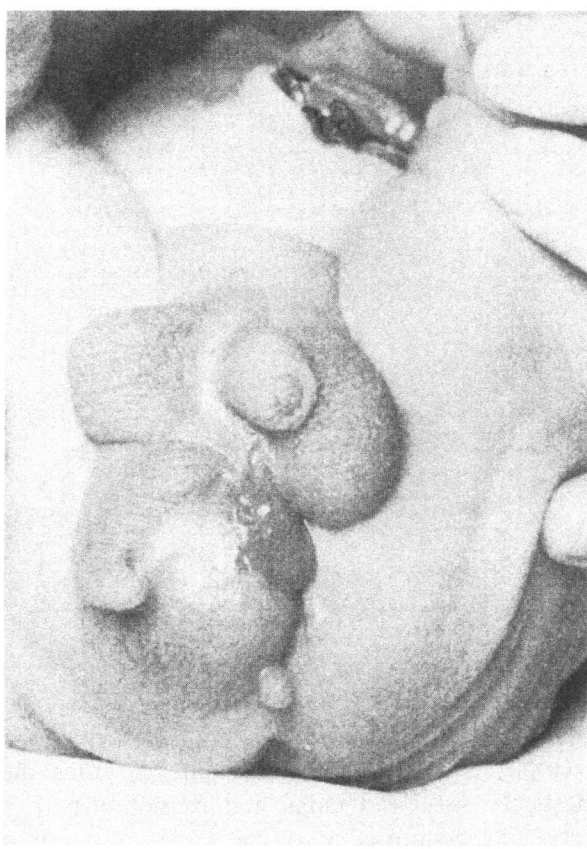

Figure 7. Picture of ectopic scrotum (from Horton 1973 p. 180).

A. Classification

There are three types of epispadias in the male, depending on the extent of the cleft in the urethra. *Balanitic*, or glandular, involves only the glans with the distal portion of the urethra open and exposed. This is the rarest form of epispadias and incontinence is generally not associated with this defect. In *penile epispadias*, the shaft of the penis and glans are affected. The urethra is displaced dorsally forming a gutter between the two corpora. This defect can be variable in length and again incon-

tinence generally does not occur. *Penopubic* or *subsymphyseal* epispadias involves the entire length of the penis and may extend a short distance up the lower abdominal wall. Depending on your perspective, this is either the most severe form of epispadias or the most minimal form of exstrophy. This defect is associated with incompetence of the bladder neck mechanism resulting in incontinence. Occasionally herniation of a portion of the bladder may occur during coughing or straining.

In the more common bladder exstrophy anomaly, the entire bladder is everted onto the lower abdomen and is always associated with epispadias. The ureters end in short tunnels on a wide trigone and will usually reflux if the bladder is closed. The pubic bones are widely separated and the penile attachments to the inferior ramus produce shortening of the urethral groove with epispadias and a stubby penis with dorsal chordee. The scrotum is broad, the testes are often palpable, and occasionally bilateral inguinal hernias are detected. There is a wide separation of the rectus muscles, even above the umbilicus (Figure 8a, b). The anal canal may be patulous and anteriorly displaced, occasionally resulting in prolapse of the rectum.

The most severe form of the exstrophy complex is cloacal exstrophy (Figure 8c). In these cases, there are two hemibladders with the cecum protruding between them. The ileum is prolapsed through the ileocecal valve but is not obstructed, and there are often duplicated appendices. The distal colon is short, opens proximally onto the cecum, and ends blindly. The ureters enter on each side of the hemibladders. This massive defect is also associated with imperforate anus, meningomyelocele, omphalocele, short small intestine and other abnormalities. The management of these children is complicated, requiring preservation of the maximal amount of functioning colon, closure of the abdominal wall and bladder if possible, with reassignment of most males to a female role.

B. Surgical Management

The surgical management of the exstrophy-epispadias complex has evolved through time to allow a moderate degree of technical success when specific attention to detail has been maintained. In the interests of brevity, we would like to divide this

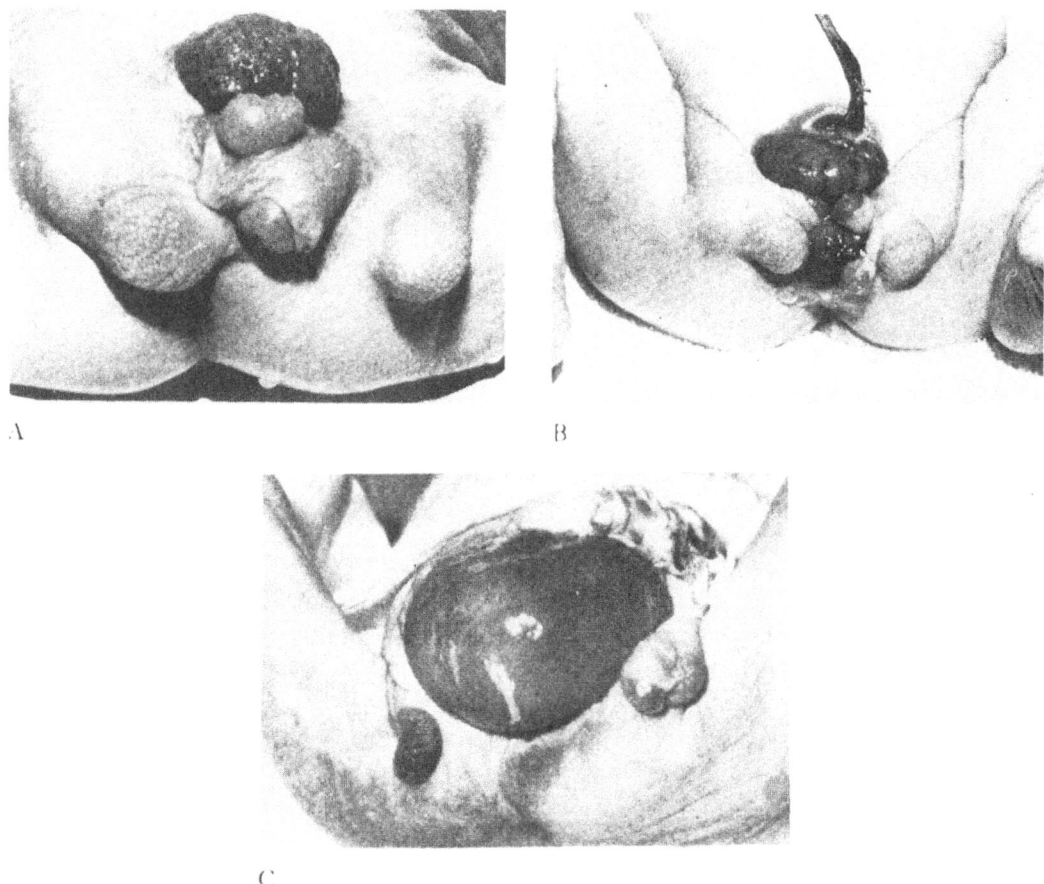

Figure 8. Photo of exstrophy patients (from Horton 1973 p. 167).

surgical management into simple epispadias without incontinence and epispadias associated with the exstrophy complex.

C. Epispadias – Simple Penile Repair

When the penis is of adequate size and without severe upper chordee, a urethral construction as described by Young (1918), may be performed from the age of two onward. With the child in the supine position and the legs slightly apart, a holding suture is placed through the glans penis (Figure 9a). A longitudinal incision is made on either side of the urethra with one side somewhat laterally eccentric to prevent overlapping suture lines. At the level of the glans, a triangular area of mucosa is excised to improve the creation of a meatus (Figure 9b). Using sharp dissection the skin flaps are widely mobilized and the urethral tube is created around the number 12 red rubber catheter. In the postero midline, the urethra is traced back to underneath the area of the

pubic arch where any tethering anterior tissue can be freed. It is usually possible to develop a second subcutaneous suture layer over the urethra which is then followed by the skin closure (Figure 9c). In most cases we use 5 or 6/0 chromic for the suture material; occasionally 4 or 5/0 nylon is used as a pullout suture for the skin. The two bared areas of the glans are brought together with a deeply placed chromic suture, care being taken to approximate the coronal sulcus as fistula formation can occur at this location (Figure 9d). We then remove the number 12 catheter and replace it with a fenestrated red rubber tube to serve only as a stent, and place a suprapubic cystotomy for approximately ten days. After an adequate trial of voiding, the catheter is removed and the child is placed on antimicrobial therapy for eight days.

D. Epispadias with Dorsal Chordee

Where epispadias is accompanied by significant

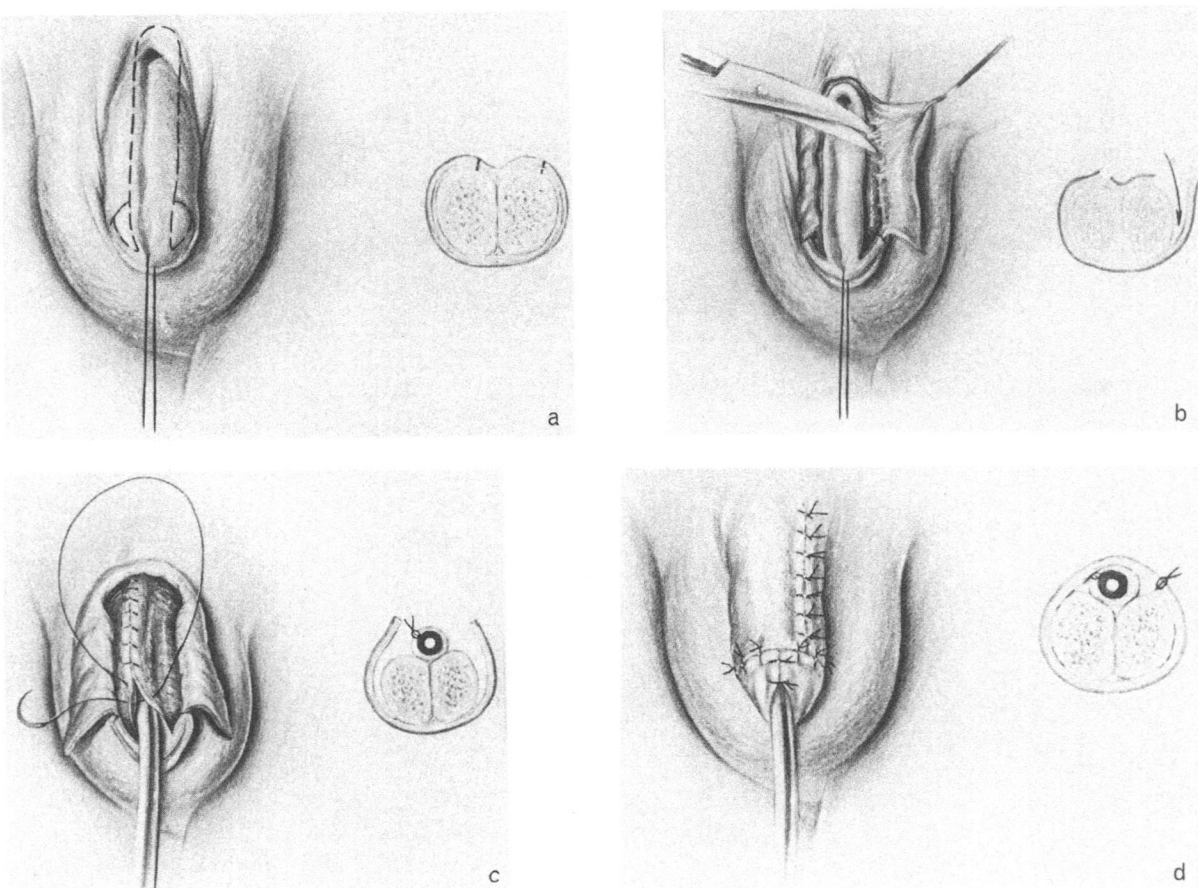

Figure 9. Young's epispadias repair (from Eckstein et al. 1977 p. 300).

dorsal chordee, the tethering anterior bands must be excised and ventral skin transferred to the dorsum for a secondary urethroplasty, much analogous to the Byars hypospadias repair (Figure 10a). Initially, an incision is made encircling the corona of the glans, and the penile skin is denuded on the shaft of the penis to a point where the corpora may be seen to splay laterally toward the pubic symphysis (Figure 10b). The upper tethering bands must be separated from the corpora with care being taken not to injure the urethra at its origin. In most cases dissection should be taken well back to the area underneath the pubic symphysis where the corpora take an inferior course toward Alcock's canal (Figure 10c). In cases where the crura are markedly divergent, they can be approximated to contribute to the overall length of the penile shaft. Throughout this entire maneuver, care should be taken to prevent damage of the neurovascular bundle entering on both portions of the crura. Next, the preputial fold of skin is opened to its full

length and a midline incision is made in this flap with the apex sutured to the frenular portion of the penis (Figure 10d). The lateral wings are brought up to cover the dorsum of the penis and sutured in the midline (Figure 10e). When the procedure is completed, a compression dressing is placed around the penis and we often leave a traction suture in the glans securing it to an overlying plastic cup for about three to four days to prevent retraction of the penile shaft. This has allowed us to obtain the maximum penile length in these patients. After a period of approximately eight to twelve months, the secondary urethroplasty is performed to advance the tube to the distal meatus.

E. Surgical Management of the Exstrophy Complex

The alternatives to managing this complex of abnormalities have varied from dressing and diapering to urinary diversion, attempts at complete functional closure, and finally, staged reconstruc-

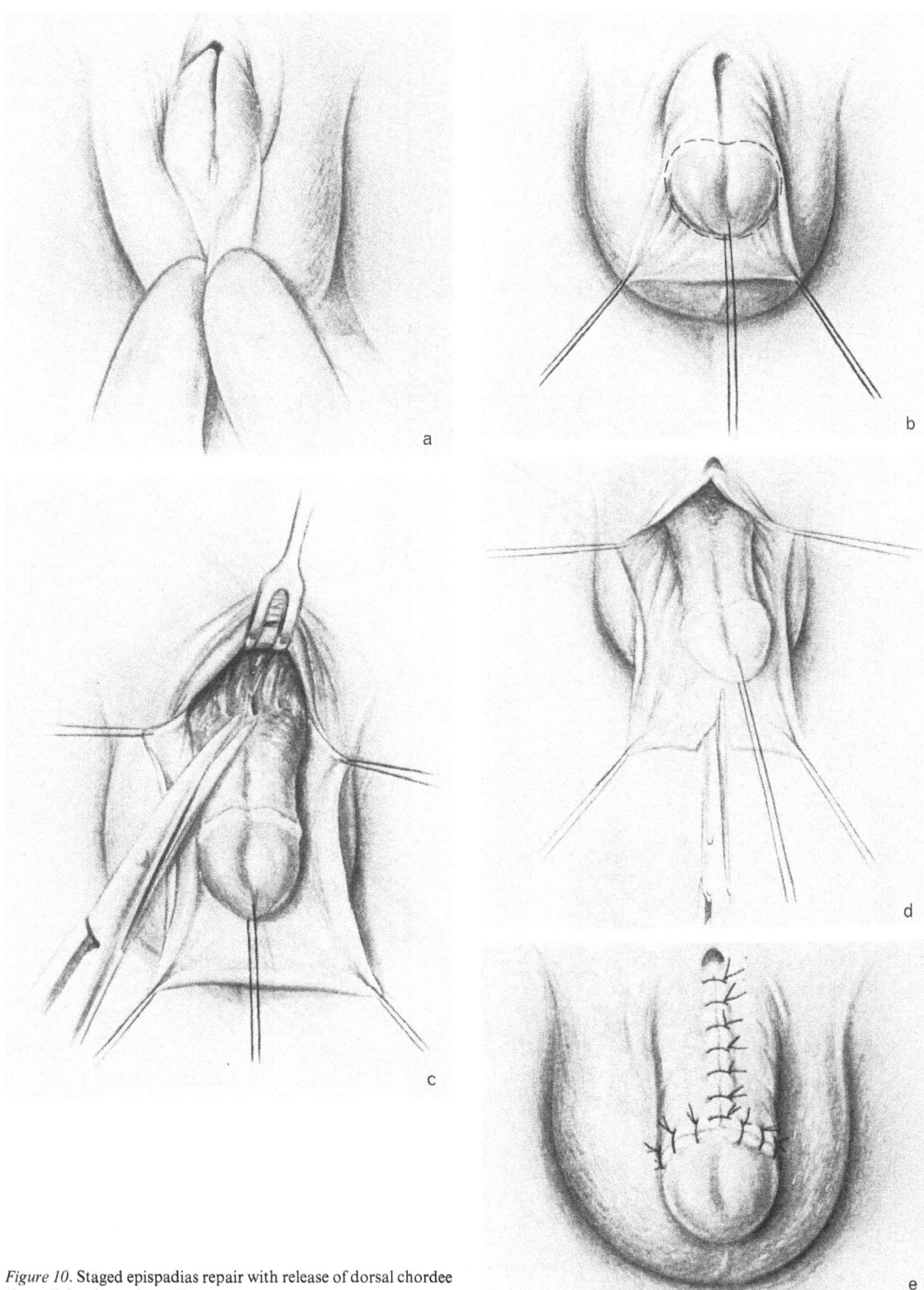

Figure 10. Staged epispadias repair with release of dorsal chordee (from Eckstein et al. 1977).

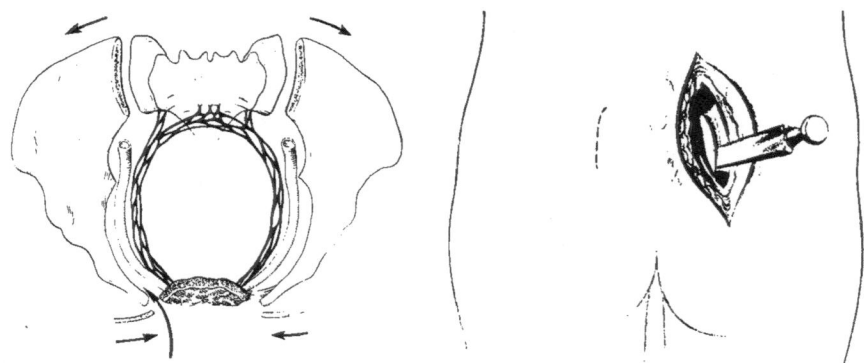

Figure 11. Iliac osteotomy for closure of the pelvic brim (from Eckstein et al. 1977 p. 311).

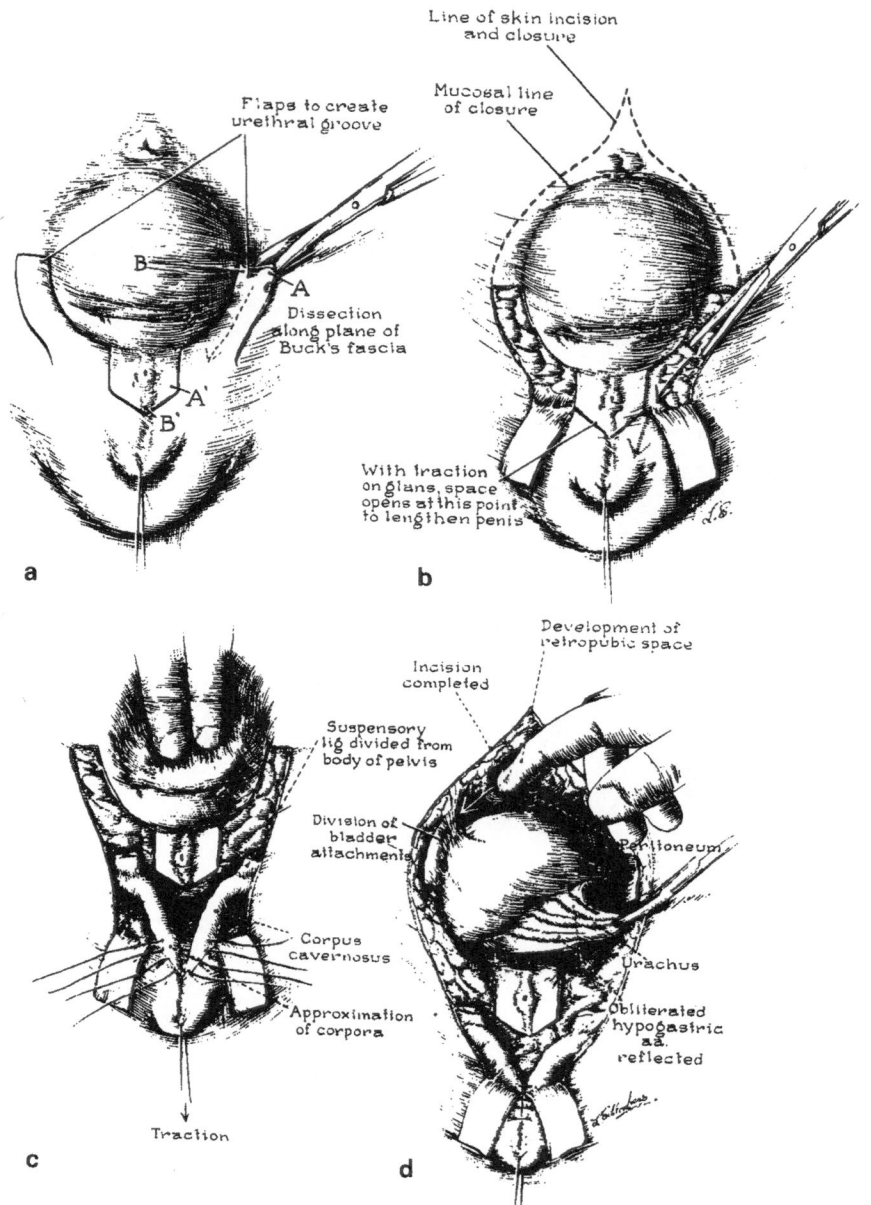

Figure 12. Vesical release and penile lengthening with division of the urethral plate (from Jeffs 1978 p. 132).

tion. In specific centers dealing with the exstrophic patients, it is now becoming apparent that staged reconstruction can result in a good cosmetic appearance and a functional urinary tract in 60-70% of the patients (Jeffs et al. 1972). The management can be divided into four separate stages:

1. Initial closure and penile lengthening.
2. The incontinent interval.
3. Bladder neck reconstruction.
4. Epispadias repair.

F. Initial Closure and Penile Lengthening

Initial closure is best performed in the neonatal period while the pelvic bones are under the influence of maternal relaxin and can be easily moulded to allow pubic closure (Ansell 1975). If the child is more than a few days of age, an iliac osteotomy must be performed in order to close the pelvic ring (Figure 11). This is essential if an adequate closure of the abdominal wall is to be obtained and additionally, it may contribute to the

eventual success in producing a continent reconstruction of the bladder neck and urethra. The bladder is approached by passing five feeding tubes up both ureteric orifices and suturing them in place with an absorbable chromic material. Using sharp dissection (Figure 12a), the bladder is separated from the surrounding skin edges down to the inferior portion of the bladder near the bladder neck where the paraexstrophy skin is found. This can be identified by putting traction on the surrounding inguinal tissue, revealing shiny mucosal type tissue. An incision (Figure 12b) is made along the medial margin of the proposed pedicle graft at the junction with the bladder mucosa. Deeper dissection into this incision identifies the intersymphyseal band which lies beneath the urethral plate. A U-shape incision is made around the verumontanum and ejaculatory ducts. This incision (Figure 12c) divides the urethral plate transversely 1 cm distal to the verumontanum at a point at which the corpora begin to diverge toward the separated pubic rami. The dissection is carried down between the crura which frees the attachment of the prostate

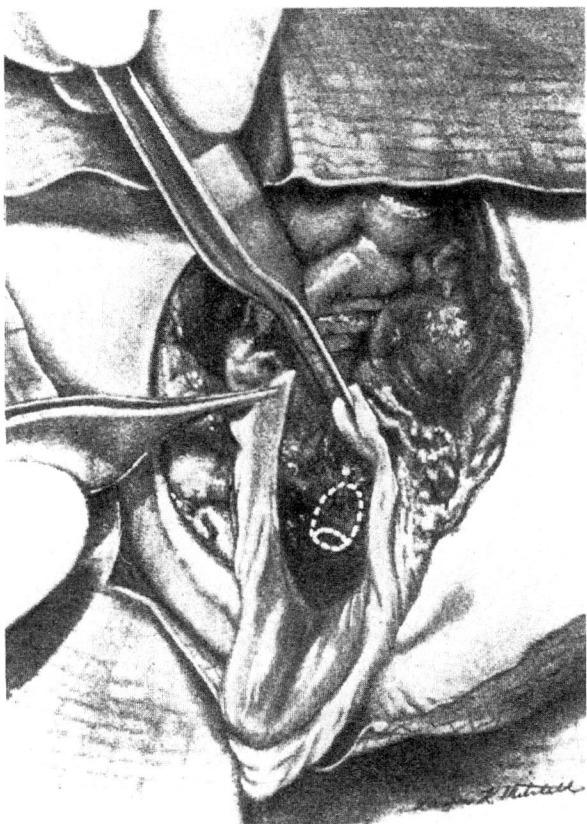

Figure 13. Formation of paraexstrophy skin flaps (from Jeffs 1978 p. 122).

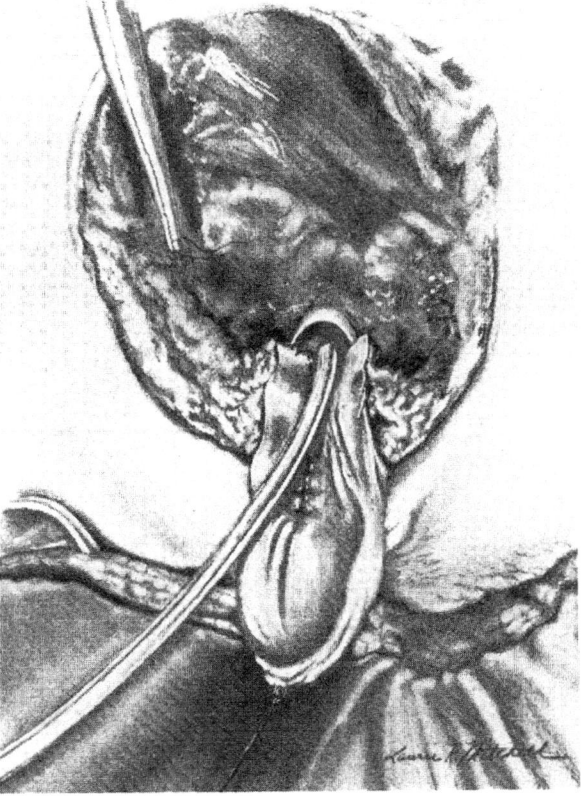

Figure 14. Construction of neourethra with paraexstrophy skin (from Jeffs 1978 p. 123).

from its intracrural position. The prostate then will retract to a more normal pelvic location maintaining its inferior vesicle blood supply. Thus the urethral plate has been transected and the prostate mobilized. Further dissection (Figure 12d) along the anterior attachment of the corpora to the inferior ramus of the pubis provides penile length and corrects the dorsal chordee. There now remains a gap of approximately 3-5 cm between the prostatic urethra and the penile portion of the distal urethra. The lateral portions of the paraexstrophy pedicle flaps (Figure 13) are then outlined and

incised laterally at their junction with the normal inguinal skin. Pedicles with a subcutaneous blood supply are mobilized sufficiently to allow for approximation of the pedicle in the midline, above the approximated crura (Duckett Jr. 1978) (Figure 14). The medial part of each pedicle forms the floor of the new urethral segment and the lateral margins are sutured anteriorly to create the roof of the urethra (Figure 15a). The bladder is closed regardless of its size, with a Malacot catheter in the dome (Figure 15b). The pubic arch is then approximated by a horizontal nylon mattress suture through the

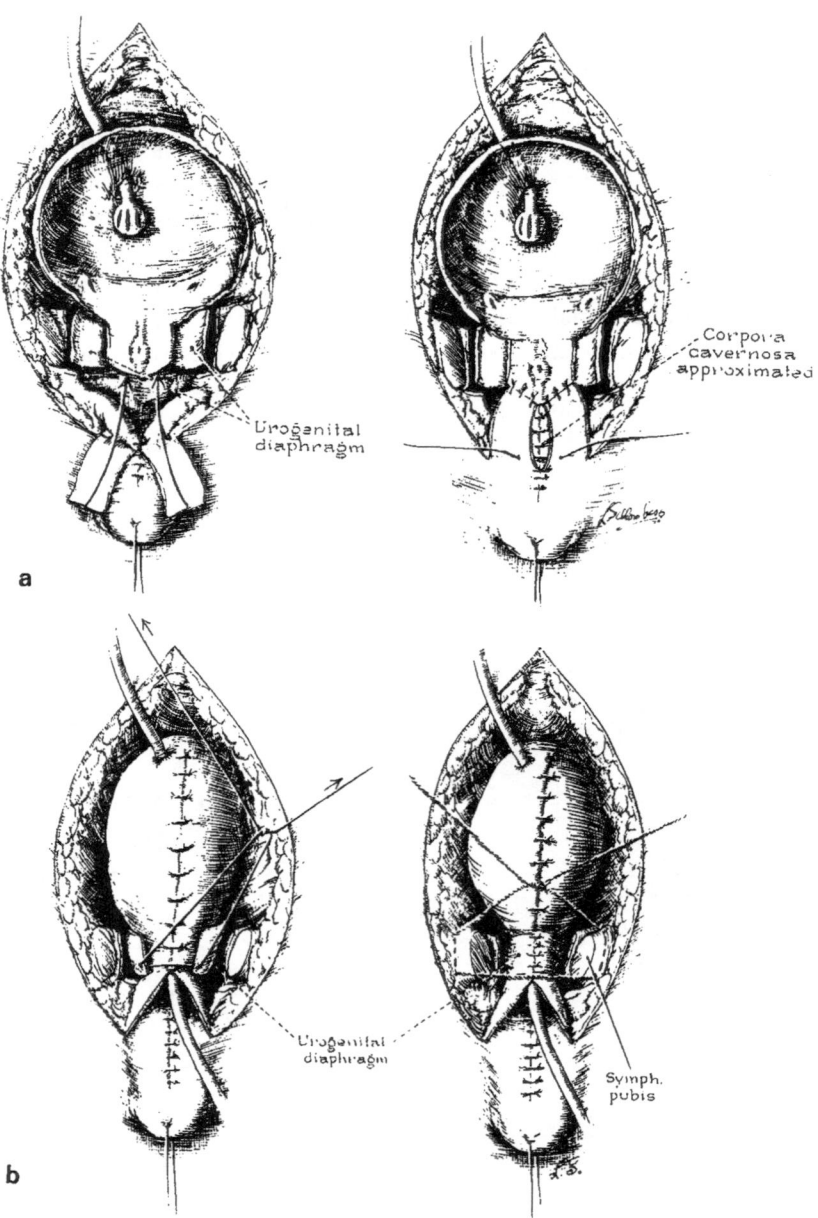

Figure 15. Vesical closure in exstrophy (from Jeffs 1978 p. 133).

pubic tubercles. In most cases, the edges of the rectus and the skin can be approximated in the midline (Figure 16). A light dressing is placed over the incision and following this, the child's legs are wrapped using moleskin padding and fluffy gauze from the thighs down to avoid external rotation and abduction of the legs. This arrangement allows the child to flex his legs at the knees, but does not allow abduction of the hip. This position is maintained for a minimum of six weeks to insure firm fixation of the pubic ring and soft tissues.

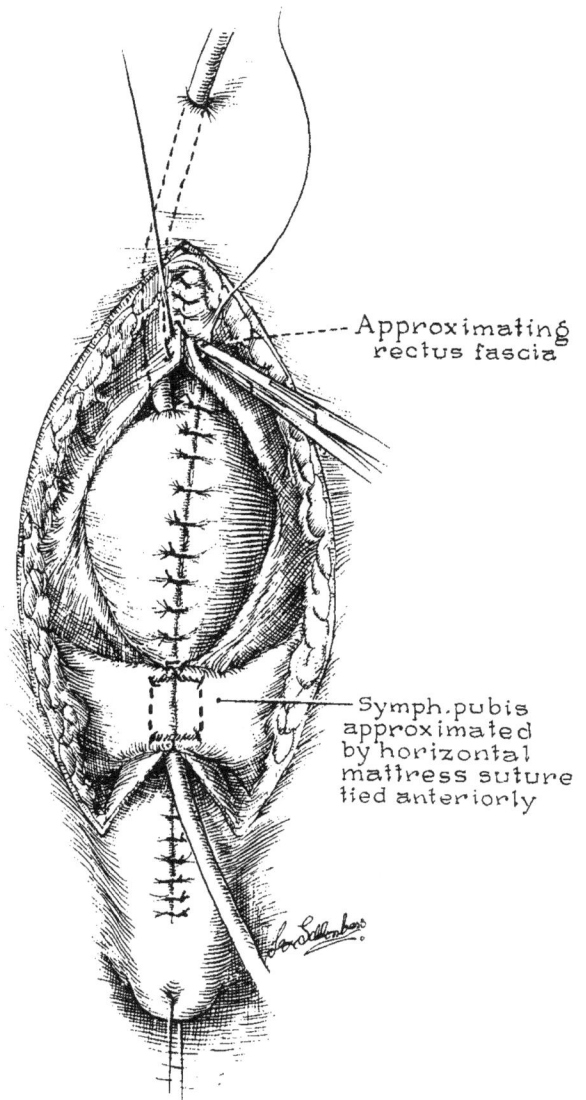

Figure 16. Symphyseal approximation and skin closure in exstrophy (from Jeffs 1978 p. 134).

G. The Incontinent Interval

Upon removal of the suprapubic tube, a sound is passed through the urethra to insure free drainage. At this point the child should be incontinent of urine and managed simply by diapering. An I.V.P. should be done at approximately six weeks to two months after surgery to insure that no hydronephrosis has occurred. If reflux is found on a cystogram, consideration can be made for a low dose suppressive antibiotic. At the end of a year, a repeat I.V.P. is carried out to assess the size of the bladder and assure protection of the upper urinary tracts.

H. The Bladder Neck Reconstruction

Between the ages of two and four in children who have a bladder capacity of 40-50 ml, the Young-Dees Leadbetter (Leadbetter 1964) procedure is performed to reconstruct the bladder neck and urethra. Vesicourethral reflux is corrected during this procedure as described by Cohen (1975) (Figure 17a-e). Following this, the new urethra and bladder neck are attached to the pubic ring and rectus fascia to create a sharp urethral vesicle angle. much in the manner of the standard Marshall-Marchetti-Krantz (Marshall et al. 1949) procedure (Figure 17f). Toguri et al. (1978), have found that continence appears to result from a combination of closure of the pelvic ring, urethral vesicle suspension and bladder neck plasty in exstrophy patients. When this procedure is omitted, continence seems to occur much later, if at all. Postoperatively, the bladder is drained suprapubically for approximately three weeks to allow for healing. Following this, continence may be delayed in onset as the child has to learn to develop an adequate capacity and detrusor control. In some cases pharmacologic manipulation with anticolinergics or alpha adrenergic stimulating agents can also improve the degree of continence.

I. Epispadias Repair

The epispadias repair required is essentially that described for a simple penile epispadias in the previous section.

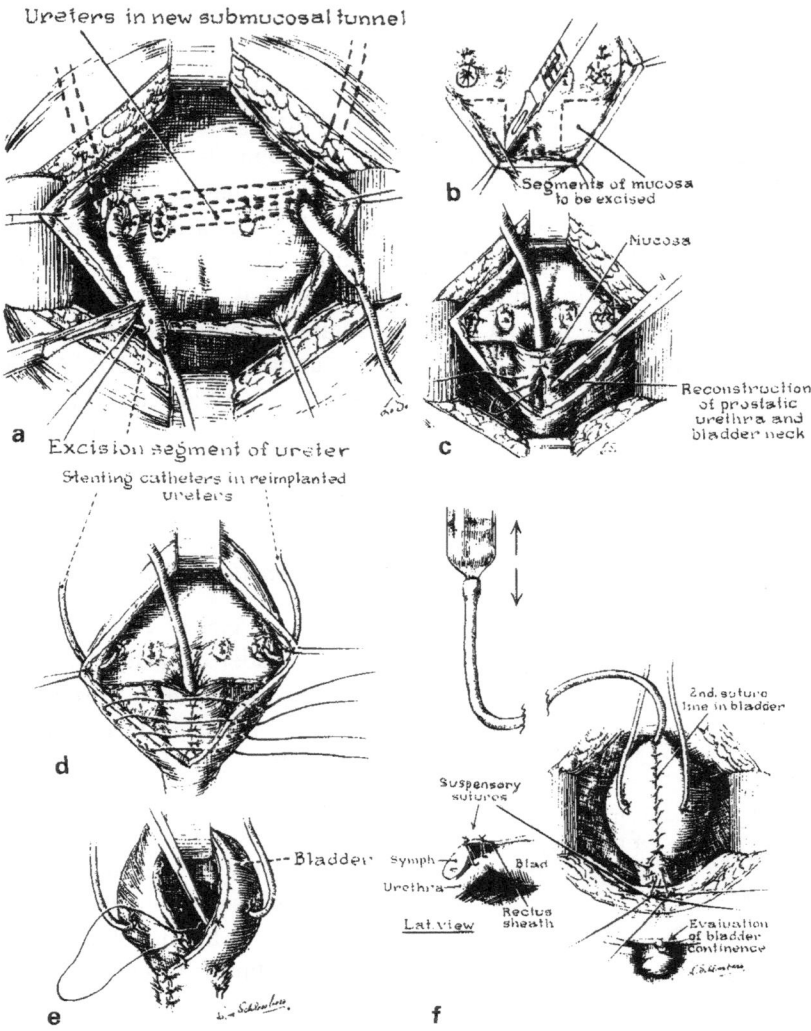

Figure 17. Reconstruction of bladder neck and antireflux procedure in the second stage of exstrophy repair (from Jeffs 1978 p. 135).

J. *Management of Exstrophy in the Nonfunctional Closure*

In some patients, bladder size does not permit a functional closure with staged technique as previously outlined. Some form of urinary diversion must be considered and historically, ureterosigmoidostomy has been the procedure of choice as exstrophy patients have normal rectal continence. Currently it is our policy to do a ureterosigmoidostomy using antireflux technique when the child is between six months and one year of age concurrent with penile lengthening and genital reconstruction. The small bladder is not removed.

Cendron (1977), has proposed a ureterocolosigmoidostomy as a means of managing this form of exstrophy. When the patient is about one year of age, a colon conduit with antireflux anastomosis is performed. An I.V.P. and loopogram are then done to insure good drainage and absence of reflux. The child is managed by external drainage for four to five years until rectal control can be tested by saline instillation. When colon conduit function and rectal continence are observed to be satisfactory, undiversion by colosigmoid anastomosis of the conduit to the rectosigmoid is performed. It is our hope in the future, as the child and hopefully the bladder increases in size, that this colosigmoid anastomosis could be secondarily taken down and anastomosed to the bladder in a procedure described by Arap et al. (1976) and urinary continuity restored.

In summary, it has become apparent that with the recent advances in plastic and reconstructive surgery of the genitalia, penile lengthening, continence and antireflux surgery, that the management of exstrophy-epispadias requires the coordinated effort of a center surgical team that appreciates the nuances in care and is committed to long term management of this devastating abnormality.

REFERENCES

Aarskog D: Clinical and cytogenetic studies in hypospadias. Acta Paediatr Scand (suppl) 203: 1, 1970.

Aleem AA: Diphallia: Report of a case. J Urol 108: 357-358, 1972.

Allen JS, Summers JL, Wilkerson JE: Meatal calibration of newborn boys. J Urol 107: 498, 1972.

Allen TD: Disorders of the male external genitalia. Clinical pediatric urology, vol 2, p 642, Philadelphia, London, Toronto, WB Saunders Co, 1976.

Ansell JS: Vesical exstrophy. In: Urologic surgery, Glenn JF (ed), Harper and Row, Hagerstown, 1975, p 316.

Arap S, Giron AM and DeGoes GM: Complete reconstruction of bladder exstrophy. Urology 7: 413, April, 1976.

Arey LB: Developmental anatomy: A textbook and laboratory manual of embryology. Seventh ed. WB Saunders Co, Philadelphia, 1965.

Belman AB: The penis, Urol Clin N America, volume 5: 17 February, 1978.

Belman AB, Duckett JW and Woodard JR: American academy of pediatrics, Urology Section, Report on Meatal Stenosis – Pediatrics, in press.

Cendron J: Bladder exstrophy from an external to an internal diversion. Birth defects: Original article series volume XIII, no 5, 197, 1977.

Cohen SJ: Ureterozysloneostomie. Eine neue Antirefluxtechnik. Aktuelle Urologie, 6: 24, 1975.

Duckett JW Jr: Epispadias, urologic clinics of north America, vol 5, no 1, 107, February 1978.

Eckstein HB, Hohenfellner R, and Williams DI (eds): Surgical pediatric urology. WB Saunders, Philadelphia, 1977.

Gee WF and Ansell JS: Neonatal circumcision: A ten year overview. Pediatrics, 58: 824, 1976.

Gleason DM, Bottaccini MR, Reilly RJ, et al: The residual stream energy as a diagnostic index of male urinary outflow obstruction. Invest Urol 10: 72-77, 1972.

Glenn JF, Anderson EE: Surgical correction of incomplete penoscrotal transposition. J Urol 110: 603-605, 1973.

Guthrie RD, Smith DW and Graham CB: Testosterone treatment for micropenis during early childhood. J Pediat 83: 247, 1973.

Hastings J: Encyclopedia of religion and ethics. Charles Scribner's Sons, New York, 1911.

Hinman F Jr: Microphallus: Characteristics and choice of treatment from a study of 20 cases. J Urol 107: 499, 1972.

Horton CE (ed): Plastic and reconstructive surgery of the genital tract. Boston, Little and Brown, 1973.

Jeffs RD (ed): Congenital abnormalities of the lower urinary tract, Urologic Clinics of North America, WB Saunders, 1978.

Jeffs RD, Charrois R, Many M and Juriansz AR: Primary closure of the exstrophied bladder. In: Current Controversies in Urologic Management, Scott R (ed), WB Saunders Co, Philadelphia, 1972, p 235.

Johnston JH and Kogan SJ: The exstrophic anomalies and their surgical reconstructions. Curr Prob Surg 1-39, 1974.

Johnston WG, Yeatman GW and Weigel JW: Congenital absence of the penis. J Urol 117: 508, 1977.

Kenawi MM: Webbed penis. Br J Urol 45: 569, 1973.

Kernahan DA: Congenital abnormalities of the scrotum. In: Plastic and reconstructive surgery of the genital area, Horton CE (ed) Little, Brown and Co, Boston, 1973.

Kossow JH, Morales PA: Duplication of bladder and urethra and associated anomalies. Urology 1: 71-73, 1973.

Leadbetter GW: Surgical correction of total urinary incontinence. J Urol 91: 261, 1964.

Lisa L, Hanak J, Cerny M, et al: Agenesis of the penis. J Pediatr Surg 8: 327-328, 1973.

Marshall VF, Marchetti AA and Krantz KE: The correction of stress incontinence by simple vesicourethral suspension. Surg Gynecol Obstet 88: 509, 1949.

Milroy E: Ectopic scrotum: a review of the literature and report of a further case. Br J Urol 41: 235-237, 1969.

Mininberg DT and Richman A: Bilateral scrotal testicular ectopia. J Urol 108: 652-654, 1972.

Muecke EC: The role of the cloacal membrane in exstrophy: the first successful experimental study. J Urol 92: 659-667, 1964.

Oster J: Further fate of the foreskin. Arch Dis Child 43: 200, 1968.

Perlmutter AD and Chamberlain JW: Webbed penis without chordee. J Urol 107: 320-321, 1972.

Preston EN: Whither the foreskin? A consideration of routine neonatal circumcision. JAMA 213: 1853-1858, 1970.

Raifer J and Walsh PC: Testicular descent, normal and abnormal. Urol Clin N Amer vol 5: 223, February, 1978.

Remzi D: Diphallia. Urology 1: 462-463, 1973.

Richart R and Benirschke K: Penile agenesis: Report of case, review of the world literature and discussion of pertinent embryology. Arch Pathol 70: 252-260, 1960.

Shulman J, Ben-hur N and Neuman Z: Surgical complications of circumcision. Am J Dis Child 107: 149-154, 1964.

Toguri A, Churchill B, Schillinger J and Jeffs RD: Continence in cases of bladder exstrophy. J Urol 119: 538, April, 1978.

Walsh PC, Wilson JD, Allen TD et al: Clinical and endocrinological evaluation of patients with congenital microphallus. J Urol 120: 90, 1978.

Wilson JD, Harrod MJ, Goldstein JL, et al: Familial incomplete male pseudohermaphroditism, type 1, New Eng J Med 290: 1097, 1974.

Wilson JSP: Diphallus – plastic and reconstructive surgery of the genital area, 163, Boston, Little, Brown and Co, 1973.

Young HH: A new operation for epispadias. J Urol 2: 237, 1918.

9. GENITAL RECONSTRUCTION FOR TRAUMATIC AND INFECTIOUS DISEASES

W.S. McDougal

Reconstruction of the genital area following traumatic injury or infectious disease not only requires a fundamental knowledge of urologic and plastic surgery principles but poses unique problems in patient management. Post injury, many patients experience fear over the possible loss of sexual potency and reproductive ability. Early counseling and supportive discussions about what can be accomplished cosmetically and functionally are critical if behavioral problems are to be minimized during the reconstructive and postreconstructive periods. In addition to psychological problems which invariably accompany these injuries, the composition of the genital tissues poses special problems in surgical management. The skin has a very thin dermis beneath which lies a layer of loose areolar tissue. These characteristics result in marked edema when the tissue is traumatized, poor capacity of sutures to hold the tissues together when they are placed under tension, and extensive hematoma formation when blood vessels beneath the skin are ruptured. There are also unique aspects of care which must be considered in the postoperative period. Erections in the immediate postsurgical period may result in bleeding and tension on the suture line. Moreover, the need to divert urine and feces away from healing wounds if their proximity will result in persistent contamination of the surgical repair must be considered.

Initial evaluation should include an appraisal of: 1) the severity of associated injuries and their effect on the stability of the patient, 2) the perineal soft tissue and cutaneous loss, 3) the competence of the urinary and rectal sphincters, and 4) the integrity of the urethra and rectosigmoid colon. In the massively traumatized patient the approach to the genital injury may have to be tailored to satisfy proper priorities of care. For example, in the stable patient in whom the trauma is isolated to the genital area, an involved surgical procedure may be appropriate; however, the same injury in the massively traumatized unstable patient often requires a less extensive procedure which can be expeditiously performed. The latter course usually necessitates further surgery at a later, more opportune time.

I. TRAUMATIC INJURIES

A. Avulsion of the Genital Skin

Extensive loss of the penile and/or scrotal skin is often the result of a degloving type injury. This injury occurs when the loose skin is caught with the clothing in a device which tears both from the patient. A moving belt on farm machinery is often the cause. Separation of the tissue occurs in the loose areolar layer which is superficial to Buck's fascia in the penis and immediately beneath the dartos muscle in the scrotum. The deeper tissues including corpora, urethra and testes are usually unharmed. The avulsion characteristically involves the circumference of the shaft of the penis from penile scrotal junction to corona. Scrotal involvement, however, does not characteristically result in the loss of the entire scrotal covering.

Immediate repair is essential for delays will result in cicatrix formation, development of contractures, and subsequent genital deformity. The wounds should be thoroughly cleansed, foreign materials sought and removed, nonviable tissue excised and the integrity of the urethra and testes confirmed.

Small noncircumferential defects in the penile skin may be closed primarily after freshening the edges provided there is no tension on the suture line. When closure cannot be accomplished without tension, either a full thickness graft taken from the foreskin in the uncircumcised or a split thickness graft is employed. In contrast, circumferential penile shaft skin losses require more aggressive debridement. All proximal viable tissue is preserved; however, the skin distal to the defect irrespective of its viability should be removed two to three millimeters proximal to the corona. Retention of the distal tissue will result in the development of brawny edema due to the interruption of lymphatic drainage (Masters and Robinson 1968). The edema may persist for months or years making both the appearance and function of the part unsatisfactory to most patients.

The defects created by extensive losses of the penile and scrotal skin are covered with thick split thickness graft and stented (Malherbe 1975). The stent is formed from cotton wadding soaked in glycerol and is held in place by leaving the sutures at the margin of the graft long and tying them over the wadding. The grafts are taken at a thickness of 0.016 to 0.018 inches in the adult. The epithelium in children is not as thick as it is in the adult and therefore, in the young, the graft is taken at a thickness of 0.010 to 0.014 inches. Circumferential wounds of the penis are covered by a single sheet of graft sewn in place utilizing the technique of an interdigitating seam located on the dorsum of the penis (Figure 1). The graft is stented for 4 to 7 days, a transurethral foley placed, and the foley taped to the abdomen so that the penis is maintained in the anatomic position. The interdigitating seam breaks the line of scar formation and the dorsal placement provides for a functional result should scar contracture occur, i.e. a slight dorsal curvature is functionally better tolerated than a ventral curvature.

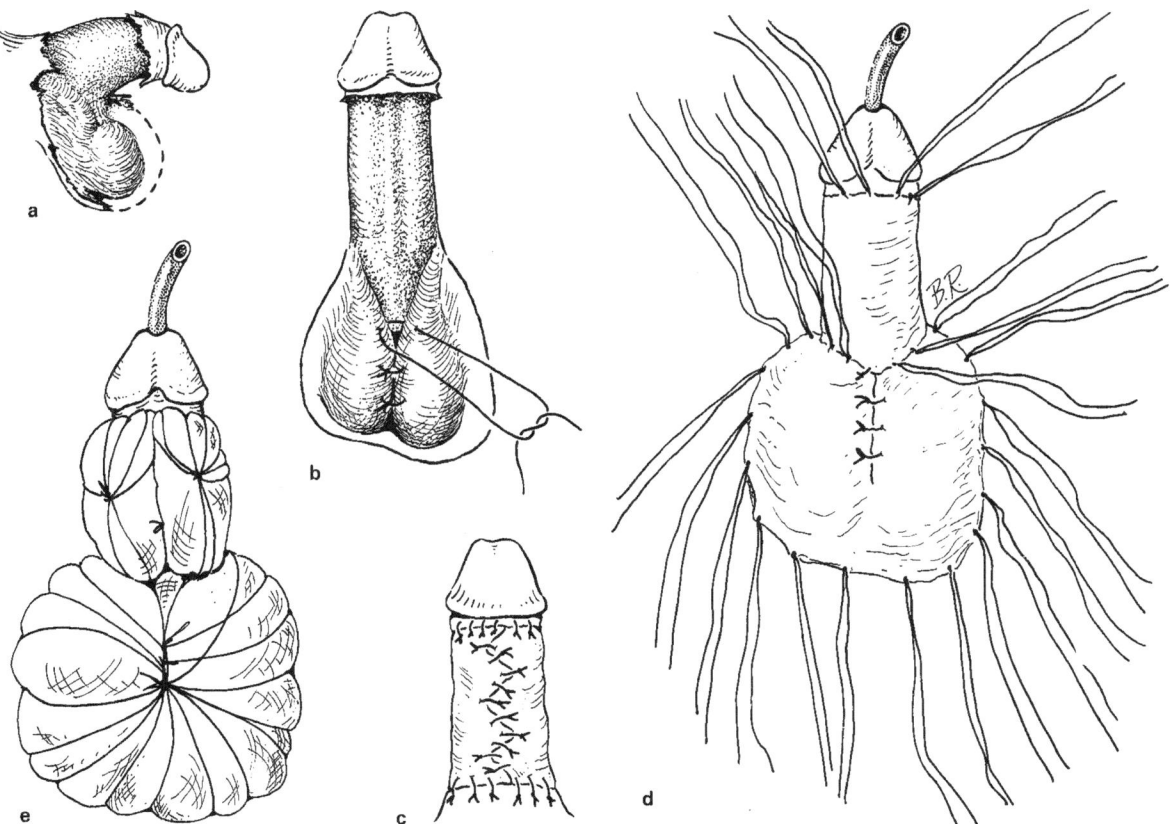

Figure 1. Avulsion injury. a. The injury which involves a circumferential skin loss from the penis and an extensive scrotal defect is illustrated. b. The skin on the distal shaft is removed. A margin of several millimeters of skin is left adjacent to the corona to which the skin graft will be sewn. The margins of the scrotal defect are debrided and the internal spermatic fascia overlying the testes is sutured together in the midline. c. The penile shaft is grafted with split thickness skin. The interdigitating seam is placed on the dorsum of the shaft. d. Split thickness graft is applied over the scrotal defect and tailored to cover the testes. The sutures used to sew the margin of the graft in place are left long. e. The grafts are stented using cotton wadding which is held in place by tying the sutures at the margin over the wadding.

All viable scrotal tissue should be preserved for its elasticity and it will often allow for complete coverage of the defect without the necessity for skin grafts. The wound margins are freshened and brought together with interrupted 3-0 reabsorbable suture. Extensive losses of scrotal skin do not allow for primary closure and result in exposure of the testes. These structures must be covered in such a way as to assure that their temperature will remain a few degrees below core body temperature if fertility is to be preserved. There are two methods of accomplishing this purpose: split thickness skin coverage (Balakrishnan 1956) and transferal to superficial subcutaneous thigh pockets (Masters and Robinson 1968). If the testes are uninjured and have a good blood supply, they are sutured together in the midline, covered with split thickness graft and stented (Figure 1e). The stent may be removed in 4 to 7 days. A very acceptable cosmetic result is obtained (Malherbe 1975), morbidity is minimized, and the thin covering results in reduced testicular

temperature thereby allowing spermatogenesis to proceed normally. If the viability of the testes is in doubt or their blood supply is marginal, each testis is implanted into the adjacent thigh. The perineal defect is closed with a split thickness skin graft and stented in place. The testes should be implanted in a superficial subcutaneous pouch so that their temperature is maintained below that of the body core temperature. The implantation should be carefully planned bearing in mind that the skin immediately overlying the testes will be used for reconstructing the scrotum. They should be placed slightly posterior and at asymmetric levels to prevent trauma during ambulation. The scrotum is reconstructed at a later date using the thigh skin and subcutaneous tissue containing the testes as pedicle flaps (Figure 2). Split thickness skin grafts will allow the patient to appreciate gross tactile sensation but generally do not provide for the finer sensations of pin prick, two point discrimination, pain and temperature.

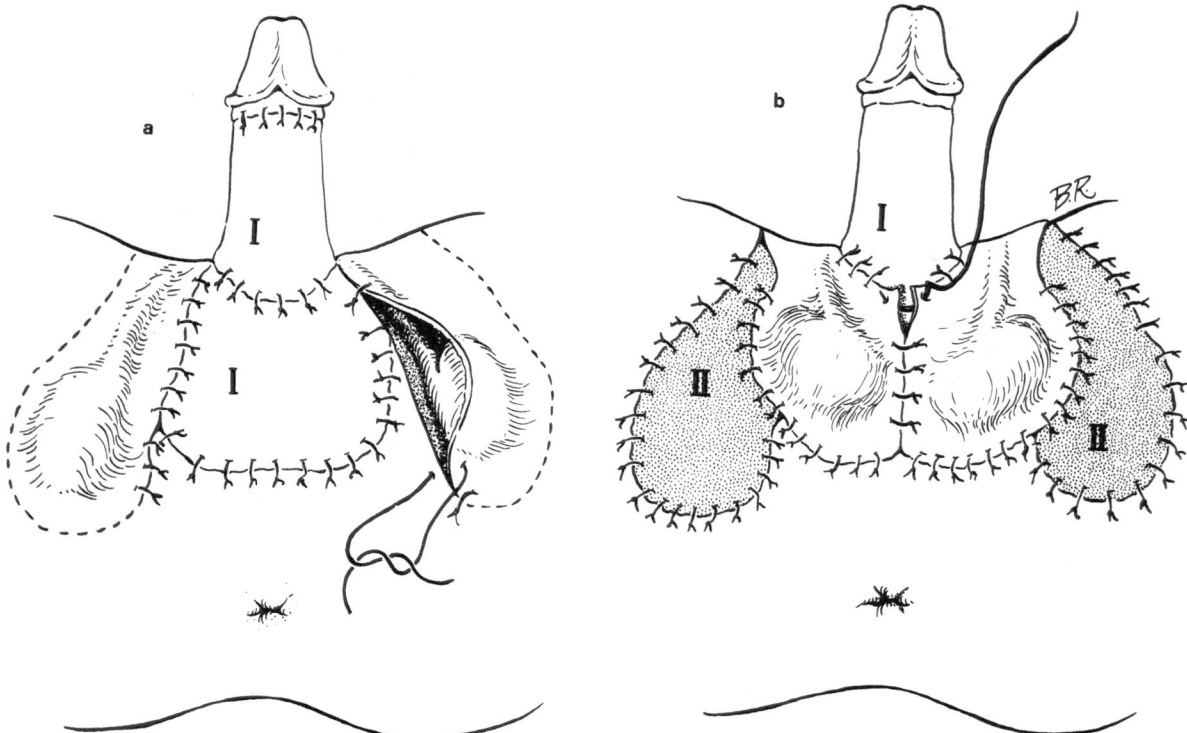

Figure 2. Implantation of the testes into the thighs with subsequent reconstruction of the scrotum from thigh pedicle flaps. a. The testes are implanted into superficial subcutaneous pockets on the posteriomedial aspects of the thighs. The denuded penile shaft and perineal defect are grafted with split thickness skin (I) and stented as described in Figure 1. b. After one to two months, the thigh pedicle flaps containing the testes are raised and rotated medially. The split thickness skin graft on the perineum is removed, and the pedicle grafts are sutured together in the midline and to the margins of the defect posteriorly and laterally. The wounds created on the medial aspect of the thighs are closed with split thickness skin grafts (II) and stented in place.

B. Penile Gangrene

Traumatic gangrene of the penis may involve only the skin and subcutaneous tissue or it may affect the full thickness of the organ. It is the result of the placement of a constriction about the penis usually as a form of masturbation, as a means of maintaining an erection, or as a form of child abuse. Many objects have been used and include nuts (Tiwari et al. 1977), pieces of pipe, string, rubber bands (Markland and Merrill 1972), wire, condoms, and hair. The latter is commonly the constricting agent in cases where the gangrene is the result of child abuse. Initially, the constricting band impedes superficial venous return but does not prevent arterial inflow or deep venous outflow. Distal skin and subcutaneous edema and necrosis result. Unchecked, the edema progresses and impedes arterial inflow. When this occurs, gangrene of the entire structure distal to the obstruction is imminent. Initially, the ability to void may be undisturbed; however, as the edema progresses, the patients may have considerable difficulty micturating. When these injuries are recognized early, before gangrene is present, metal bands may be cut and removed, or slipped off by threading a string through the band, wrapping the distal penis with the string after several puncture holes have been made in the distal skin to allow edema fluid to escape, and unwrapping the string from the proximal aspect of the band. Occasionally, the metal band cannot be cut nor can it be removed by the string technique. Under these circumstances the penile skin and subcutaneous tissue should be surgically excised to the level of Buck's fascia from object to corona (Schellhammer and Donnelly 1973). The object can then be slid off and the penile shaft grafted as described for avulsion injuries (Figure 1). String, wire, rubber bands and hair may be very difficult to find once edema has become significant. These objects tend to become buried and if they cannot be appreciated, the penis should be anesthetized and a longitudinal slit should be made beginning in the normal skin and extending onto the area of edema. This will result in severance of the band.

After the constricting agent is removed, an assessment of the extent of necrosis must be made. If the gangrene extends to the deep tissues, a suprapubic cystostomy should be placed and the lesion should be treated with twice daily applications of a topical antimicrobial preceded by thorough cleansing with an iodophor. Mafenide acetate and silver sulfadiazine are both acceptable topical antimicrobials; however, mafenide acetate is preferred due to its better penetrability of the eschar. This therapy is continued until demarcation is unequivocally established. The gangrenous area is removed with an attempt to preserve as much penile length as possible. The procedure is identical to a standard partial penectomy.

C. Amputation of the Penis with Retention of the Transected Part

Amputation of the penis may be a result of a self-inflicted injury, an act of violence to the individual, a blast injury, or other mechanical trauma. Massive bleeding and shock are common sequelae. Hemostasis should be achieved by compression and not by indiscriminate ligation of bleeding vessels until blood pressure is restored to normal. This is important in order to assure the best possible chance for a successful microvascular repair. The amputated part is placed in iced Ringer's Lactate containing penicillin and streptomycin. The dorsalis penis and profunda arteries and corpora cavernosa are flushed with cold heparinized saline until the venous effluent is clear. If the transection has occurred distal to the penile scrotal junction a tourniquet may be applied to the proximal retained portion to achieve hemostasis. The proximal arteries and veins are identified, cannulated with polyethylene catheters and flushed with heparinized saline. When brisk arterial bleeding is obtained the vessels are occluded with noncrushing microvascular clips. The wound is irrigated and loose nonviable tissue removed. A suprapubic cystostomy or perineal urethrostomy is performed, the former being preferred since it may be accomplished without manipulation of the proximal penile stump. A foley catheter is placed through the urethra of the severed part and thence through the proximal urethra into the bladder. This serves to align the structures to be sutured (Figure 3). The urethra is the first structure to be anastomosed and is sutured together in an oblique manner with 4-0 atraumatic chromic suture. The corpora cavernosa are then sutured together with interrupted 5-0 Proline. These two structures must be sutured together first for they provide the necessary stability required for the subsequent microvascular anastomosis. It should be noted that some surgeons prefer to anastomose the profunda arteries in which case this must be accomplished following the urethral anastomosis and prior to the corpora anastomosis. These arteries are often impossible to find in the severed part and are not critical to an acceptable result. Using the operative microscope, the deep dorsal and superficial dorsal veins are each anastomosed with 9 or 10-0 nylon suture. Usually only one of the two

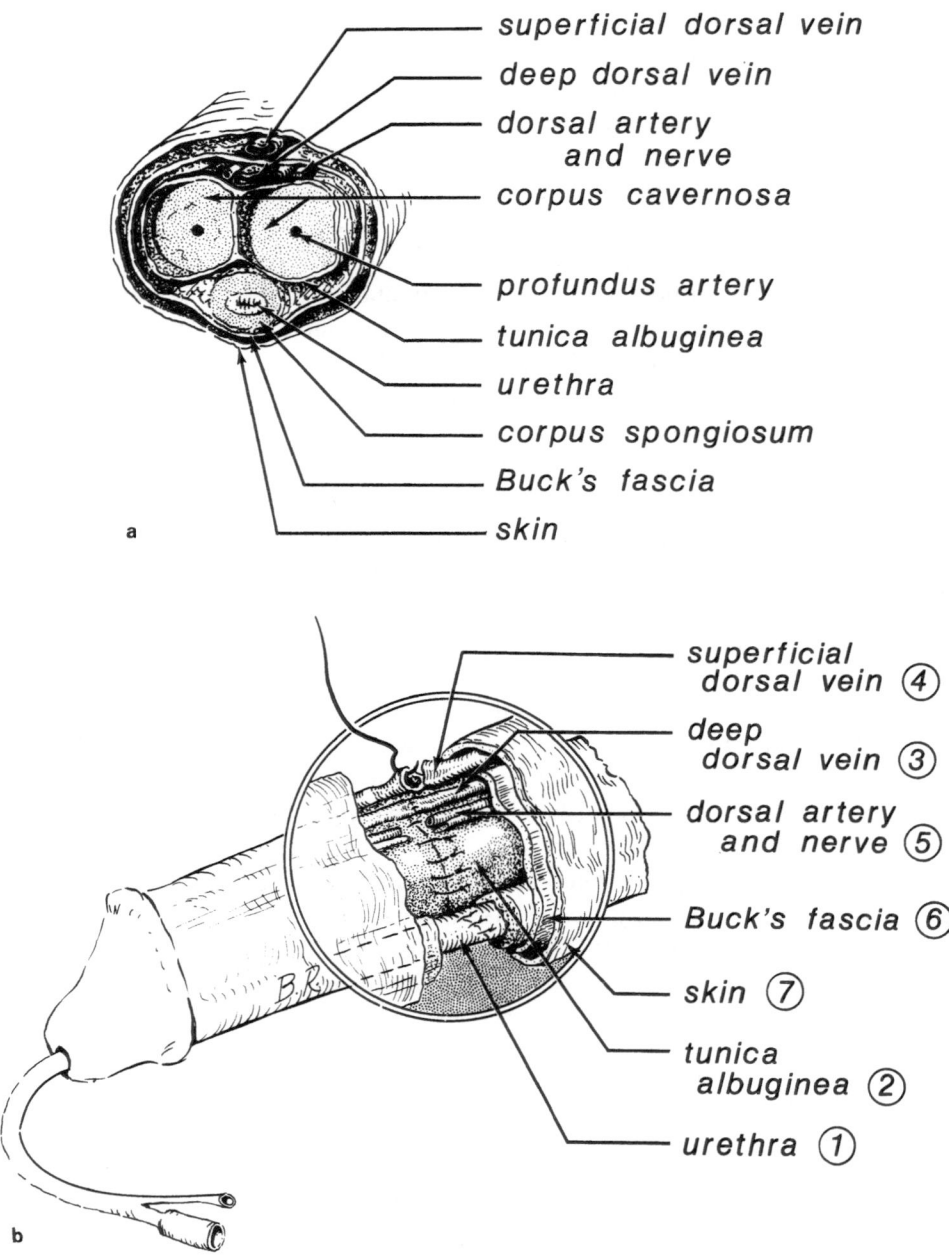

Figure 3. Microvascular repair of the amputated penis. a. Cross sectional anatomy of the penile shaft. b. The urethra has been repaired in an oblique fashion over a stenting catheter (1) and the tunica albuginea of the corpora cavernosa have been reapproximated (2). Using a microvascular technique the deep dorsal vein has been repaired (3) and the superficial dorsal vein is being reanastomosed (4). The dorsal arteries and nerves (5) are subsequently reapproximated. Finally, Buck's fascia (6) and the skin (7) are loosely sutured together.

veins can be found in which case one anastomosis is generally adequate. Attention is then turned to the two dorsal arteries which are sutured together with interrupted 10-0 nylon. The two dorsal nerves are identified and reapproximated with 10-0 nylon. The penis and glans should immediately 'pink up' after release of the microvascular clamps. Bleeding points from the severed edges may now be individually ligated. When adequate hemostasis has been achieved, Buck's fascia is loosely sutured together with 5-0 Proline. The skin is loosely brought together with 4 or 5-0 nonreabsorbable suture. A bulky dressing is placed on the penis and it is taped to the abdominal wall (Tamai et al. 1977; Cohen et al. 1977).

The use of anticoagulants in the postoperative period is controversial. Bleeding into the penis with large hematoma formation has been reported with the use of heparin. Urokinase and low molecular weight dextran have also been employed with some success (Cohen et al. 1977). Edema invariably occurs postoperatively but generally subsides by two to three weeks. Some superficial skin loss may occur which will require the application of split thickness skin as described in the section on avulsion injuries. Slight scarring and contracture of the corpora cavernosa at the level of the anastomosis is to be expected but has little consequence (Tamai et al. 1977). Sensation to light touch and pin prick returns by three months. The cosmetic and functional result is excellent, many patients reporting satisfactory erections and ejaculations. Successful microvascular replantations have been reported up to 18 hours post injury. Complications include urethral strictures, urethral fistulae, distal skin necrosis, poor sensation and inability to obtain or maintain erections (Heymann et al. 1977). These complications are much less common when the microvascular technique described above is employed than they are when the vessels are ligated and the amputated part is sutured in place using the urethra, corpora cavernosa, Buck's fascia and skin (Engelmann et al. 1974). Indeed, skin necrosis is so common with the latter method that it has been suggested that the penile skin should be removed from the severed part. Following the anastomosis the penis is buried in the scrotum (Figure 4). The shaft is released at a later date (McRoberts et al. 1968).

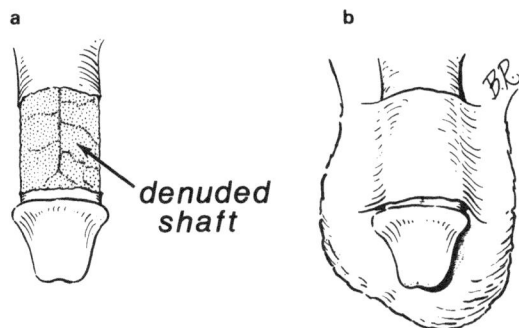

Figure 4. Scrotal flap technique for covering a denuded penile shaft. The denuded penile shaft, A, is placed beneath a scrotal flap, B. The glans is exposed.

D. Amputation of the Penis with Loss of the Transected Part

This injury occurs as a result of amputation for malignancy, gun shot wounds, blast injuries, mechanical trauma and self-inflicted injury. Loss of the scrotum may often accompany this injury. The wounds should be debrided and the defect closed either primarily or with split thickness skin (the former is preferred since it makes subsequent surgery less complicated). The reconstructive procedures are begun one to three months post-injury to allow for adequate healing of the perineal wounds.

When the scrotum is present, a nonfunctional, purely cosmetic appendage may be created from the scrotal tissues (Figure 5). Over the long term this structure is prone to shrinkage, atrophy, and deformity. In an attempt to prevent these complications, one testis and its cord have been translocated into the scrotal appendage. Initial results are encouraging (Taguchi et al. 1977). The procedure seems appropriate for the patient who has had a total penectomy for cancer and is troubled by the appearance of his external genitalia. Voiding is performed through a perineal urethrostomy.

A more functional structure may be created by constructing the penis from a tubed pedicle graft as originally described by Gilles (Gilles and Harrison 1948) and subsequently modified by others (Figure 6). The structure allows the patient to void in the standing position, is cosmetically acceptable, and may be used for coitus provided cartilage or a silastic rod has been implanted in it. The cartilage or silastic prosthesis is implanted on either side of the pedicle tube in the fatty tissue between the skin and neourethra three to four months following final attachment of the pedicle. The proximal part of the rigid stent is anchored to the corpora bodies. The prosthesis should extend along the entire length of the pedicle for if it falls short, a floppy end will result which will make intromission difficult. Complications of the reconstructive procedure include tissue slough, strictures and urethral fistulae (Fleming 1970; Evans 1963). A modification has been described in which an epithelialized channel is created by suturing the pedicle so that the epithelium forms a tube on the inside. Split thickness graft covers the exterior surface. This allows the patient to place a silastic tube in the channel and thereby transform the flaccid organ to a rigid one at will (Noe et al. 1974). If absent, the scrotum is reconstructed with thigh pedicle flaps as illustrated in Figure 2.

E. Fracture of the Penis

Fracture of the penis occurs as a result of a forcible tear in one or both cavernous bodies during an erection. The wall of the corpora in the flaccid state is normally 2 mm thick; however, during an erection, it has a thickness of 0.25 to 0.5 mm thereby making it much more susceptible to injury. The tear occurs as a result of blunt trauma and is usually located in the distal third, central part, or rarely at the root of the penis (Ovrum 1978). The urethra is involved in 30% of the cases (Hudson 1975). A urethral injury should be suspected when blood is present at the meatus. A cracking noise is heard at the moment of injury and is followed by rapid detumescence. Pain may be severe. The penis appears contorted, echymotic and edematous.

Two forms of therapy have been advocated

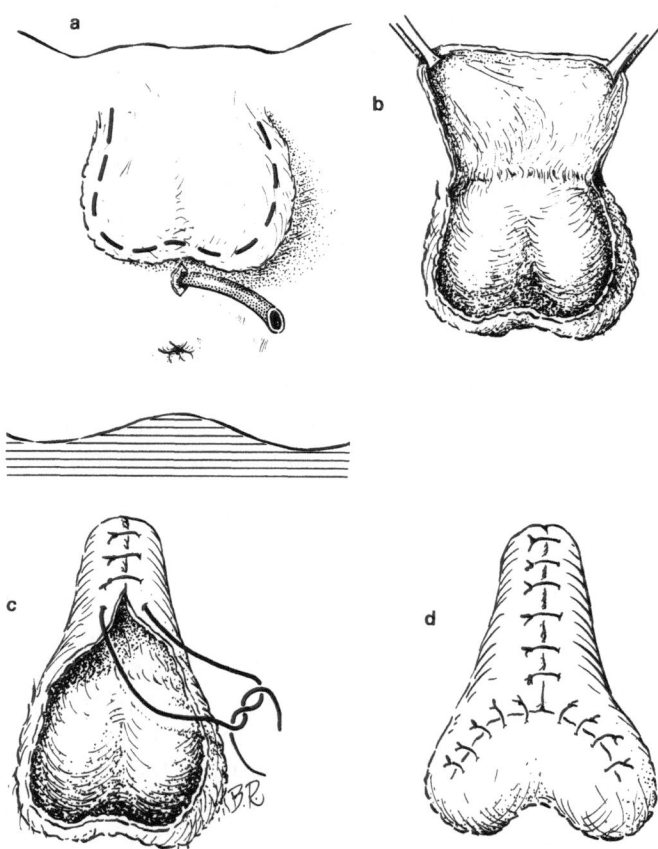

Figure 5. Reconstruction of the penis from scrotal tissues. a. The penis has been amputated and a perineal urethrostomy has been created. These wounds have been allowed to heal for several months. The incision to be made in the scrotum is outlined. b. A scrotal flap is raised with meticulous attention to hemostasis. c. The lateral margins of the scrotal flap are sutured together to create a cylinder. d. The scrotal defect is closed.

provided the urethra is uninjured: conservative and surgical. Conservative therapy involves application of ice packs to the area, elevation of the part, injection of enzymatic agents and subsequent hematoma evacuation if they become troublesome (Davies and Mitchell 1978). This management provides an acceptable result in 90 percent of patients so treated. Others suggest that the surgical approach affords better functional results with reduced morbidity (Gross et al. 1971). The tear is usually longitudinal and is repaired with interrupted 3-0 Prolene suture. The hematoma is evacuated, the wound closed, a compression dressing applied, and antibiotics administered. Irrespective of the method of treatment erections must be prevented during the healing period. This may be accomplished by the oral administration of stilbestrol. It should be noted that patients who have sustained a concomitant urethral injury require a surgical approach (Gross et al. 1977). The corpora are repaired before the urethral injury is approached.

F. Testicular Rupture

Rupture of the testes occurs as a result of blunt or penetrating trauma. Following injury a large intrascrotal hematoma develops. Occasionally, the hematoma follows the plane of Colles' and Scarpa's fascia and extends onto the anterior abdominal wall. These injuries require early surgical exploration. The necrotic tissue should be debrided, viable extruding seminiferous tubules returned to the testis and the tunica albuginea sutured together with interrupted 3-0 chromic. Rarely, a portion of the tunica albuginea is lost and the defect cannot be primarily reapproximated. It may be covered with a free graft of tunica vaginalis.

The necessity for early exploration and repair is apparent when the results of nonintervention are compared to early surgical therapy. Eighty percent of patients explored early and repaired maintain viable testes whereas only thirty-three percent of patients treated conservatively are found to have viable testes on followup examination.

G. The Burned Perineum

Burns of the perineum are rarely isolated injuries but rather occur in patients who have sustained major total body surface area burns (McDougal et al. 1979). Although treatment must be integrated with the care of the patient as a whole, two general principles apply to perineal burns: 1) preservation of as much tissue as possible is the goal, and therefore, there is no place for radical debridement in these injuries, and 2) wound coverage should be obtained as rapidly as possible. Initial therapy of the perineal burn is dependent upon whether it is due to a thermal, chemical or electric injury. All clothing is removed. Thermal injuries, if of limited extent, may be cooled (frost bite is rapidly rewarmed) and chemical injuries are copiously irrigated with water or saline. The use of neutralizing agents for chemical burns has no place in perineal injuries. Electric injuries are deceptive for a small area of skin injury may belie an extensive soft tissue necrosis below. In all types of injury, the loose tissue is removed and the hair overlying and adjacent to the area is shaved. The wound is gently washed with an iodophor and a topical antimicrobial is applied (mafenide acetate, silver sulfadiazine, or 0.5 percent silver nitrate soaks). Twice daily thereafter the wound is washed with an iodophor and the antimicrobial reapplied. Mafenide acetate is preferred because of its broad spectrum coverage and its ability to penetrate beneath the eschar. With its use, however, staphylococci and fungi may emerge as a significant problem in the burn wound.

Burns are classified according to the depth of injury as first, second, or third degree. A first degree injury involves only the epidermis, has an erythematous appearance and is painful. First degree injuries of the perineum, particularly when accompanied by a large fluid resuscitation, often result in massive swelling of the genital tissues. These injuries are treated by elevation and exposure (application of a topical antimicrobial is optional). The swelling subsides in two to six days post injury and healing is complete by six to ten days. Second degree or partial thickness injuries involve the epidermis and part of the dermis. They are red in appearance, may blister, are sensitive and will spontaneously heal if burn wound sepsis does not supervene. These injuries are treated by twice daily iodophor washes and topical antimicrobial application. A urethral catheter is usually necessary early

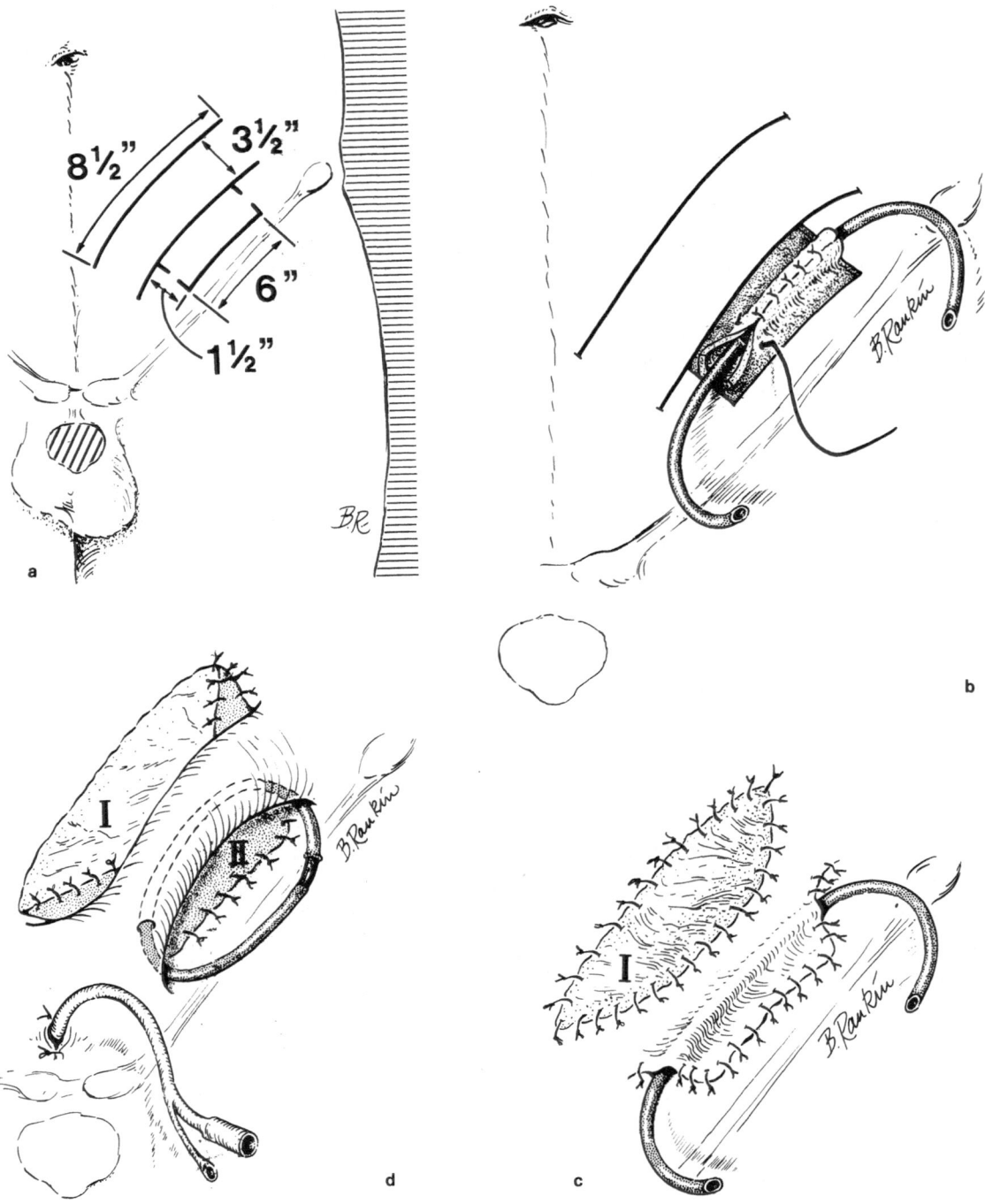

Figure 6. Reconstruction of the penis utilizing a tubed pedicle graft. a. The lines of incision, their position, and their dimensions are illustrated. b. A neo-urethra is constructed by raising two thin flaps and suturing the margins together with fine interrupted chromic over a stenting catheter so that the skin lies adjacent to the catheter. Care must be taken not to undermine the central one-half inch strip of skin for the neo-urethra is dependent upon this attachment for its blood supply. c. The bipedicle flap is mobilized, placed over the neo-urethra and sutured laterally to the margin of the wound. Excellent hemostasis must be obtained and the pedicle must not be placed under tension. The medial defect is covered with a split-thickness skin graft (I) which may be stented in place. Frequent postoperative checks are necessary to prevent hematoma formation. d. After three to four weeks, the bipedicle graft is tubed to include the neo-urethra. The skin edges of the pedicle tube must be brought together on the posterior surface without tension. Excision of fat may be required at this stage to achieve a tension free suture line. The defect created beneath the tube is covered with a split thickness skin graft (II). After several weeks, the stenting catheter may be removed, the neo-urethra flushed with saline and a new catheter placed. A suprapubic cystostomy for urinary diversion is placed lateral to the midline on the contralateral side. e. After one to

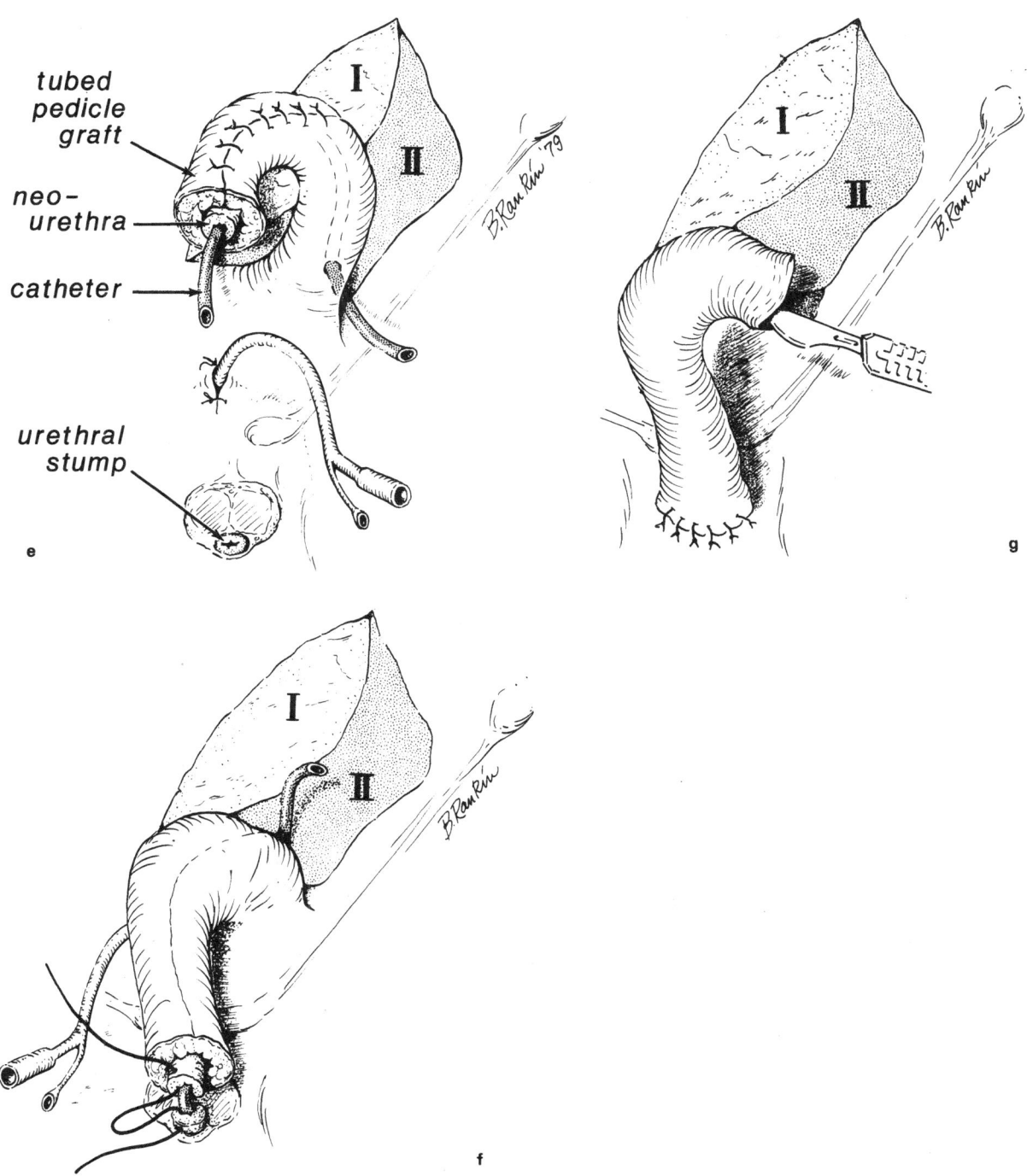

three months, an incision is made across one half of the cephalad end of the pedicle. One week later the cephalad end is completely transected and the pedicle is rotated to the area of the urethral stump. Care must be taken not to kink or twist the base of the pedicle which remains attached to the abdominal wall for the viability of the pedicle is dependent upon the blood supply received through this portion of the graft. Supportive dressings may be required to assure a gentle curve. If the pedicle does not lay as desired and more length is required, two parallel incisions made at the base which extend toward the pubis will lengthen the graft. f. The neo-urethra is sutured in an oblique fashion to the urethral stump over a stenting catheter with fine interrupted chromic. The pedicle tube is sutured to a broad based defect made in the skin of the perineum. g. One to two months later, the abdominal attachment is severed. This may also be delayed by making an incision across one half of the attachment followed one week later by complete transection. The skin margins on the end of the pedicle tube are sutured to the skin margins of the neo-urethra. Tip reconstruction, meatoplasty and implantation of cartilage or silastic prostheses are performed three to six months later after the vascular supply to the pedicle has become well established (adapted from Evans 1963).

in the course but may be removed as healing commences. Healing is complete in two to three weeks. Contracture formation, particularly in deep second degree injuries, is a common sequela in the

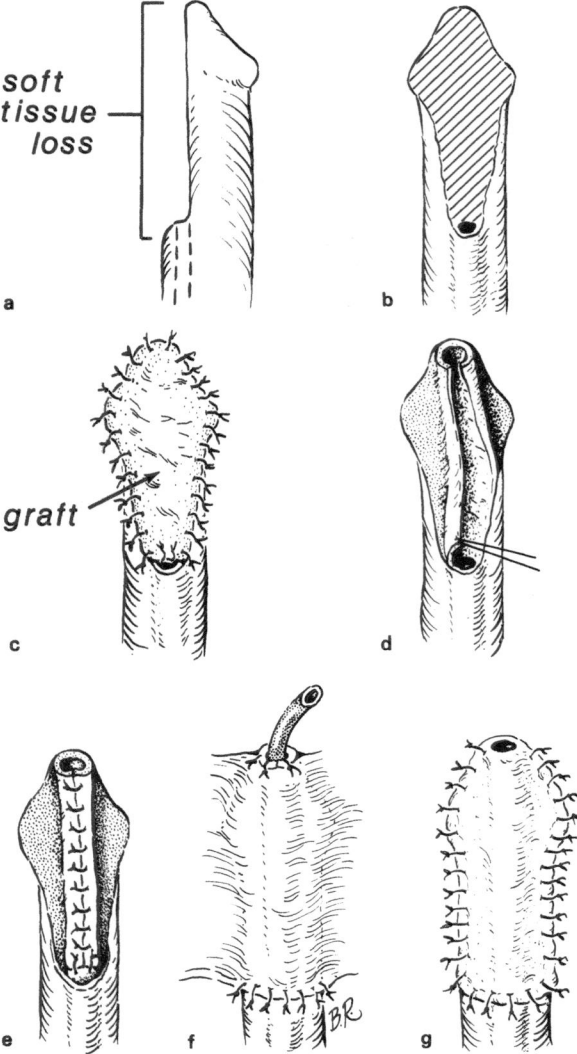

Figure 7. Repair of a penile soft tissue loss associated with a penile scrotal hypospadias. a. The injury viewed from the lateral aspect of the penis. b. The ventral aspect of the penis. c. A suprapubic cystostomy is placed and a full thickness skin graft taken from a non hair bearing area is sutured over the defect and stented in place. d. After four to six weeks, the margins of the graft are raised being careful not to undermine the central strip of skin. e. A neo-urethra is constructed by suturing the margins together with fine interrupted chromic. The urethra is mobilized and sutured to the neo-urethra over a stenting catheter. f. The distal shaft is placed beneath a superficial abdominal flap. g. After one to two months, the flap may be severed from the abdominal wall and its margin sutured to the shaft of the penis. (A delayed technique is preferred. One side of the graft is transected and sutured to the penis. Several weeks later, the opposite side is severed.)

ensuing months. Third degree or full thickness injuries involve all of the epithelium, dermis and deep dermal structures. They appear white to charred, are insensitive and will not heal. These injuries must be grafted. Treatment involves twice daily iodophor washes followed by application of a topical antimicrobial and conservative debridement. Conservative debridement of the eschar involves the daily removal of loose and separating tissue. This process takes two to three weeks for complete eschar removal. Granulation tissue covers the defect and when it bleeds readily and is red in appearance, the wound is ready for the application of split thickness graft. If the granulation tissue is gray in appearance or does not bleed readily, it may be prepared by the application of wet dressings for several days, or it may be covered with homograft (cadaver skin) or xenograft (pig skin). The latter are removed at five to seven day intervals until a healthy base of granulation tissue which will accept a split thickness graft is formed. The shaft of the penis should be grafted with sheet split thickness skin (0.16 to 0.18 inches thick) as depicted in Figure 1 and stented for four to six days. The scrotum may be grafted with either sheet or meshed graft. The latter is meshed 1.5 to 1 and has the advantage of allowing drainage through the interstices of the graft. It provides a cover which looks very much like scrotal skin when healing is complete.

Urethral catheters are routinely employed in those with either perineal or large total body surface burns. They should be removed as early as possible and replaced only during periods of perineal grafting. Indeed, patients who have sustained full thickness burns to the ventrum of the penis must have the catheter removed within 48 to 72 hours post injury and a suprapubic cystostomy placed. If this is not accomplished, the ventral portion of the penis and urethra will slough, often resulting in a large soft tissue loss and a penile scrotal hypospadias (McDougal et al. 1979). This injury is repaired as indicated in Figure 7 six to eight months post injury.

The most common long term complication of perineal burns is contracture formation. Contractures develop slowly and therefore a surgical repair should not be performed for eight to twelve months post burn at which time maturation of the scar is usually complete. The contracture is released by an incision placed perpendicular to the line of stress (Figure 8). Darts are fashioned at each end of the incision to minimize development of margin contractures. A thick split thickness graft is obtained after the release for often the size of the defect created is much larger than anticipated. The graft is sutured in place and stented for five to seven days.

H. Radiation Injury

Radiation injury of the perineum is usually a complication of radiotherapy to the pelvis for malignant disease. The acute injury is manifested by erythema and edema. Chronic changes include atrophy of the skin, telangiectasias, hyperpigmentation, excoriation, and compromise of the small blood vessels in the skin and integument. The lesion is painful, itches and occasionally progresses to frank ulceration. Conservative therapy is indicated initially; however, when skin loss and ulceration occur, it is rarely of any benefit. Split thickness grafts enjoy minimal success due to the poor vascu-

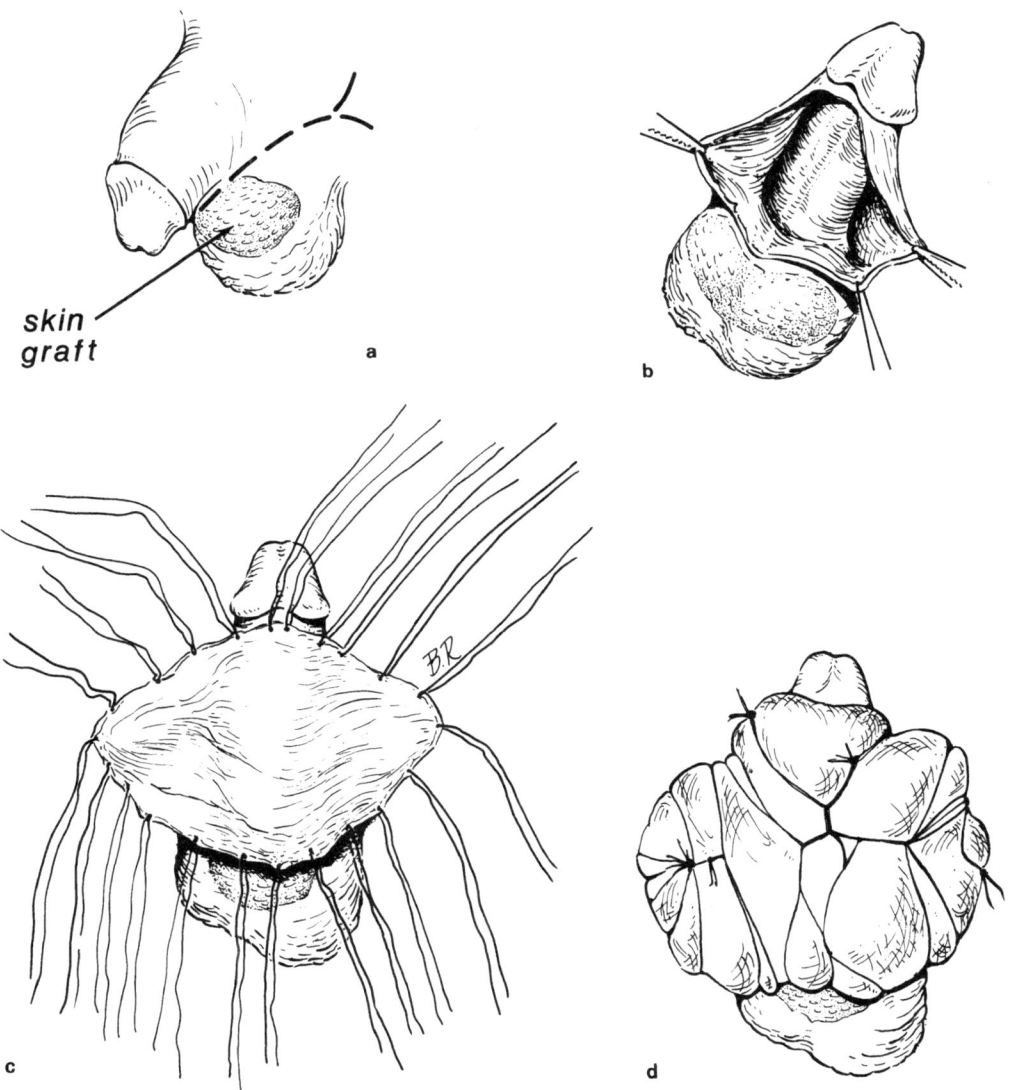

Figure 8. Release of genital contractures. a. The contracture has resulted in a short penile shaft which is immobile. A full thickness injury of the scrotum which required a split thickness skin graft in the immediate post burn period is illustrated. The incision to be made is outlined and is placed perpendicular to the line of the contracture. It extends beneath the penis to the opposite of the scrotum (not depicted). Darts are placed at either end of the incision. b. The defect created is extensive. The penis is released and assumes its normal length. c. Thick split thickness skin is applied to the defect and sutured in place. d. The graft is stented by tying the sutures placed at the margin of the graft over cotton wadding.

larity of the underlying tissues. Defects created by radiation are best treated by excision and primary closure or by rotating uninjured tissue into the area to close the defect (Barnes et al. 1964; Beare 1962). The latter may be accomplished with either myocutaneous or arterialized pedicle flaps.

I. Circumcision Injuries

These injuries may involve the glans penis, the urethral meatus or the penile shaft. Trauma to the glans is treated by primarily suturing the defect with fine reabsorbable suture. Small superficial skin losses will re-epithelialize spontaneously if the wound is kept uninfected. Large full thickness skin losses from the glans require the application of a split thickness skin graft. Meatal injuries may eventually result in scar formation with severe stenosis. A meatoplasty is then required. Excessive skin loss of the penile shaft is treated by the application of split thickness skin as described for avulsion injuries (Figure 1). The proper technique for circumcision is illustrated in Figure 9. It is essential that the foreskin be separated from the glans before crushing clamps are applied or incisions are made. Failure to do this is the single most common cause of the complications described above.

II. INFECTIOUS DISEASES

A. Hidradenitis Suppurativa

Hidradenitis suppurativa occurs as a result of a chronic indolent infection of the apocrine sweat glands which are located in the axilla, areola of the nipple, perianal, periumbilical, and perineal areas. The infecting organisms are usually hemolytic staphylococcus and Aerobacter aerogenes. The disease is more common in negroes than it is in whites, is rare in orientals, has a peak incidence between the ages of 20 and 40 years, is three times more prevalent in women than in men, is often associated with a history of acne, and appears to be more common in patients who have abnormalities of steroid metabolism. Hidradenitis suppurativa presents as painful small nodules which become fluctuant, rupture and discharge pus. Progression of the

disease results in the formation of multiple sinus tracts with extensive scarring and fibrosis of the skin and subcutaneous tissue. The pathologic process does not usually extend into the muscle of the perineum or beneath the tunica vaginalis in the scrotum. Mechanical irritation, poor hygiene, chemical depilatories, shaving and tight clothing have all been implicated in contributing to its development. Hidradenitis must be differentiated from tuberculosis, lymphogranuloma venerium, granuloma inguinale, actinomycosis, diabetes mellitus, perineal abscess, perineal fistula, infected sebaceous cyst and furunculosis. Skin tests (PPD, Frei Test), cultures for fungi, anoscopy, and tissue biopsy confirm the diagnosis. Complications of the disease include renal disease amyloidosis, interstitial keratitis, fistulas to the peritoneal cavity, and squamous cell carcinoma (Masson, 1969).

If the process is localized conservative therapy will suffice. Improved hygiene, antibiotics, wet soaks, and incision and drainage will limit the inflammatory process. Ultraviolet treatments and x-ray therapy have also been successfully employed. Unfortunately, the disease is usually a progressive one and conservative efforts often fail to control the process. Many patients are totally incapacitated as the disease involves larger areas, and a more aggressive approach is required if these patients are to return to a useful life. The involved area is excised to normal tissue at the margins and to a level which will assure removal of all sinus tracts. The latter usually requires excision to fascia (Vickers 1975). Urinary and/or stool diversion should be considered if the anticipated excision will cause the wound to be bathed in excrement (Chalfant and Nance 1970). Split thickness skin meshed 1.5 to 1 may be placed unspread directly on the fascia to achieve wound closure. An alternative method which is particularly applicable to wounds which are not ideally prepared is to place homograft or xenograft (physiologic dressings) over the wound. The former is preferred because, unlike the latter, it becomes vascularized thereby resulting in lesser wound bacterial counts and more rapid production of granulation tissue. The physiologic dressings are removed at 5 to 7 day intervals and replaced as often as is necessary to achieve a healthy bed of granulation tissue. Once the wound has been prepared, one may anticipate an excellent autograft

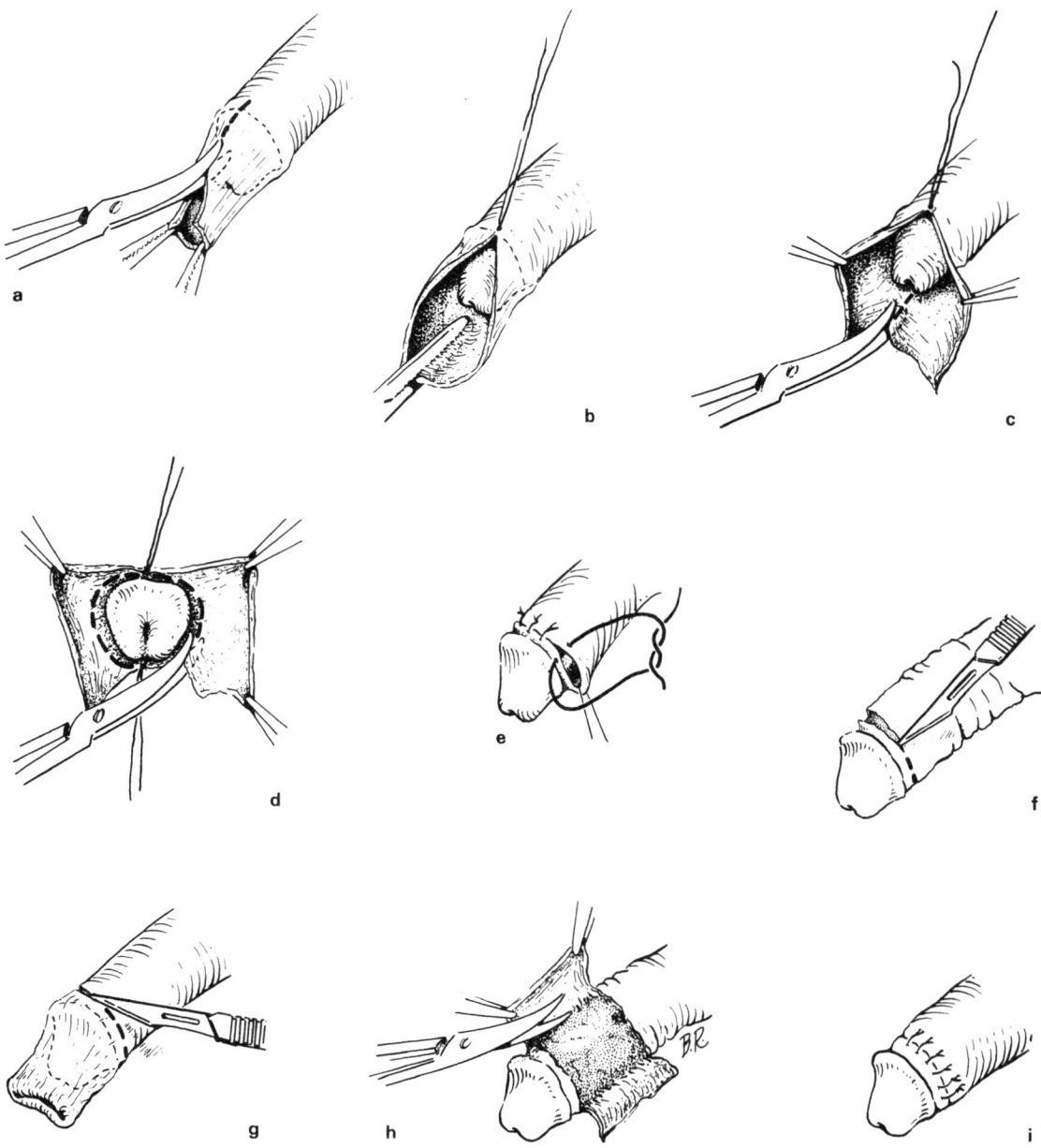

Figure 9. Techniques of circumcision. The dorsal slit method is the preferred procedure when the circumcision is performed for phimosis. a. If adhesions between the foreskin and glans are present, they are taken down. A small dorsal slit may be required to gain exposure so that the glans may be freed from the foreskin. The dorsal foreskin is crushed and cut to the level of the corona as illustrated by the dotted line. b. A suture is placed at the apex of the incision which brings the cut edges together, and the ventral foreskin is crushed. c. The ventral foreskin is cut to the level of the corona. The frenular artery on the ventrum should be ligated. It may be incorporated into the second suture (depicted in d) which brings the skin margins on the ventral aspect together. d. By holding the lateral halves of the foreskin at right angles to the penile shaft, the redundant tissue is excised several millimeters proximal to the corona. e. Bleeding vessels are ligated and after meticulous hemostasis has been achieved,

the skin margins are sutured together with 3 or 4-0 reabsorbable suture. When paraphimosis is present, puncture wounds are made in the edematous skin (which will be removed by circumcision) and the foreskin is brought back over the glans. The edema is allowed to subside before a circumcision is performed. Patients whose foreskin can be retracted with ease may be circumcised by either the dorsal slit method or the sleeve resection method described below. f. The foreskin is retracted and a circumferential incision is made 2-3 mm below the corona. The frenular artery is identified on the ventrum and ligated. g. The foreskin is brought back over the glans and a second circumferential incision is made using the corona lying beneath as a landmark. h. The tissue between the two incisions is removed by sharp dissection. Bleeders are individually ligated. i. The skin margins are sutured together with reabsorbable suture after hemostasis has been established.

'take'. Antibiotic soaks have also been used to prepare these wounds; however when the excision is to fascia, either homo-, xeno- or autografts should be employed, for the fascia will desiccate with other methods of therapy.

B. Elephantiasis of the Penis and Scrotum

Elephantiasis is classified as either primary or secondary. Primary causes include congenital hypoplasia and congenital aplasia of the lymphatics. The etiology of secondary elephantiasis includes: 1) inflammatory lesions such as tuberculosis, lymphogranuloma venerium, and other bacterial infections, 2) parasitic infestations of which Onchoceria volvulus, Wuchereria bancrofti and schistosoma are the most common, or 3) noninfectious lesions such as malignancy and radiation (Fogh-Anderson and Sorensen 1962). The lymph stasis which occurs results in enhanced subcutaneous fibroblastic activity. The skin overlying the genitalia becomes thickened, woody and may contain warty excrescences and has an increased susceptibility to fungal and bacterial infections. The disease process involves the dermis and subcutaneous tissue but does not penetrate beneath the deep fascia (Buck's fascia in the penis and the internal spermatic fascia in the scrotum).

The primary cause must be sought and treated when possible. However, the lymphedema usually persists despite treatment thereby making a surgical procedure necessary in order to reduce the bulk of the genitalia. All of the involved skin and subcutaneous tissue must be removed. The dissection is begun just distal to the corona and carried down to Buck's fascia. After the tissue is excised from the penis, attention is turned to the external inguinal rings where the cords are identified. Identification of the cords at this level minimizes the chances of injury to them and the testicles. All tissue superficial to the internal spermatic fascia is removed. The shaft of the penis and scrotum are covered with split thickness graft as described for avulsion injuries (Figure 1).

Portions of the penile or scrotal skin should not be used for resurfacing since the continued presence of lymphatic obstruction in this tissue will result in a high incidence of recurrent edema. The inner layer of the prepuce, however, may be used since its

lymphatics drain deep and are often uninvolved by the disease process (Raghavaiah 1977). Postoperative complications include hematoma and seroma formation and skin slough. Meticulous hemostasis, small stab wounds placed in the graft for drainage, antibiotics, the use of stents and urethral catheter drainage will minimize complications.

C. Necrotizing Gangrene of the Perineum

Necrotizing synergistic gangrene of the perineum was originally described by Fournier in 1884 (Fournier 1884). The source of the infection was thought to be the periurethral glands; however, as more cases have been reported, it has become clear that the infection can originate from either the genitourinary tract or the gastrointestinal tract. When the genitourinary tract is the source, the site of infection is often not obvious; however, when the gastrointestinal tract is the source an ischiorectal abscess, carcinoma of the rectum or a perforated colon diverticulum often precedes the process. Microaerophilic streptococcus and staphylococcus aureus are classically the responsible organisms when the genitourinary tract is the source whereas Pseudomonas aeruginosa, Escherichia coli, and Bacteroids sp. are the causitive organisms when the colon is the source (Flanigan 1978). This disease occurs more commonly in diabetics, cirrhotics and chronically debilitated patients. The process is very aggressive and begins as a localized discoloration on the perineum which over a period of a few hours rapidly progresses to involve the penile, scrotal and finally the abdominal wall skin in the gangrenous process. The patient becomes toxic and his cardiovascular system becomes unstable. This disease entity is a surgical emergency for even under the best of circumstances the mortality is exceedingly high (Rosenberg et al. 1978). The blood pressure must be supported and broad spectrum antibiotics need to be given intravenously. The regimen should include a penicillin, an aminoglycoside and an agent active against anaerobes (particularly if the bowel is the source). The patient is taken directly to the operating room where a radical debridement is performed. If the bowel is the source, a diverting colostomy may need to be performed. Often large cutaneous defects are created and the penis and testes are denuded. Due to their separate blood supply, the deep tissues of these structures are invariably viable. The wounds should be left open and packed. The patient is returned to the operating room, anesthetized and debrided on a daily basis until no more necrotic tissue can be found on two consecutive days. At this point, the testes are implanted in the thighs and the defect covered with autograft, or homograft followed by autograft. Reconstruction of the scrotum may be performed at a later date as described in Figure 2.

REFERENCES

Balakrishnan C: Scrotal avulsion: a new technique of reconstruction by split-skin graft. Br J Plast Surg 9: 38, 1956.

Barnes WE, Hoffman GW and Pickrell K: Surgical treatment of irradiation injuries of the perineum. Surg Gynecol Obstet 118: 1067, 1964.

Beare RLB: Irradiation injuries of the perineum. Br J Plast Surg 15: 22, 1962.

Chalfant WP and Nance FC: Hidradenitis suppurativa of the perineum: treatment by radical excision. Am Surg 36: 331, 1970.

Cohen BE, May JW Jr, Daly JSF et al: Successful clinical replantation of an amputated penis by microneurovascular repair. Plast and Reconstr Surg 59: 276, 1977.

Davies DM and Mitchell I: Fracture of the penis. Br J Urol 50: 426, 1978.

Engelman ER, Polito G, Perley J, et al: Traumatic amputation of the penis. J Urol 112: 774, 1974.

Evans AJ: Buried skin-strip urethra in a tube pedicle phalloplasty. Br J Plast Surg 16: 280, 1963.

Flanigan RC, Kursh ED, McDougal WS et al: Synergistic gangrene of the scrotum and penis secondary to colorectal disease. J Urol 119: 369, 1978.

Fleming JP: Reconstruction of the penis. J Urol 104: 213, 1970.

Fogh-Anderson P and Sorensen B: Surgical treatment of genital elephantiasis. Acta Chir Scand 124: 539, 1962.

Fournier FA: Etude clinique de la gangrène foudroyante de la verge. *Semaine Med* 4: 69, 1884.

Gilles H and Harrison RJ: Congenital absence of the penis with embryological considerations. Brit J Plast Surg 1: 8, 1948.

Gross M, Arnold TL and Waterhouse K: Fracture of the penis: rationale of surgical management. J Urol 106: 708, 1971.

Gross M, Arnold TL and Peters P: Fracture of the penis with associated laceration of the urethra. J Urol 117: 725, 1977.

Heymann AD, Bell-Thomson J, Rathod DM et al: Successful reimplantation of the penis using microvascular techniques. J Urol 118: 879, 1977.

Hudson MJK: Rupture of the corpus cavernosum of the penis. Br J Clin Pract 29: 191, 1975.

Malherbe WD F: Injuries to the skin of the male external genitalia in Southern Africa. S Afr Med J 49: 147, 1975.

Markland C and Merrill D: Accidental penile gangrene. J Urol 108: 494, 1972.

Masson JK: Surgical treatment for hidradenitis suppurativa. Surg Clin North Am 49: 1043, 1969.

Masters JW and Robinson DW: The treatment of avulsions of the male genitalia. J Trauma 8: 430, 1968.

McDougal WS, Peterson HD, Pruitt BA et al: The thermally injured perineum. J Urol 121: 320, 1979.

McRoberts WJ, Chapman WH and Ansell JS: Primary anastomosis of the traumatically amputated penis: case report and summary of the literature. J Urol 100: 751, 1968.

Noe JM, Birdsell D and Laub DR: The surgical construction of male genitalia for the female-to-male transsexual. Plast and Reconstr Surg 53: 511, 1974.

Ovrum E: Rupture of the penis. Scan J Urol Nephrol 12: 83, 1978.

Raghavaiah NV: Reconstruction of scrotal and penile skin in elephantiasis. J Urol 118: 128, 1977.

Rosenberg PH, Shuck JM, Tempest BD et al: Diagnosis and therapy of necrotizing soft tissue infections of the perineum. Am Surg 187: 430, 1978.

Schellhammer P and Donnelly J: A mode of treatment for incarceration of the penis. J Trauma 13: 171, 1973.

Taguchi H, Saito K and Yamada T: A simple method of total reconstruction of the penis. Plast and Reconstr Surg 60: 454, 1977.

Tamai S, Nakamura Y and Notomiya Y: Microsurgical replantation of a completely amputated penis and scrotum. Plast and Reconstr Surg 60: 287, 1977.

Tiwari VS, Raydan JL and Yadav VNS: Strangulation of the penis by a metallic nut. Intern Surg 62: 558, 1977.

Vickers MA: Operative management of chronic hidradenitis suppurativa of the scrotum and perineum. J Urol 114: 414, 1975.

10. THE INFLATABLE PENILE PROSTHESIS FOR TREATMENT OF ERECTILE IMPOTENCE

F.B. SCOTT and I.J. FISHMAN

Erectile impotence is defined as the inability of the male to attain and sustain an effective penile erection in order to accomplish sexual intercourse to the satisfaction of both partners. Erection in the normal human male results from a stimulatory input from the various natural senses resulting in an autonomic, mostly parasympathetic, discharge causing the engorgement of the spongy tissue of the corpora cavernosa with blood. The net result is the distention of the tunica albuginea, a resilient fibrous elastic tissue containing the corpora cavernosa producing a tumescent penis. Disease or injury directly to the penile erectile tissue or to its blood or nerve supply results in erectile impotence.

Stafford-Clark (1954) estimated that psychogenic factors are the cause of impotence in approximately ninety percent of patients. However, with the advent of more sophisticated evaluation of these patients with monitoring of nocturnal penile tumescence and penile blood pressure recordings, organic causes for impotence exceeded an incidence of thirty percent (Karacan et al. 1978).

I. TREATMENT

Surgical treatment of erectile impotence by implantation dates back to 1936 when Bogoras reported on the implantation of a segment of rib cartilage into the penile shaft. Within one and one half years, the cartilage began to bend on itself and within several years it was almost totally reabsorbed. Subsequent investigations carried this form of treatment a step farther by implanting penile stiffeners made of various synthetic materials (Beheri 1960; Goodwin and Scott 1960; Leoffler 1960).

In 1960, Beheri described a polyethylene penile stiffener that he used in 700 cases of impotence. In 1967, Pearman utilized a single penile prosthesis made of silicone rubber. In 1973, Morales et al. described a double polyethylene penile prosthesis, implanting one unit in each corpus cavernosum. Subsequently, in 1975, Small, Carrion, and Gordon employed a paired prosthesis which consisted of a medical grade silicone exterior with a silicone sponge interior. Again, the latter prosthesis consisted of two rods, one for each corpus cavernosum.

Since all the above prostheses are either rigid or semirigid, the penis remains permanently erect. This causes problems of concealment and makes endoscopic procedures difficult and at times impossible. Also, because of the constant pressure exerted by the rigid and semirigid prosthesis there is a greater danger of pressure necrosis leading to extrusion of these devices. In a recent survey of the female sexual partners of men who underwent implantation of the Small-Carrion prosthesis, Sonja Kramensky-Binkhorst (1978) found that only 42 percent of the women were totally satisfied with the results of the operation. The most serious complaints, 16 percent of the cases, involved the size and rigidity of the penis. It was believed to be too short, too thin, too flexible and it buckled at the tip making vaginal penetration or effective continued vaginal containment impossible.

In 1973, as an outgrowth of work on a hydraulic urethral sphincter, Scott, Bradley, and Timm described an inflatable hydraulic penile prosthesis. This original device consisted of two silicone cylinders which were inplanted in the corpora cavernosa, a reservoir filled with isotonic fluid which was implanted extraperitoneally beneath the rectus muscles, and two pumps which were implanted in the scrotum, one for inflation and the other for deflation. The various components of the system are interconnected with silicone tubing. Since 1973 multiple improvements have been made in the device. Presently, the inflatable penile prosthesis consists of two silicone rubber cylinders which are both inflatable and expandable; they are connected via silicone rubber tubing to a seamless reservoir, and to a single dacron reinforced pump that has both an inflate component and a deflate valve built into one unit (Figure 1). The system is filled with a 12.5 percent radiopaque dye in a lactated Ringer's solution. On compression of the inflate portion of the pump, fluid is transferred from the reservoir to the cylinders within the corpora cavernosa. Finger pressure against the deflate valve releases the fluid to return from the cylinders to the reservoir, resulting in a normally flaccid penis. The deflate valve activating button is sufficiently small (2-4 mm^2) to prevent accidental release of the fluid. In addition, the pump is freely movable inside the scrotum.

The main advantage of the inflatable corporal cylinders is that they simulate the physiologic erectile process when fluid is transferred into these cylinders. The fluid causes distention of the tunica albuginea simulating the engorgement of the cor-

pora during a natural erection. Another advantage is that the patient can control the timing and the turgidity of his erection. On deflation of the cylinders the penis resumes a normally appearing flaccid state.

II. SURGICAL PROCEDURE FOR IMPLANTATION OF THE INFLATABLE PENILE PROSTHESIS

Since 1973, when the inflatable penile prosthesis was first introduced, a variety of implantation techniques has been used. The main objectives of all these techniques were to give the surgeon adequate exposure of the corpora cavernosa, the prevesical space, and the scrotum. The procedure is planned to take into account the anatomy of the patient, be it normal or distorted by previous radical surgery or trauma.

The original surgical technique has been described (Scott et al. 1973). Dissection through the lower part of a small midline incision extending from the base of the penis to a point above the symphysis pubis isolates the corpora cavernosa.

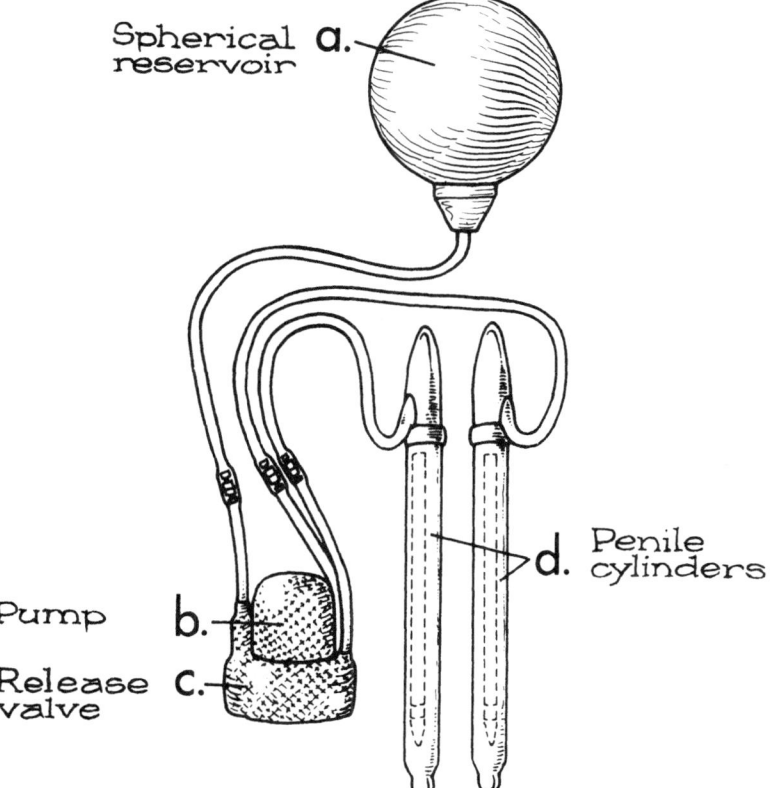

Spherical reservoir **a.**

Pump **b.**

Release valve **c.**

d. Penile cylinders

Figure 1. Inflatable penile prosthesis unit.

Incisions in the tunica albuginea at the base of the penis allow dilation of the corporal spongy tissues with Hegar's dilators. A Furlow insertion tool measures the length of the corporal spaces and permits placement of the cylinders in the distal corpora beneath the glans penis and, therefore, reduces operating time. Incision of the midline abdominal fascia allows placement of the reservoir in the prevesical space. Also, blunt dissection creates a pocket in the scrotum for placement of the pump. Stainless steel tubing connectors placed subcutaneously connect all components. Nonabsorbable sutures are best for closing the incision in layers.

Since all the components of this prosthesis are hollow and, therefore, quite compressible, it is now possible to implant the whole system via a small 3 cm longitudinal incision in the scrotal raphe near the penoscrotal angle (Figure 2). The corpora cavernosa are identified and the tunica albuginea is incised at a point lateral from the midline to avoid injury to the urethra. A Foley catheter in the

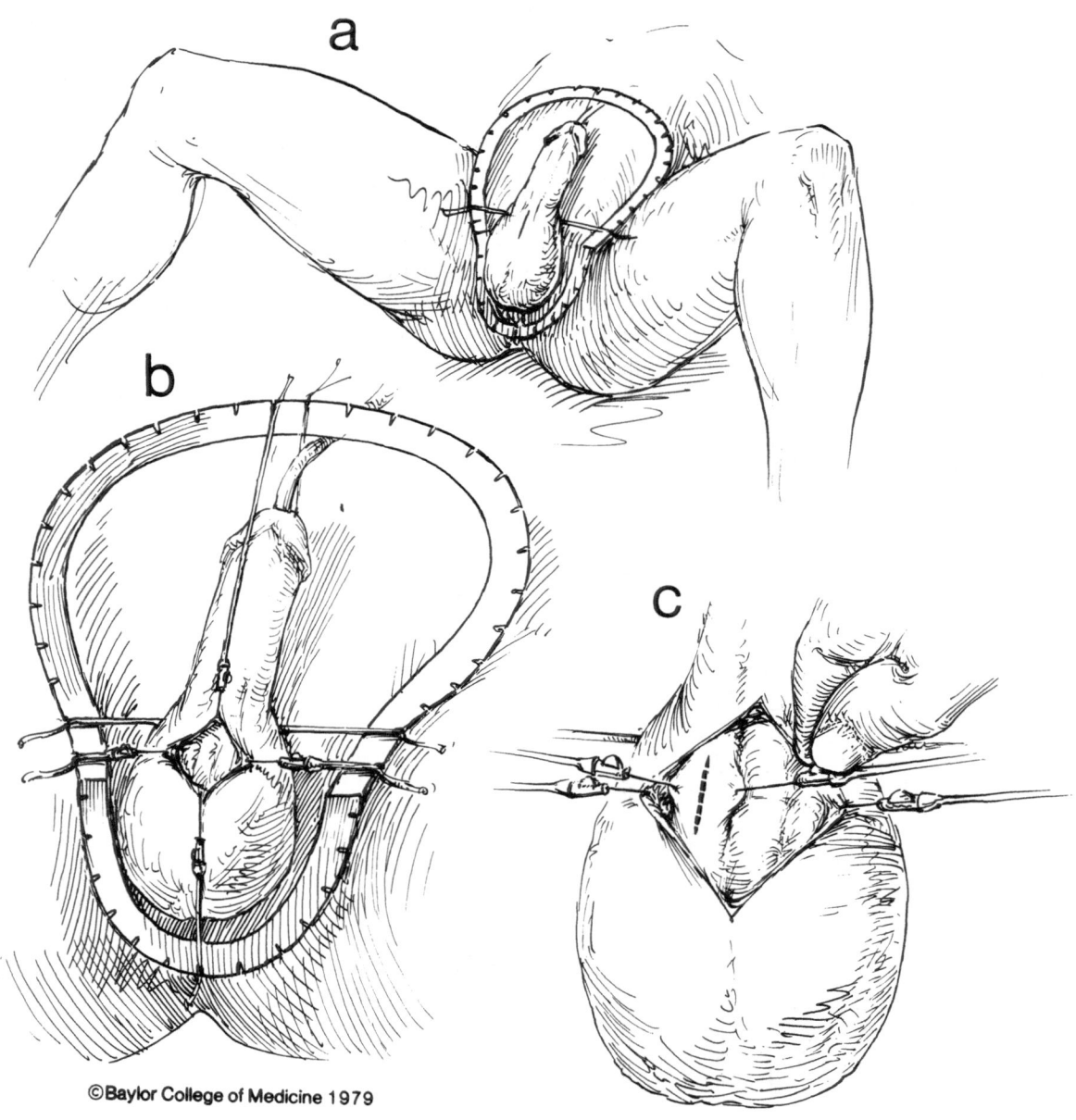

©Baylor College of Medicine 1979

Figure 2a, b, and c.

pendulous and bulbous urethra helps to define and to avoid urethral injury. In similar fashion to that described previously in the pubic approach, the corpora are dilated to accommodate the cylinders which are inserted with the aid of a Furlow insertion tool. The incision in the tunica albuginea is closed with a running horizontal mattress suture of 3-0 prolene. Next, the dip-coated silicone rubber reservoir is introduced into either the right or left paravesical space via the corresponding external inguinal ring. In order to accomplish this, traction is exerted on the ipsilateral testis (Figure 2h) to displace the cord structures laterally. The external inguinal ring is palpated via the same scrotal incision and by gentle blunt dissection the transversalis fascia is perforated and the paravesical space is entered. With the aid of an Army-Navy retractor, or a specially designed extended nasal speculum, the paravesical space can be visualized and the reservoir introduced into this space. It is then inflated with 65 cc of 12.5 percent Hypaque lactated Ringer's solution. A pocket is next developed

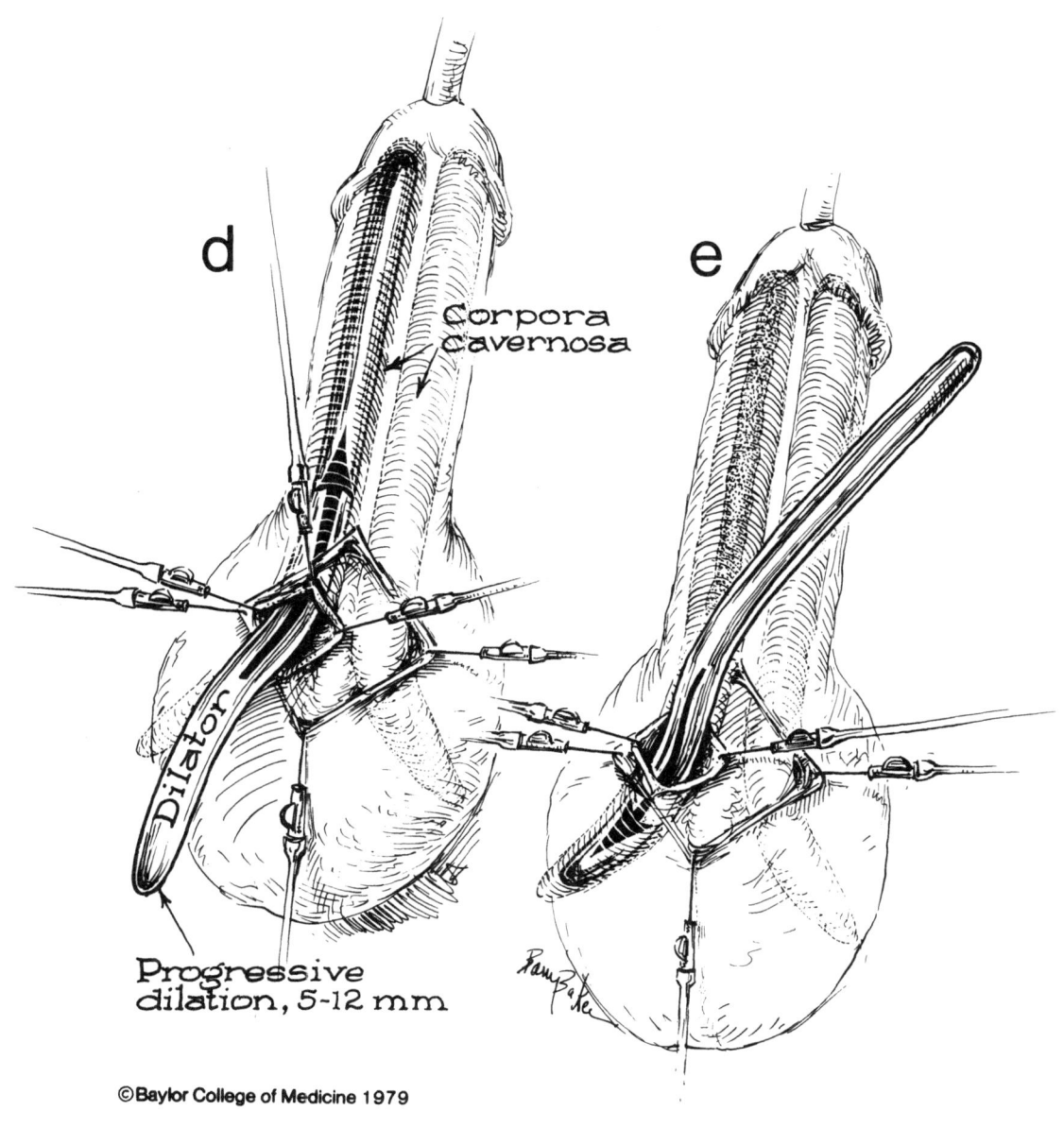

© Baylor College of Medicine 1979

Figure 2d and e.

in the ipsilateral side of the scrotum (Figure 2k) wherein the pump is positioned so that the deflate valve is palpable in the lateral aspect of the scrotum. In order to secure the pump in this position and to prevent it from rotating, one of the silicone tubes that will conduct the fluid to the cylinders is directed through the scrotal septum with the aid of a curved blunt 'knitting' needle that is provided

with the set (Figure 2m). In similar fashion the silicone tubings coming from the cylinders are passed through the deep connective tissue so that they lie in a more superficial plane. This tubing is routed so that it aligns with the tubing from the pump avoiding any sharp curves where the tubing might subsequently become kinked inside the tissues. The appropriate tubes are then con-

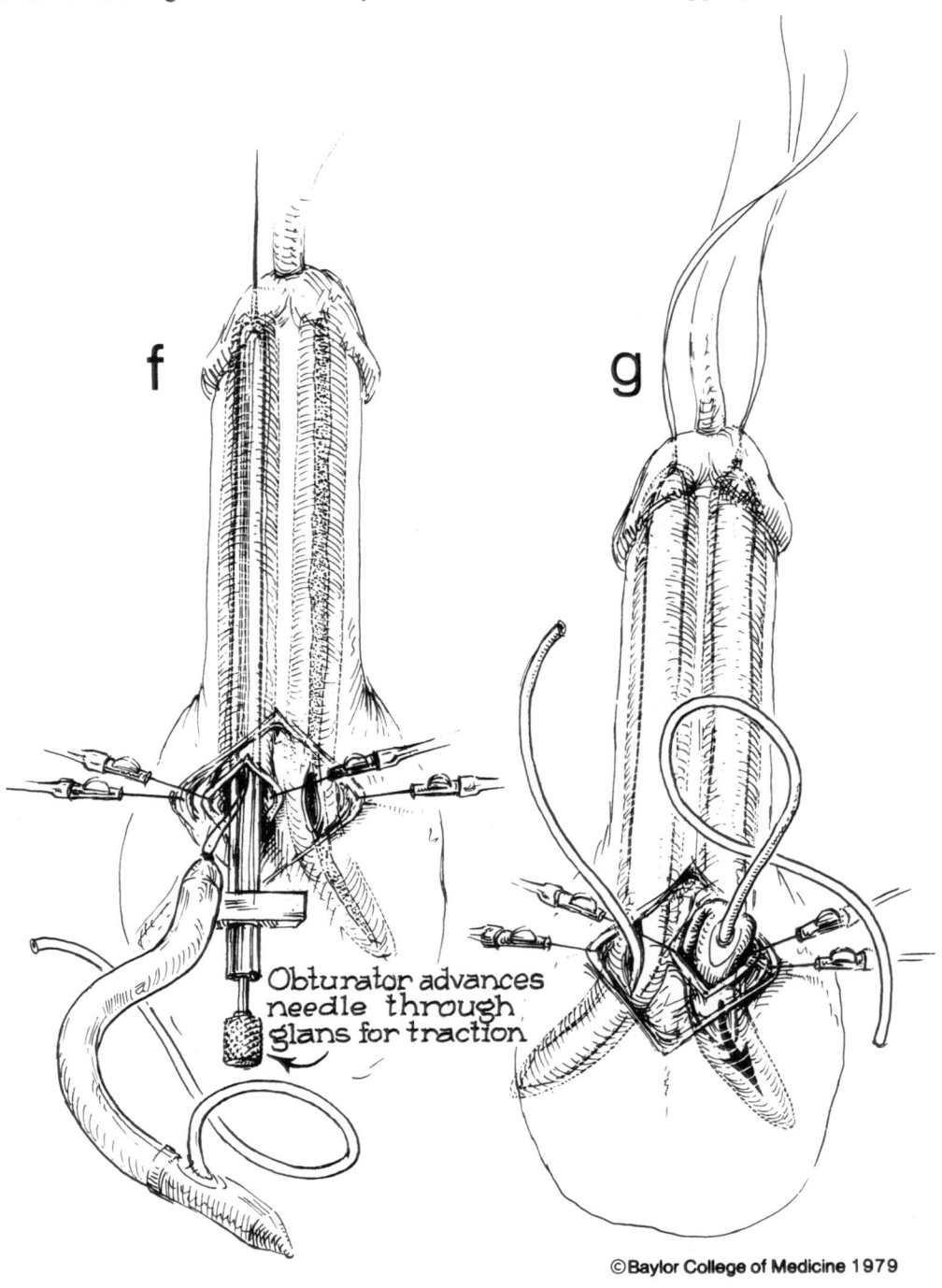

Figure 2f and g.

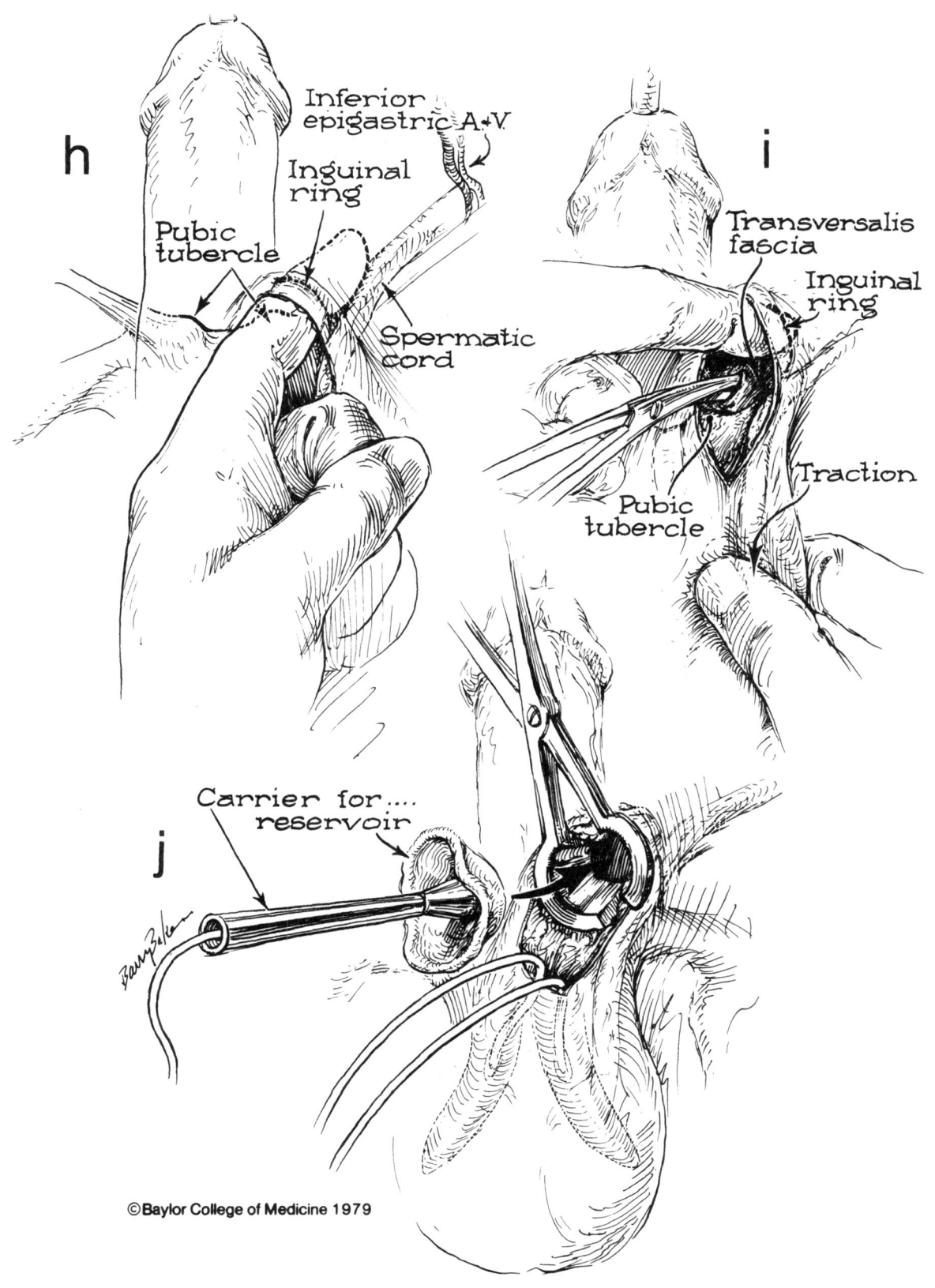

Figure 2h, i, and j.

nected by means of stainless steel metal connectors after redundant tubing is removed. The incision is then closed in layers using careful surgical technique and avoiding the use of drains (Figure 2o-p). The scrotal skin edges are closed with a continuous subcuticular 4-0 polyethylene suture.

The prerequisites that must be met in order that the scrotal approach technique be applied are the following:

1) The patient must have an adequate sized scrotum under normal room temperature conditions.
2) There is no history of any pelvic or abdominal surgery or trauma which might distort the normal anatomy in the paravesical area.

One advantage of this technique is that there is no evident scarring. Also, since minimal dissection is

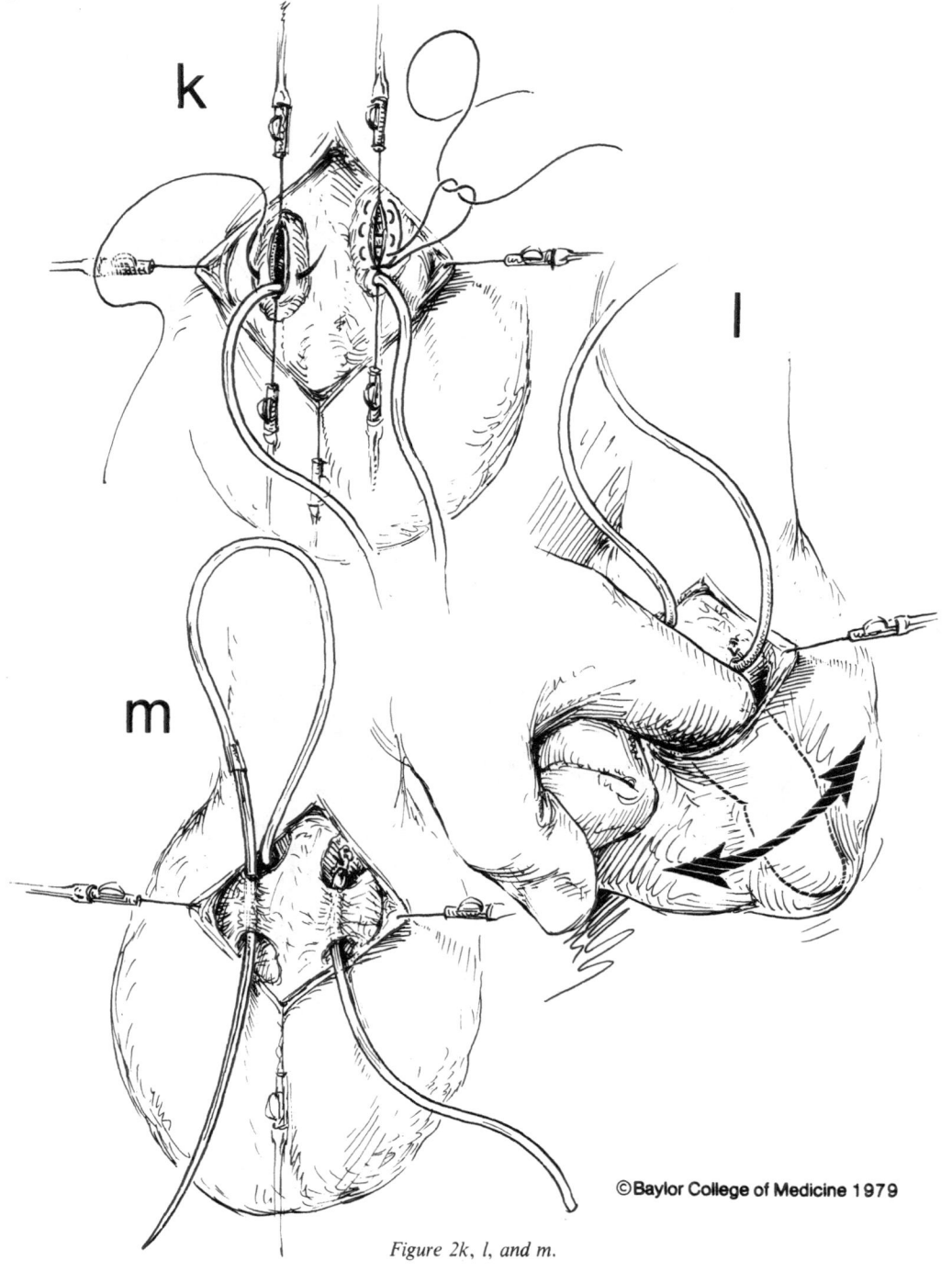

Figure 2k, l, and m.

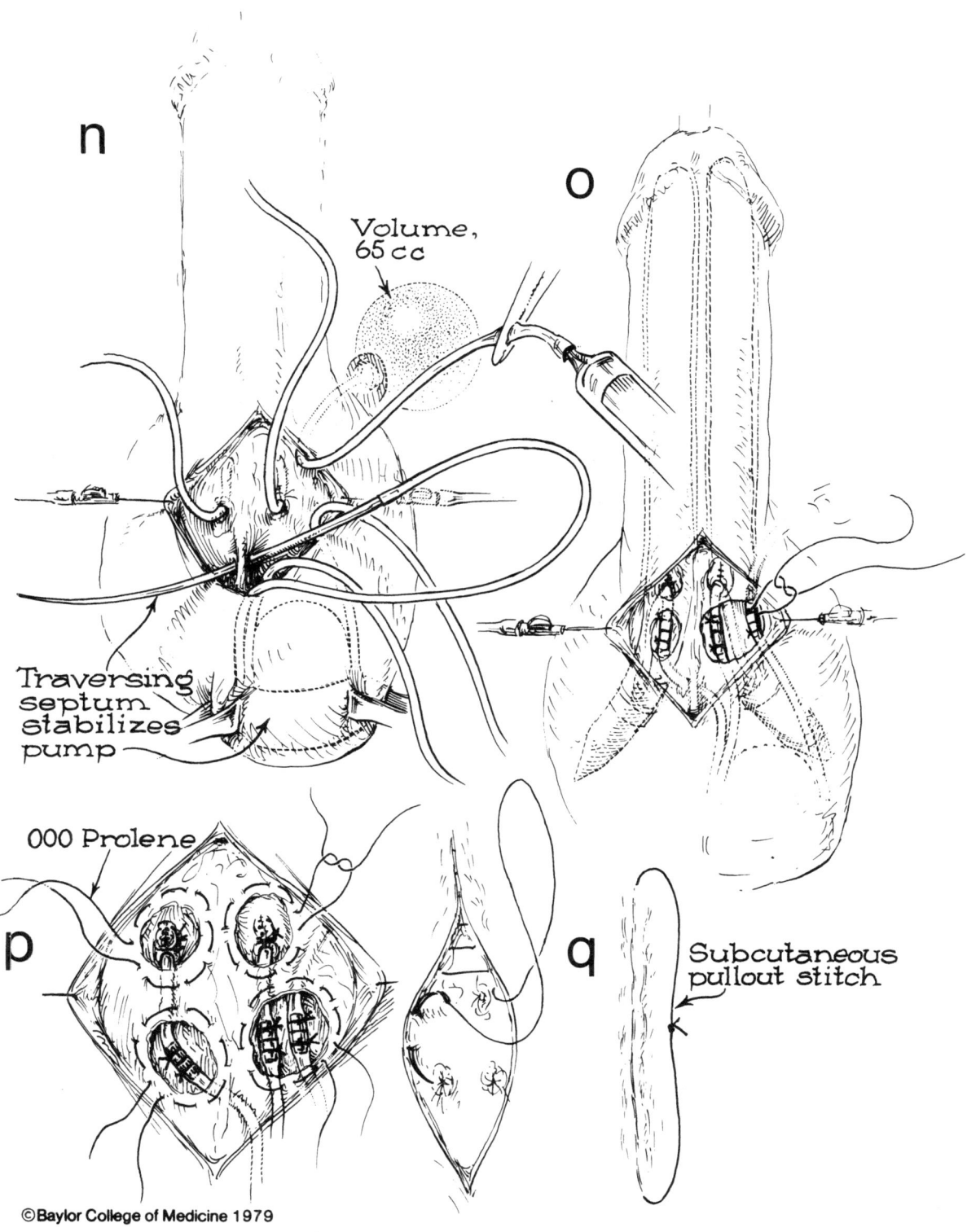

n

Volume, 65 cc

o

Traversing
septum
stabilizes
pump

000 Prolene

p

q

Subcutaneous
pullout stitch

Figure 2n, o, p, and q.

necessary, the amount of postoperative pain and swelling is usually less than with the other techniques. This operative procedure has been done on six occasions as outpatient procedures under local anesthesia. One of the patients drew an analogy between the scrotal approach and the building of a ship in a bottle.

No matter which technique is applied, a Foley catheter is left in place for a 24 hour period. The cylinders are left partially inflated at the conclusion of the surgery. The sutures are removed on the seventh postoperative day and the patient is instructed in the operation of the prosthesis. Sexual intercourse is permitted three weeks after implantation. In the interim he is advised to inflate the penis to a full erection once a day. By six weeks postoperatively the majority of the patients state that inflation of the penis is associated with a very pleasurable sensation. The patient is warned against overinflating the device as this results in an excessively rigid penis that is a source of discomfort to his partner and eventually to himself. He is, therefore, instructed as to the degree of erection for a natural effect. It is also suggested to the patient that at the conclusion of the sexual act he deflate the penis as much as possible as chronic overdistension of the cylinders leads to overexpansion of the intracylinder volume resulting in a relative insufficiency of fluid to provide a rigid erection.

III. COMPLICATIONS

The most dreaded complication of any form of prosthesis surgery is infection, since it accounts for the highest number of prosthesis failures necessitating complete removal. In order to avoid this complication the following stringent precautions are taken at the time of implantation. The urine is cultured and must be sterile preoperatively. Immediately prior to surgery, in the operating room, the skin is shaved and the area thoroughly scrubbed with an antiseptic iodine solution for at least ten minutes. Since the distal urethra is known to contain bacterial flora, it too is flushed with an antibiotic solution. The surgeon's hands are also sprayed with an iodine solution immediately after scrubbing and before donning gloves. As mentioned earlier, the wound is periodically irrigated

with an antibiotic solution throughout the operation. The patient is also started on prophylactic antibiotics 24 hours before surgery and maintained on these medications for 48 hours postoperatively. As a result of these precautions the incidence of infection is extremely low (1.5 percent).

As in any other operative procedure, good surgical technique is essential. Complications resulting from lack of adherence to prescribed technique include kinking of the tubes when excessive tubing is left in the body. Improper placement, twisting, or folding of the cylinders results in uneven expansion of the prosthesis and the patient will not get a normally expanding penis on erection. If the tunica albuginea is overstretched as a result of excessive dilation, weakening of the tunica albuginea can occur with resultant bulging of the penile shaft on inflation. Great care must be taken in handling of the silicone rubber since any scratch at the time of surgery can weaken the material and act as a focus for a leak at a later time.

With the advent of the dip-coated silicone reservoir and improvement in quality control the main source of manufacture associated defects has been eliminated and at the moment it is very rare to find faults in material or workmanship. Fortunately, however, should the prosthesis malfunction, the source of the problem can be easily identified and the affected component is replaced by relatively minor surgery.

Since implantation of the device does not involve cutting into any major organs or cavities, muscular relaxation is not necessary. Both implantation of the device as well as any revision can be done under either regional or local anesthesia on an outpatient basis.

IV. SELECTION OF PATIENTS

An important consideration of the surgical treatment of erectile impotence is the ability to objectively select the candidate for this type of surgery. The evaluation of patients who present with a complaint of inability to perform sexually because of inadequate or total absence of erection must include a complete review of the patient's past medical history looking for some predisposing causes such as diabetes, ingestion of antihypertensive medication, atherosclerosis, previous surgery or trauma to his spine or lower abdomen, alcoholism, etc. Inquiries should be made about the presence or absence of nocturnal penile erections as well as about the patient's ability to achieve orgasm and ejaculation. Also, it is important to establish whether his impotence is limited to only one sexual partner. A thorough physical examination is then performed with emphasis on the evaluation of the genitalia, of the peripheral vasculature, and the neural reflex arcs. Should there be any question of testicular atrophy, serum testosterone levels are measured. In order to qualify and quantify the patient's erectile abilities he is subjected to a three night course of nocturnal penile tumescence (NPT) monitoring with simultaneous EEG recordings of REM sleep activity under the supervision of a sleep researcher. The patient's penile blood pressure is also recorded during these sessions. Karacan et al. in a study of thirty-six patients noted a good correlation between diminished penile blood pressure and poor NPT (Karacan et al. 1978).

Psychological evaluation via the administration of the Minnesota Multiphasic Personality Inventory (MMPI) is a simple screening analysis of a patient's personality which can provide both an initial suggestion of organic or psychological etiology and a preliminary evaluation of psychological conflicts (Beutler et al. 1976). It is also very useful in helping the investigator to decide if more elaborate evaluation is necessary.

Psychiatric evaluation of the patient is a standard part of the impotent patient evaluation (Scott et al. 1979). The psychiatrist is not given any information on the patient other than the fact that he would like to have a penile prosthesis. During the interview emphasis is placed on evaluation of the patient's personality, his sexual relations, and the personality of his sexual partner. Based on this the psychiatrist can determine the patient's mental stability and his ability to adapt to his postoperative state. The psychiatrist also tries to detect any evidence of marital descord.

Another important aspect of the patient evaluation is a discussion of the inflatable penile prosthesis, its function, and possible complications of the surgery. This interview should be held preferable in the presence of the spouse or sexual partner. It is important that the patient not have any unrealistic expectations. He must realize that the length of the penis will probably not be as long in the erect state with the prosthesis in place as it was when he was capable of having spontaneous erections. He should be aware that he will be able to have normal orgasm postimplantation of the prosthesis if he had orgasms preoperatively. Observation of the female partner's reactions and participation during the interview gives the physician an idea of her acceptance of this form of therapy.

The majority of patients can be fairly accurately classified into either psychogenic or organic etiologies and treated accordingly. The patients who are organically impotent but are medically fit to undergo surgery and have been cleared by the other members of the evaluation team undergo implantation of the penile prosthesis. The patients who are found to have erectile impotence of psychogenic etiology are usually referred for psychiatric and/or behavior modification therapy. Should this fail to achieve any successful results then, with the agreement of the psychiatrist, psychologist, and urologist, these patients may become candidates for implantation of the penile prosthesis.

Thus, complete objective evaluation of impotent patients ideally requires a team approach involving a urologist, psychologist, psychiatrist, and sleep researcher.

V. RESULTS

A recent review by the American Medical Systems (AMS) statisticians of the experiences of 21 physicians involving the implantation of the inflatable penile prosthesis into 1,243 patients between 1973-1979 indicated an overall success rate of 91.5 percent (American Medical Systems 1979). Revision rate as a result of mechanical problems was initially about 25 percent. However, as a result of improvements in the prosthesis itself, as well as in the technique of its implantation, especially if great care is taken to remove redundant tubing thereby preventing kinks, the incidence of revision has been decreased to 4 percent in recent years (Furlow 1979). The overall success rate in our institution is over 95 percent. Based on a recent review of our own patient population the patient and partner satisfaction was very positive in all of our surgically successful implants.

The incidence of infection in the AMS study ranged between one and four percent. Meticulous surgical technique, liberal application of antibiotic solution during surgery, in addition to pre- and postoperative prophylactic antibiotics are believed to account for this low infection rate.

VI. SUMMARY

Surgical implantation of the inflatable penile prosthesis effectively treats erectile impotence. This device restores penile erections, simulates a natural erection and, therefore, can help the patient suffering from impotence caused by trauma, diabetes mellitus, atherosclerosis, Peyronie's disease, cancer surgery, and psychogenic factors. However, in order to objectively select the candidate for this surgery, the impotent patient should ideally undergo a team oriented evaluation that includes a urologist, psychiatrist, psychologist, and sleep researcher.

REFERENCES

American Medical Systems: A summary of clinical experience to date with the AMS inflatable penile prosthesis. May 13, 1979. American Medical Systems, Inc, 3312 Gorham Avenue, Minneapolis, Minnesota 55426, U.S.A.

Beheri GE: The problem of impotence solved by a new surgical operation. Kasr el aini. J Surg 1:50, 1960.

Beheri GE: Surgical treatment of impotence. Plastic Reconstr Surg 38: 92, 1966.

Beutler LE, Scott FB and Karacan I: Psychological screening of impotent men. J Urol vol. 116: 193-197, 1976.

Bogoras NA: Über die volle plastische Wiederherstellung eines zum Koitus fähigen Penis (peniplastica totalis). Zentralbl Chir 63: 1271, 1936.

Furlow WL: Inflatable penile prosthesis: Mayo Clinic experience with 175 patients. Urology vol XIII no 2, 1979.

Goodwin WE and Scott WW: Phalloplasty. J Urol 84: 559, 1960.

Karacan I, Ware H, Pervant B, Altinel A, Thornby JI, Williams RL, Kaya N and Scott FB: Impotence and blood pressure in the flaccid penis: relationship to nocturnal penile tumescence. Sleep I (2): 125-132, 1978.

Kramarsky-Binkhorst S: Female partner perception of Small-Carrion implant. Urology vol XII no (5): 545-548, 1978.

Leoffler RA and Sayegh ES: Perforated acrylic implants in management of organic impotence. J Urol 84: 559, 1960.

Morales PA, Suarez JB, Delgado J and Whitehead ED: Penile implant for erectile impotence. J Urol 109: 641, 1973.

Pearman RO: Treatment of organic impotence by implantation of a penile prosthesis. J Urol 97: 716, 1967.

Scott FB, Bradley WE and Timm GW: Treatment of urinary incontinence by implantable prosthetic sphincter: preliminary report. Urology 1: 252, 1973.

Scott FB, Bradley WE and Timm GW: Management of erectile impotence: use of implantable inflatable prosthesis. Urology 2: 80, 1973.

Scott FB, Byrd GJ, Karacan I, Olsson PO, Beutler LE and Attia SL: Erectile impotence treated with an implantable inflatable prosthesis: five years of clinical experience. JAMA 241 (24): 2609-2612, 1979.

Small MP, Carrion HM and Gordon JA: Small-Carrion penile prosthesis: new implant for management of impotence. Urology 5: 479-486, 1975.

Stafford-Clark D: The etiology and treatment of impotence. Practitioner 172: 397, 1954.

11. GRAFTS AND PROSTHESES FOR PEYRONIE'S DISEASE

E. HOUTTUIN and I.S. HAWATMEH

During the zenith of the French court, in an age of strict manners and loose morals (Durant and Durant 1963), François de la Peyronie first recognized the condition that now bears his name. In 1743 this physician to the Sun King, Louis XIV, described localized indurations in the wall of the cavernous bodies in three men. He suspected venereal transmission. The first detailed description of the disease in American medical literature was in 1874 by Van Buren and Keyes, and for many years the disease was known as 'Van Buren's Disease'. Although other more descriptive names, such as chronic cavernositis, fibrous sclerosis of the penis and plastic induration of the penis have been used, the name Peyronie's disease remains the most popular term today. Peyronie's disease in clinically recognizable form is rare; most urologists see no more than two or three cases per year and over a 20-year period at the Mayo Clinic the diagnosis was made in only 177 patients (Furlow et al. 1975). Medical interest in this disease exceeds its clinical significance and over 3,000 cases have been reported. English language medical literature during the period 1966 through 1975 contains at least 94 publications dealing with Peyronie's disease, including two excellent reviews (Billig et al. 1975; Chesney, 1975).

I. ETIOLOGY

No single causative factor can be found for Peyronie's disease. Many contributing factors have been considered and the most important of these are discussed briefly. Peyronie himself believed that a relationship existed with gonorrhea and syphilis, but more recent studies do not support this view (Smith 1966). Frequent association with chronic urethritis of nonvenereal origin is noted. Major trauma to the penis such as previous surgery or straddle injury can be elicited in only a small minority of cases. Recurrent minor injuries such as occur during sexual intercourse and with masturbation cannot easily be excluded as a contributing factor. Of interest is the frequently reported association with other forms of nonspecific fibrosis. There is an approximate 10 percent coexistence with Dupuytren's contracture. Patients with carcinoid syndrome, some of whom have fibrosis of the cardiac structures and retroperitoneum, also have a high incidence of Peyronie's disease (Bwens et al. 1973). These associations suggest systemic rather than local factors. No increased incidence exists in keloid-forming individuals.

II. PATHOPHYSIOLOGY

Microscopically Peyronie's disease starts as a perivasculitis with lymphocyte and plasma cell infiltration in the loose connective tissue located just inside the tunica albuginea of the corpus cavernosum (Smith 1969). As the disease progresses the adjacent intercavernous septum and dorsal tunica albuginea show increased thickness and fibrosis. In some cases cartilage and bone are present. The area of fibrosis appears grossly as a well delineated plaque, usually in the dorsal or dorsolateral mid-shaft position and extending into the intercorporal septum. Proximal extension may be into the crura. The corpus spongiosum is not involved.

Fibrosis may surround the dorsal neurovascular bundle but the artery remains patent and decreased sensation distal to the plaque due to nerve compression usually does not occur. Deep to the plaque the spongiosa can be scraped off the fibrotic tissue and the deep penile artery does not appear involved even in impotent patients. The pathogenesis of erectile failure therefore remains unresolved but it may be caused by disruption of the venous outflow regulating mechanism rather than disturbed arterial inflow.

III. PRESENTATION

Commonly patients with Peyronie's disease come to their physician after noticing a swelling in the penile shaft and because of concern about possible malignancy. Penile angulation usually does not concern the patient until pain during sexual intercourse or difficulty with vaginal intromission prevents the patient from having coitus. Sometimes it is pain in the female partner during intercourse that causes the patient to seek medical attention. In our liberated society masturbation and orolingual gratification are alternatives to which some patients resort. Penile erections in these men rarely are painful and ejaculations are normal.

As is the case at other clinical centers that attract large numbers of patients for surgical correction of erectile failure, the diagnosis of Peyronie's disease is made frequently at St. Louis University when a corpus cavernosogram is performed just prior to the insertion of a penile prosthesis. Severe angulation then poses an additional technical surgical problem. Although the somatic nature of erectile failure can be documented in these patients with the nocturnal tumescence meter, usually no definite etiology for impotence such as diabetes mellitus or atherosclerosis can be established. Peyronie's disease should be suspected in each patient presenting with impotence.

Most patients presenting with penile curvature or a palpable plaque are in their late forties or early fifties. Symptoms may occur as early as age 23 (Winter and Khanna 1975) but are rarely reported over age 70.

IV. DIAGNOSIS

Where presentation is typical the diagnosis can be made with near certainty by telephone. Palpable induration of the penis is located in the dorsal or dorsolateral position and should be differentiated from the ventral induration seen in patients with urethral stricture. The penile skin remains freely movable over the plaque. Calcifications in the plaque can be seen on a soft tissue radiograph. The amount of penile curvature cannot be appreciated in the flaccid state. Objective evaluation requires a corpus cavernosogram. This can be performed preoperatively with local anesthesia or under general anesthesia on the operating table. We rapidly inject 50 ml of Renografin via a No. 19 scalp vein needle into one corpus cavernosum without the use of a tourniquet (Figure 1a). If a tourniquet around the base of the penis is used, less than 20 ml of contrast material usually suffices. The degree of angulation and the exact location of the lesion are

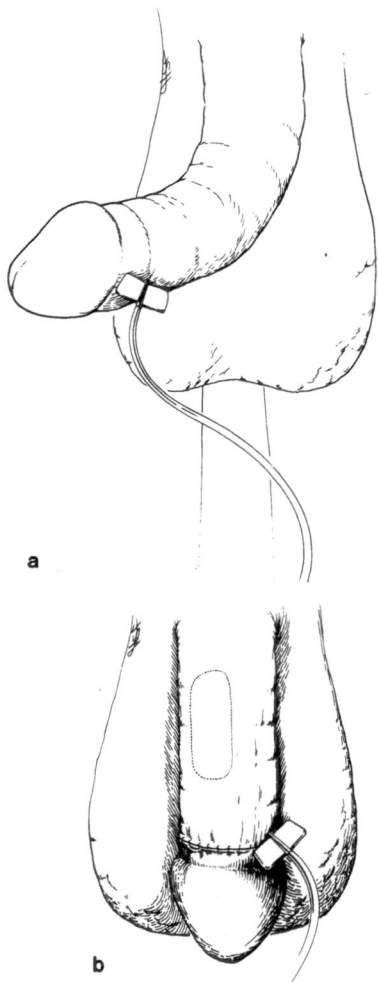

Figure 1. a. A corpus cavernosogram before surgery can be obtained with or without tourniquet at the base of the penis. b. Postoperative corpus cavernosogram documents complete operative correction of penile angulation.

readily appreciated. A repeat cavernosogram upon completion of the surgical procedure documents complete correction of the angulation and rules out significant extravasation and hematoma formation at the site of plaque excision (Figure 1b). In patients in whom erectile ability is in question nocturnal penile tumescence can be documented with the nocturnal tumescence meter (American Medical Systems, Inc., Minneapolis, Minnesota) to aid in the decision whether a penile prosthesis should be inserted.

V. CHOICE OF TREATMENT

Patient management should be based on presenting symptoms and natural progression of the disease. Long term followup of patients without treatment shows that slow improvement (Bystrom et al. 1973; Poutasse 1972), no change (Furlow et al. 1975), or progression with loss of erectile function (Ashworth 1960) may occur. Asymptomatic patients presenting with palpable induration of the penis require explanation and reassurance only. It should be explained to these patients that future loss of erectile function may occur due to progression of this disease and that surgical treatment is now available. This explanation may save some of these patients considerable future expense for ineffective psychotherapy.

Patients complaining of painful erections which interfere with their usual sexual activities require treatment. The large number of nonsurgical therapeutic modalities available suggests their limited effectiveness. Results of most treatment regimens are little different from those observed without treatment. Oral vitamin E has the advantage of low cost and produces no undesirable side effects. Ultrasound treatments are completely safe but require many return visits. Surgery is the only treatment available for patients with impotence and has

the advantage of rapid excellent results in patients with severe sexual disability. Excision of the plaque using dermal graft or vein patch to fill the defect with or without simultaneous insertion of a penile prosthesis is the treatment of choice in these patients.

VI. MEDICAL TREATMENT

A. Systemic Therapy

The frequent association of Peyronie's disease with other forms of fibrosis suggesting systemic etiologic factors can be considered a reason for systemic treatment (Table 1). In the absence of severe symptoms, patients usually prefer noninvasive therapy even if this requires oral medication for at least three to six months. Vitamin E, 100 mg three times daily, combines the advantages of low cost and lack of undesirable side effects. This regimen can be maintained even if subsequent surgical treatment becomes necessary (Devine and Horton 1974).

Potassium para-aminobenzoate (Potaba), 12 gm per day in divided doses (Zarafonetis and Horrax 1959), may produce nausea and vomiting and has no advantages over vitamin E. Serious side effects prohibit the long term use of systemic corticosteroid hormones. The combination of vitamin E with potassium iodide, 5 minims daily in a glass of water, is now rarely used (Hand 1970).

B. Local Therapy

Ultrasound treatments of symptomatic Peyronie's disease have the advantage of being completely noninvasive with minimal side effects. Daily treatments for five minutes with an intensity of 1.5 watts per cm^2 may provide symptomatic improvement after only a few days, but occasionally require several prolonged courses (Frank and Scott 1971).

Table 1. Systemic therapy.

Treatment	Daily oral dose	Duration	Reference
Vitamin E	100 mg × 3	3-6 months	Devine & Hortin 1974
Potassium para-amino-benzoate (Potaba)	4 gm × 3	Many months	Zarafonetis & Horrax 1959
Potassium iodide (with vitamin E)	5 minims × 1	Many months	Hand 1970

Orthovoltage therapy with doses between 250 and 600 roentgens to the entire penile shaft in a single or occasionally repeated doses appears to be a safe (Furlow et al. 1975) but not very effective form of treatment. Improvement of symptoms occurs no more frequently but possibly earlier than if no treatment is given.

Iontophoresis, a method whereby electrical current is used to promote transcutaneous transport of drugs to the site of the plaque, is used in conjunction with steroids (Rothfield and Murray 1967) and histamine (Whalen 1960). Early permanent improvement of symptoms seems to be the usual result.

Percutaneous injection of steroids into the plaque with a standard syringe (DeSanctis and Furey 1967) or percutaneous dermojet (Winter and Khanna 1975), as well as injection after surgical exposure of the plaque (Taranger et al. 1975), probably results in a rather uneven distribution of the drug. Some patients require subsequent plaque excision. Similarly, injections of parathyroid hormone into the plaque at weekly intervals for eight weeks (Morales and Bruce 1975) have been tried (Table 2).

VII. SURGICAL TREATMENT

A. Surgical Approach

Longitudinal incisions on the penis are undesirable as they leave a palpable scar. Usually access to the fibrotic plaque is gained via a circumferential incision 0.5 cm proximal to the coronary sulcus. Dissection of the loose subcutaneous connective tissue allows the sleeve of penile skin to be pushed upward in accordion fashion (Figure 2). The extent of the plaque usually can be palpated more easily than seen. If the plaque is in the usual dorsal and septal location, elevation of the dorsal neurovascular bundle is necessary and requires sharp dissection with a number 15 knife blade. A heavy stay suture through the glans at this time facilitates manipulation (Figure 3). A considerable amount of connective tissue should be left with the bundle to avoid injury to vessels and nerves. Venous branches are doubly ligated with fine absorbable sutures before they are divided. Nonabsorbable sutures will remain palpable through the thin penile skin. Electrocoagulation easily injures the nerves.

At the end of the procedure the skin is returned to its original position and closed with interrupted absorbable sutures. Repeat injection of saline or contrast material as in a cavernosogram will confirm complete operative correction of penile angu-

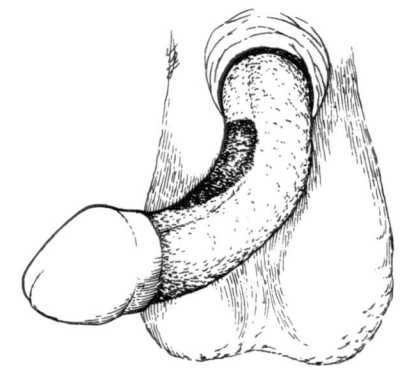

Figure 2. Following a circumferential skin incision 0.5 cm proximal to the coronary sulcus, blunt dissection of loose subcutaneous tissue allows the penile skin to be retracted in an accordion fashion.

Table 2. Local therapy.

Treatment	Dose	Route	Duration	Reference
Ultrasound	5 minutes daily 1.5 watts per cm^2	Direct application	One month	Frank & Scott 1971
Orthovoltage radiotherapy (250 kV)	450-550 roentgens	Entire penis	1-3 monthly doses	Furlow et al. 1975
Steroid	Dexamethasone 2 ml	Percutaneous injection	Weekly (as many as 62 injections)	DeSanctis & Furey 1967
Steroid	Dexamethasone 0.4% 0.6-1.0 ml	Percutaneous dermojet	6 monthly injections	Winter & Khanna 1975
Steroid	Hydrocortone, 0.3 ml	Iontophoresis	13 triweekly	Rothfield & Murray 1967
Parathyroid hormone	50 units	Percutaneous injection	8 weekly treatments	Morales & Bruce 1975
Histamine	Imadyl ointment, 1%	Iontophoresis	3-4 minutes 3× daily 6-8 treatments	Whalen 1960

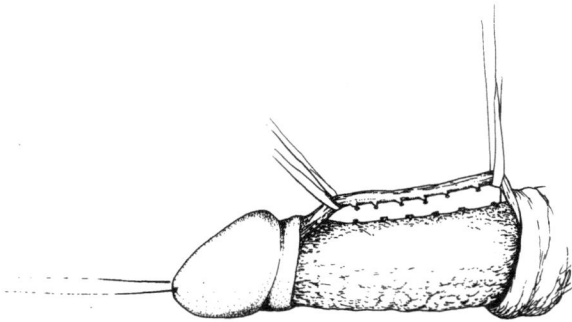

Figure 3. Elevation of dorsal neuro-vascular bundle following sharp dissection. Small venous branches are ligated before they are divided.

lation (Figure 1b). An elastic pressure dressing is applied loosely for 24 hours, leaving the glans exposed. A catheter is not used routinely. Our preference in gaining access to the penile shaft is for a curved infrapubic incision at the base of the penis (Figure 4). Blunt subcutaneous dissection around the root of the penis and in a distal direction make possible the delivery of the entire shaft as far distally as the coronary sulcus (Figure 5). Better access is gained to the proximal shaft and crurae than with a circumcising incision. Insertion of a rigid penile prosthesis, if required, is also convenient with this approach. The incision is later closed with interrupted absorbable sutures in the infrapubic fat and fine monofilament nylon in the skin. Skin sutures are removed one week post-

operatively. Pressure dressing around the penis is the same as used with a circumcising incision. A urethral catheter is rarely necessary.

B. Excision of Plaque

With extensive and severe fibrosis, excision rather than simple incision of the plaque is advisable. Palpable thickening and calcification are not likely to disappear following incision of the plaque and may remain symptomatic even if severe angulation is corrected. Incision of a calcified plaque is technically almost impossible. Instability of the penis following incision alone has been reported (Raz et al. 1977). We advise liberal excision of the plaque well into normal tunica albuginea and the intercavernosal septum.

The erectile tissue is scraped from the undersurface of the plaque with a scalpel blade. Damage to the deep penile artery is thus avoided. Bleeding from the spongious tissue in the absence of anesthesia-induced erection is amazingly little. There is no need for the routine use of a tourniquet at the

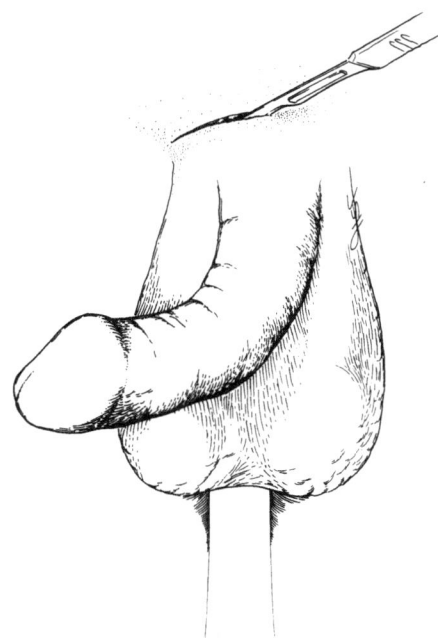

Figure 4. Preferred incision for access to penile shaft.

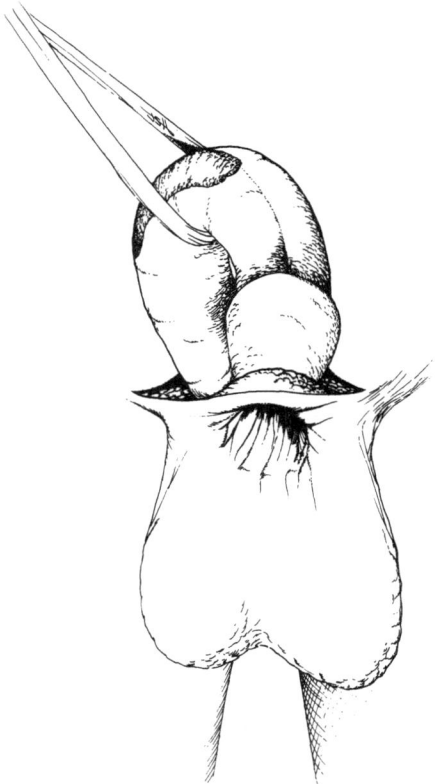

Figure 5. Excellent exposure of entire penile shaft is gained via a small infrapubic incision.

base of the penis. Following complete excision of the plaque the created fascial defect usually measures between 3 and 6 cm in length and no more than 2 cm in width. The penile angulation should now have been completely corrected (Figure 6). The fascial defect is now closed with the selected material.

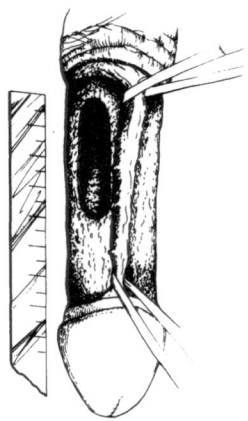

Figure 6. Following excision of the plaque penile angulation is completely corrected. Bleeding from the erectile tissue is little. No tourniquet is required.

C. Selection of Patch Material and Techniques

Following complete excision of the penile plaque local response depends on surgical trauma, continuation of the original pathological process and the material used to fill the defect. Given gentle handling of the tissue during surgery, selection of patch material remains the main variable.

Free fat and fascia are no longer used to fill the defect. Lyophylized dura gave excellent results in an experimental study in dogs (Kelami et al. 1975) but clinical results have not yet been reported. In recent years dermal grafts have been popular and reported results are excellent (Bystrom et al. 1973; Bevine and Horton 1974; Hall and Turner 1977; Hecks et al. 1978; Melman and Holland 1978; Wild et al. 1979). The dermal graft is usually obtained from the lower abdominal wall. An area at least 1.5 times the size of the penile defect is marked. Epidermis 12/1000 of an inch thick is removed with a dermatome (Figure 7). The underlying dermis with very little fat attached to its deep surface is then harvested and placed with the deep side toward the erectile tissue into the penile defect. Excess dermal graft is trimmed away. Fine continuous nonabsorb-

able sutures are used to approximate graft and fascial margins. The knot is buried in the corpus cavernosum so it will not remain palpable later. The penile skin is replaced and closed as described earlier. The skin defect on the abdominal wall is covered with a sterile nonadherent dressing until healed completely, usually about four weeks. Alternatively the epidermis is used as a free graft, using fine interrupted nylon sutures for approximation of the edges.

Our dissatisfaction with dermal grafts is based on theoretical and practical considerations. The corpora cavernosa are modified vascular spaces lined with endothelium. Defects in the vascular wall are ideally replaced with a patch lined on the inside with endothelium and on the outside with connective tissue. Autogenous vein wall in most patients is readily available from the saphenous vein. In the immediate postoperative period most discomfort originates from the site where the dermal graft was obtained. Although results from dermal patches generally are good, some patients have required repeat grafting (Devine and Horton 1974).

A 14 cm long segment of greater saphenous vein (Sachse 1976) can easily be obtained via two small

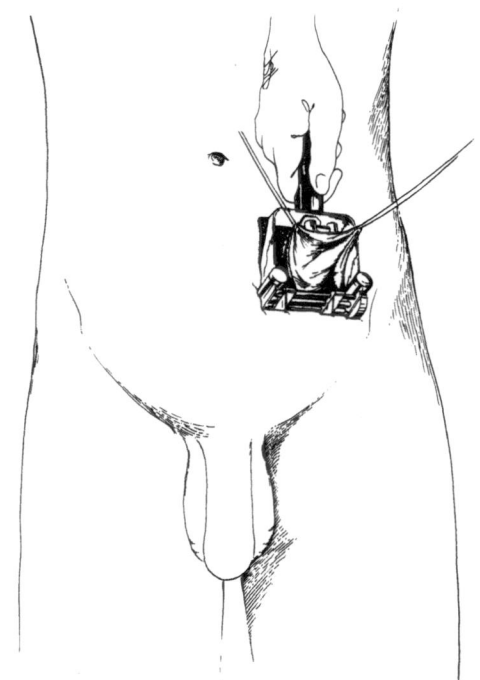

Figure 7. With a dermatome, epidermis is removed from the lower abdominal wall before harvesting the dermal patch.

incisions that cause little postoperative discomfort. Through a 4 cm long oblique incision just below the groin, extending medially from the femoral artery, the junction of the greater saphenous vein and the femoral vein is identified (Figure 8). Four venous branches are usually present and are doubly ligated and divided. The surgeon's index finger creates a tunnel along the saphenous vein and a small counter incision in the skin is made over the finger tip. Here the saphenous vein is ligated with 2-0 silk and transected above the ligature. The free vein is pulled out through the upper incision. The upper end of the saphenous vein, near its entry into the femoral vein, is doubly ligated with silk 2-0 before removing the vein segment. With a scissors, this vein is opened longitudinally (Figure 9) and depending on the size of the defect to be covered the vein patch can be cut into two shorter segments equal to the length of the penile defect. Appropriate trimming to the correct length is done at this time to avoid later cutting of the continuous 5-0 vascular suture used to sew the segments side by side (Figure 10).

The vein patch so obtained has been of sufficient size to cover any defect encountered to date. The vein patch, with endothelium toward the cavernous tissue is sutured in place using continuous 5-0 vascular sutures and burying the knots (Figure 11). Excess width can be trimmed accurately after sutures on three sides are completed. No attempt is made to sew the vein patch into any existing septal defect. Hemostasis can and should be perfect and postoperative pressure dressing is usually not required.

In the absence of suitable autogenous vein, prosthetic material such as a Dacron or Teflon velour patch can be used.

D. Penile Prostheses

Since 1972 surgical treatment of erectile failure with rigid or inflatable penile prostheses has become increasingly popular (Pearman 1972; Scott et al. 1973; Small et al. 1975; Raz and Kaufman 1976; Furlow 1978). In several large series approximately 4 percent of patients with organic impotence were thought to have Peyronie's disease (Small 1978; Study Group Report 1978). In impotent patients with minimum angulation, insertion of Small-Car-

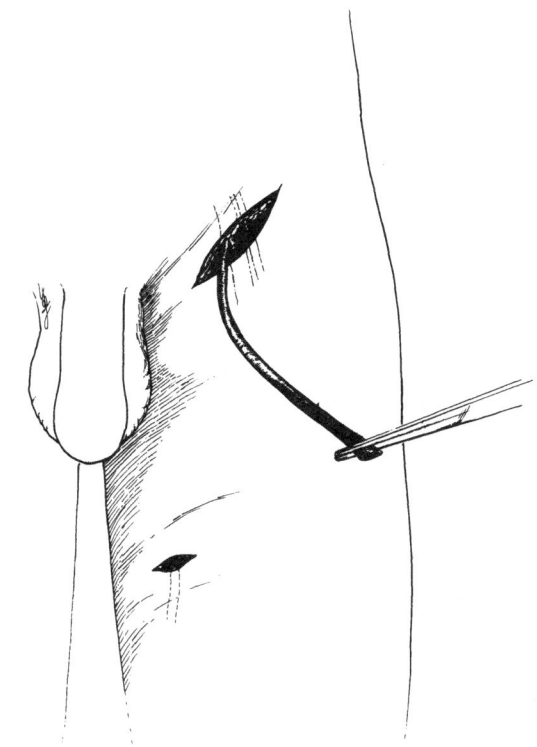

Figure 8. A segment of saphenous vein is harvested through two small incisions.

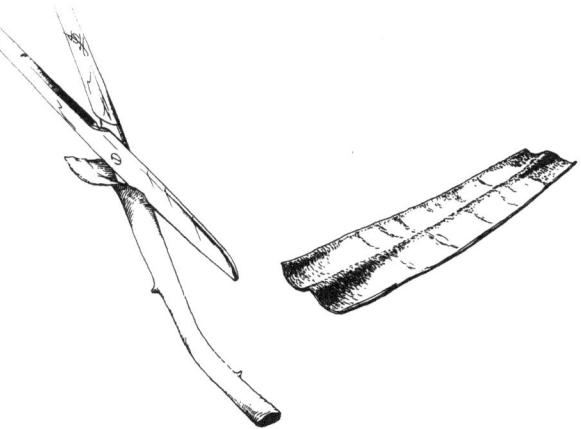

Figure 9. The vein segment is opened longitudinally.

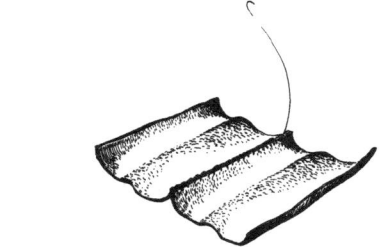

Figure 10. If needed the vein is cut transversely and sutured side-to-side to obtain a wider patch.

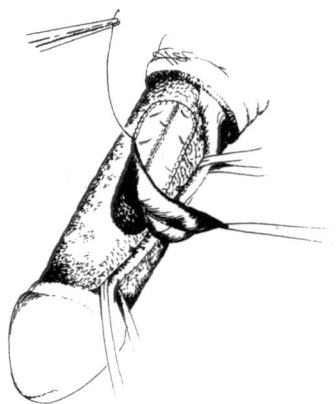

Figure 11. The saphenous vein patch is sutured into place with continuous vascular sutures. The knots are buried into the corpus cavernosum.

rion rigid prostheses (Heyer-Schulte Corporation, 600 Pine St., Goleta, CA) or of Scott inflatable prostheses (American Medical Systems, Inc., 3312 Gorham Ave., Minneapolis, Minnesota) will suffice. If severe angulation exists or if a palpable plaque seems bothersome, additional incision of the plaque (Raz and Kaufman 1977) or excision with closure of the defect as described in the previous section is necessary.

If a corpus cavernosogram is routinely performed before insertion of a penile prosthesis, severe angulation will be apparent and excision of the plaque with patch closure should be performed first. Insertion of the Small-Carrion penile prosthesis is then performed through short, paired, longitudinal incisions in the dorsolateral aspect of each corpus cavernosum as proximal as conveniently possible. Dilatation of the cavernous spaces with Hegar dilators is done in both directions, being careful to dilate the entire length without perforating the tunica albuginea or the patch. Selection of the correct cylinder size is based on the total distance of dilator insertion. Several sizes may have to be tried before an optimal fit is obtained (Figure 12). Usually identical sizes can be used on both sides. Excessive length and diameter should be avoided. The most frequently used sizes have a diameter of 1.1 cm and a length of 15.8 or 17.0 cm, but a full range of sizes should be available in the operating room. The incisions for prosthesis insertion are closed with running sutures of 5-0 monofilament nylon, carefully burying the knots. If no preoperative corpus cavernosogram was performed, the

severity of penile angulation may have been underestimated and only become apparent after insertion of the penile prosthesis. Plaque excision or incision is now best accomplished using electro-cautery to avoid injury to the penile prosthesis, an essential technique if inflatable cylinders were used. After removal of the plaque, the penile prosthesis on the same side frequently needs to be replaced with a larger size.

The technique for insertion of the inflatable prosthesis is described by Scott and Fishman (in the previous chapter). If plaque incision or excision is combined with the inflatable prosthesis, the cylinders are best kept in semi-inflated condition for about three weeks.

Special precautions to avoid infection of the penile prosthesis are recommended. Selection of the incision site, special intraoperative precautions (Schuster 1976) and broad spectrum antibiotic coverage starting the night before surgery and for several days postoperatively (Small 1978) are important. We advise the patient to abstain from sexual intercourse until after the first postoperative visit, four weeks following surgery.

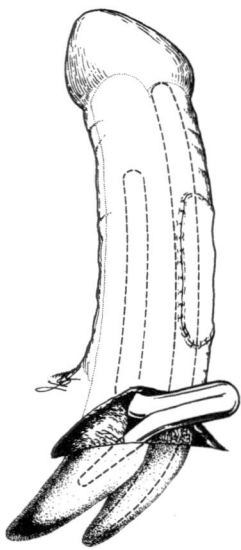

Figure 12. Insertion of Small-Carrion prosthesis following excision of Peyronie's plaque. Defect is filled with autogenous saphenous vein patch.

E. Complications

Complications following surgical excision of the fibrotic plaque and dermal or vein patch replacement are remarkably few. Minimal penile swelling, present on the first postoperative day, rapidly subsides. Pain is easily controlled with mild analgesics even if erections occur. Decreased sensation in the glans penis may result from excessive traction on the dorsal neurovascular bundle. This is quite distracting to the patient but is usually temporary and disappears gradually over several months.

Superficial infection in the absence of prosthetic material is of no consequence, but infection of the prosthesis will require removal of the prosthesis and thus results in complete failure of the procedure. Protrusion of the Small-Carrion prosthesis through the urethra or glans usually results from insertion of too large a cylinder and requires removal of that cylinder. Reinsertion of a new prosthesis at a later time may be successful.

Late development of erectile failure in patients who did not have a penile implant at the time of surgery is not considered a complication, but rather evidence of natural progression of the disease. This can be treated by the insertion of a penile prosthesis.

VIII. RESULTS

Immediate complete correction of penile angulation results from wide plaque excision and replacement with dermal or vein patch. If potent, the patient is extremely grateful. A major disturbance to the patient may be the palpable suture knot if this was not buried deeply. Progression of the disease is not halted by excision of the fibrotic plaque. In patients with already decreased penile tumescence, complete erectile failure may gradually develop over several months or years. We have not observed the recurrence of a palpable fibrotic plaque or penile angulation following wide excision and the use of a vein patch but this certainly could occur if excision was insufficient or if the dermal patch graft was too small.

In view of the excellent surgical results obtained, we have gradually abolished complicated, costly and time consuming modes of therapy and recommend surgical treatment for disabling degrees of penile angulation not improved after oral vitamin E treatment, and for patients with erectile failure.

REFERENCES

Ashworth A: Peyronie's disease. Proc R Soc Med 53: 652, 1960.

Billig R, Baker R, Immergut M and Maxted W: Peyronie's disease. Urology 6: 409, 1975.

Bwens CH, Maricek RL and Feldman JM: Peyronie's disease: A presenting complaint of the carcinoid syndrome. N Engl J Med 289: 844, 1973.

Bystrom J, Alfthan O, Johansson B and Korlof B: Induratio penis plastica (Peyronie's disease): Result after excision and dermo-fat grafting. Scand J Plast Reconstr Surg 7: 137, 1973.

Chesney JL: Peyronie's disease. Br J Urol 47: 209, 1975.

DeSanctis PN and Furey CA Jr: Steroid injection therapy for Peyronie's disease: A 10 year summary and review of 38 cases. J Urol 97: 114, 1967.

Devine CJ and Horton CE: Surgical treatment of Peyronie's disease with a dermal graft. J Urol 111: 44, 1974.

Durant W and Durant A: The story of civilization. Part VIII: The age of Louis XIV. New York, Simon and Schuster, 1963, p 27.

Frank IN and Scott WW: The ultrasonic treatment of Peyronie's disease. J Urol 106: 883, 1971.

Furlow WL: The current status of the inflatable penile prosthesis in the management of impotence: Mayo Clinic experience updated. J Urol 119: 363, 1978.

Furlow WL, Swenson HE and Lee RE: Peyronie's disease: A study of its natural history and treatment with orthovoltage radiotherapy. J. Urol 114: 69, 1975.

Hall WT and Turner RW: Experience with Devine-Horton dermal patch graft for Peyronie's disease. Urology 9: 407, 1977.

Hand JR: Surgery of the penis and urethra. In: Urology, Volume 3, third edition, Campbell MF and Harrison JH (eds), Philadelphia, WB Saunders Company, 1970, p 2541-2647.

Hicks CE, O'Brien DP III, Bostwick J III and Walton KN: Experience with the Horton-Devine dermal graft in the treatment of Peyronie's disease. J Urol 119: 504, 1978.

Kelami A, Gross U, Fiedler U, Richter-Reichhelm M and Tsaoussidis N: Replacement of tunica albuginea of corpus cavernosum penis using human derma. Urology 6: 464, 1975.

Melman A and Holland RF: Evaluation of the dermal graft inlay technique for the surgical treatment of Peyronie's disease. J Urol 120: 421, 1978.

Morales A and Bruce AW: The treatment of Peyronie's disease with parathyroid hormone. J Urol 114: 901, 1975.

Pearman RO: Insertion of a silastic penile prosthesis for the treatment of organic sexual impotence. J Urol 107: 802, 1972.

Peyronie F de la: Sur quelques obstacles qui s'opposent à l'éjaculation naturelle de la semence. Mém de l'acad roy de chir 1743: 425-434.

Poutasse EF: Peyronie's disease. J Urol 107: 419, 1972.

Raz S, DeKernion JB and Kaufman JJ: Surgical treatment of Peyronie's disease: A new approach. J Urol 117: 598, 1977.

Raz S and Kaufman JJ: Small-Carrion operation for impotence: Improved technique. Urology 7: 68, 1976.

Rothfield SH and Murray W: The treatment of Peyronie's disease by iontophoresis of [21]C esterified glucocorticoids. J Urol 97: 874, 1967.

Sachse H. Venenwandplastik bei Induratio penis plastica. Urologe A 15: 131, 1976.

Schuster K: Operating room protocol in implantation of the inflatable penile prosthesis. Mayo Clin Proc 51: 339, 1976.

Scott FB, Brandley WE and Timm GW: Management of erectile impotence: Use of implantable inflatable prosthesis. Urology 2: 80, 1973.

Small MP: Small-Carrion penile prosthesis: A report on 160 cases and review of the literature. J Urol 119: 365, 1978.

Small MP, Carrion HM and Gordon JA: Small-Carrion penile prosthesis: New implant for management of impotence. Urology 5: 479, 1975.

Smith BH: Peyronie's disease. Am J Clin pathol 45: 670, 1966.

Smith BH: Subclinical Peyronie's disease. Am J Clin Pathol 52: 385, 1969.

Study Group Report: Inflatable penile prosthesis. Urograms 2: 10, 1978.

Taranger LA, Robson CJ and Barkin M: The surgical approach to Peyronie's disease. J Urol 114: 404, 1975.

Van Buren WH and Keyes EL: Practical treatment of the surgical disease of the genito-urinary tract. New York, Appleton-Century-Crofts, Inc, 1874.

Whalen WH: A new concept in the treatment of Peyronie's disease. J Urol 83: 851, 1960.

Wild RM, Devine CJ Jr and Horton CE: Dermal graft repair of Peyronie's disease: Survey of 50 patients. J Urol 121: 47, 1979.

Winter CC and Khanna: Peyronie's disease: Results with dermo-jet injection of dexamethasone. J Urol 114: 898, 1975.

Zarafonetis CJ and Horrax T: Treatment of Peyronie's disease with potassium paraaminobenzoate (Potaba). J Urol 81: 770, 1959.

12. CORPORAL SHUNTS FOR PRIAPISM

H.W. Schoenberg and J. Banno

Priapism is defined as an abnormally prolonged painful erection in the absence of sexual excitation or desire. It is a rare condition with a variety of known and suspected etiologies that is associated sporadically with a large number of disease states. It may occur at any age because the lesions with which it is associated present throughout the entire life span. The untreated course of the disease varies markedly from individual to individual, thus making difficult the evaluation of various therapeutic maneuvers. The many medical and surgical methods of management attest to the fact that even for priapism related to a single underlying cause, no single method of treatment is always successful, although it is becoming apparent that some are more efficacious than others. A review of the literature indicates that in more than half of the reported cases of priapism, no specific etiologic factor can be identified (Nelson et al. 1977). Sickle cell disease accounts for about 25 percent of the reported cases, thus being the most important demonstrable lesion causally related to priapism (Larocque and Cosgrove 1974).

I. ETIOLOGY

The largest group of cases of priapism reported in the literature are generally classified as idiopathic. Into this group fall those patients for whom prolonged sexual stimulation or continuous masturbation seems to be related to the onset of priapism. The use of drugs to enhance sensation may also lead to a variety of actions during which penile trauma may occur. The combination of prolonged stimulation and trauma may increase the likelihood of the development of priapism. Attempts by the patient to relieve priapism by continuing intercourse are painful and do not promote subsidence of the erection. Where a specific cause or frequently related disease state can be identified, it usually falls into one of several groups. Hematologic diseases with which priapism is associated include sickle cell anemia, leukemia and glucose phosphate isomerase deficiency (Goulding 1976). Irritative problems involving the lower urinary tract include prostatitis, urethritis, phimosis and trauma to the urethra. Neurological causes for priapism are most notably multiple sclerosis, infectious myelitis, and traumatic lesions of the spinal cord. Tumors associated with priapism are primarily those of the prostate, penis and kidney (Weisman et al. 1969; Narayana et al. 1977). A miscellaneous group of suspected etiologic factors includes pharmacologic agents, toxic agents and congenital problems such as Fabry's disease (Wilson et al. 1973). Stein has proposed a classification system which is useful in approaching the problem of priapism (Stein and Matin 1974).

II. PATHOPHYSIOLOGY

A normal erection depends upon both an increased blood flow into the corpora cavernosa and a closing down of the shunts which direct blood away from the corpora cavernosa when the penis is flaccid. Erection occurs in response to either psychic or tactile stimuli and seems to be primarily a parasympathetic function, although the sympathetic system may play some part in the vascular alterations. The sympathetic system is considerably more important in the process of detumescence (Hinman 1960). When an erection is maintained longer than a reasonable period of time for completion of intercourse or when it is maintained in the absence of physical or psychic stimuli, then priapism is deemed to be present. Although the association of priapism with some disease states and some activities seems clear, the mechanisms that trigger priapism in many cases (idiopathic priapism) remain obscure. However, with a prolonged erection, blood stagnating in the corpora cavernosa loses its oxygen content and develops a rising carbon dioxide tension. In this circumstance, sludging of the blood occurs along with local acidosis. The sludged blood further obstructs the venous outflow and perpetuates the erection. Ultimately, if the priapism is not relieved, engorgement and inflammation lead to fibrosis of the fine structure of the corpora and the ultimate development of erectile impotence.

A. Hematologic Disease

In patients with sickle cell anemia who develop priapism, the corpora cavernosa become engorged with irreversibly sickled erythrocytes. The stasis results in a local hypoxia acidosis and further sickling. The incidence of priapism in male patients hospitalized for complications of sickle hemoglobinopathies is approximately 5 percent. Precipitating factors include mild acidosis with hypoventilation during sleep, normal erection during REM sleep, masturbation, intercourse, infection and local trauma. In patients who have leukemia and subsequently develop priapism, four causes for developing priapism have been proposed: (1) a sludge of leukemic cells in the corpora cavernosa, (2) direct central nervous stimulation, (3) leukemic infiltrates along or adjacent to the sacral nerves, and (4) splenomegaly resulting in mechanical obstruction of the abdominal veins and nerves (Schreibman et al. 1974). Recently a case of priapism associated with glucose phosphate isomerase deficiency has been reported (Goulding 1976). This condition is one of the erythroenzymopathies. Altered membrane deformation, particularly in the presence of relative acidosis, may account for the priapism encountered. Only about 20 cases of this disease have been reported thus far in the literature.

B. Neurologic Disease

Central nervous system disease is often associated with priapism. Cervical and complete lesions of the cord are more often associated with priapism than are lower or incomplete lesions. In one group of 67 patients, 40 percent developed priapism (Austin 1972). Priapism occurs in infectious myelitis and multiple sclerosis, spinal cord injury and in the presence of leukemic infiltrates and metastatic tumors. The exact mechanism is unknown, but it may be related to decreased sympathetic vasoconstrictor tone, which is known to increase engorgement of the corpora cavernosa. Priapism may also be related to a mass reflex or irritative involvement of the parasympathetic pathways.

C. Irritative Lesions

Infectious lesions involving the urethra and prostate, traumatic lesions of the urethra such as straddle injury, phimosis, urethral polyps and vesical calculi are all occasionally noted in association with priapism. In these cases the priapism is usually of short duration and responds rather promptly to treatment of the primary lesion.

D. Solid Tumors

Cancer of the penis with infiltration of the corpora cavernosa, cancer of the prostate with extension into the penis, and metastatic lesions, particularly from the kidney, may sufficiently interfere with venous drainage from the corpora cavernosa, resulting in priapism.

E. Drugs

A number of drugs have been implicated in the development of priapism. Although it seems somewhat paradoxical, heparin has been associated with the onset of priapism (Duggan 1970). Since thromboembolic phenomena seem to play an important role in the development of priapism, the explanation of heparin's role in producing priapism is difficult to understand. There are a number of possible explanations but none have been established with any certainty. Some antihypertensive medications, particularly hydralazine, have been associated with priapism and reported in the literature (Becker and Mitchell 1965; Rubin 1968). The action by which these drugs produce priapism seems to be a suppression of sympathetic activity which removes vasoconstrictor tone and permits the development of a parasympathetic predominance. The phenothiazines also have been associated with priapism (Dorman 1976). These drugs also have an alpha-adrenergic blocking capability as well as a hypotensive effect.

III. DIAGNOSIS

The diagnosis of priapism is made readily by history and observation. The importance of further diagnostic studies is to identify the underlying cause, if one exists; therefore, further studies should be directed toward uncovering any of the lesions mentioned above. Hematologic studies and those which demonstrate the vasculature of the pelvis are generally the most rewarding.

IV. TREATMENT OF PRIAPISM

Many urologists and physicians working in other fields have demonstrated ingenuity in devising methods of treatment for priapism. Assessment of methods is complicated by the variety of causes of this affliction and its relative rarity. Furthermore, spontaneous detumescence usually occurs within 1 to 11 days and further complicates the evaluation of therapeutic measures (Nelson and Winter 1977).

Many of the methods employed in the past are of historical interest only. Medical management has fallen by the wayside in favor of early surgical intervention with the exception of priapism related to hematologic disorders. Adjunctive medical measures such as sedation, protection of the penis from contact stimulation and local cooling may be of some benefit during the early phases of management. Compression dressings alone, hypotensive anesthesia, general anesthesia, pudendal nerve block, ganglionic blocking agents, heparin, estrogens, enemas and fibrinolytic agents have generally been abandoned as primary methods for managing priapism. The management of idiopathic priapism today is primarily surgical. For the urologist dealing with the patient with priapism, certain specific precautions must be taken. After successful therapy, recurrent priapism is not uncommon and the patient must always be aware of this possibility, just

as he must be informed that successful shunting procedures may be accompanied by erectile impotence for as long as the shunt remains patent. Most important, of course, is the fact that impotence secondary to fibrosis of the corpora cavernosa remains a serious sequela in many patients with priapism. This type of impotence will be permanent. Impotence may develop regardless of the rapidity of the response to therapy. The patient must be informed of this unfortunate possibility before any measures are undertaken; otherwise, he may associate the subsequent impotence with the therapeutic measures used to control priapism.

Patients developing priapism secondary to hematological disorders, such as sickle cell anemia, leukemia and multiple myeloma can be successfully treated by using a rational therapeutic program aimed at relieving the initiating lesion.

Transfusion was first suggested in 1962 as a treatment for priapism secondary to sickle cell anemia (Hasen and Raines 1962). It was not until nine years later that Seeler popularized the concept that by diluting the obstructing cells with normal red cells, drainage of the corpora cavernosa would improve and resolution might occur (Seeler 1973). Her concept was supported by the frequent observation of a dramatic reduction in splenic size following packed red cell transfusion in patients suffering from a sickle cell crisis. Hydration, alkalinization and analgesics are used to correct the dehydration, acidosis and pain associated with priapism. Intensive packed red cell transfusion causes the release of entrapped red cells, thus leading to detumescence. Baron and Leiter in 1978 proposed a schedule for treating priapism secondary to sickle cell anemia which includes hydration, alkalinization and analgesics initially. If no response is seen in the first 12 hours, then hypertransfusion using packed red cells is given to double the hematocrit over a 4-6 hour period. The patient is observed for 36-48 hours, and if detumescence is not achieved, then an exchange transfusion is given to lower the hemoglobin S to 30 percent. A shunting procedure should be seriously considered if the above medical regimen does not relieve the priapism.

In Seeler's series, 8 out of 11 patients responded within 2 to 3 days, and 7 of these 11 patients had documented post-therapy potency (Seeler 1973).

Radiation therapy to the spleen and penis and chemotherapy are specific modalities used to treat the leukemic patients with priapism (Schreibman et al. 1974). In 1960 the use of chemotherapy was first mentioned (Haar et al. 1960). A 24 year-old man was given an alkoxyl derivative of ethyleneimine and this relieved his priapism. A number of patients with priapism secondary to chronic granulocytic leukemia have been successfully treated with intravenous cytosine arabinoside or hydroxyurea (Schreibman et al. 1974).

Priapism associated with multiple myeloma and hyperviscosity has been successfully treated with plasmapheresis (Rosenbaum et al. 1978). At the conclusion of the 90-minute procedure, there was a complete resolution of the priapism which had been present for 28 days.

When priapism is associated with malignant tumors involving the penis or its venous drainage, direct attack upon the priapism will only be palliative and recurrence after shunting is to be expected. The primary attack, therefore, should be directed toward the tumor using surgery, radiation therapy, chemotherapy and immunotherapy, singly or in combination, as dictated by the nature of the malignant process.

While some authors proceed immediately to vascular shunting, the majority of experienced urologists reporting in this area recommend a trial of through-and-through irrigation of the corpora using a 10 percent heparin solution followed either by intermittent compression with a blood pressure cuff or a compression dressing which places the now flaccid penis against the perineum (Harlow 1969). If a circular compression dressing is used, frequent inspection of the glans is essential to be alert to any symptoms of necrosis of the distal portion of the penis (Weiss and Ferguson 1974). Because of the real danger of this sequela, circular compression dressings probably should be avoided. Irrigation may be tried two or three times over a period of 24-36 hours before it is abandoned (Figure 1).

If, after 36 hours, resolution of the erection has not been achieved, shunting should be undertaken.

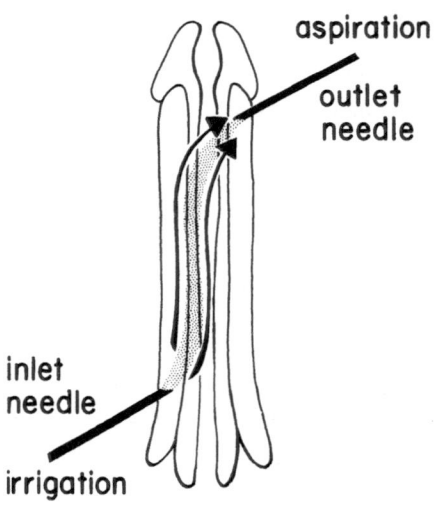

Figure 1. Technique of aspiration and irrigation of the corpora cavernosa using a heparin-saline mixture.

The saphenocavernosus shunt was first described in 1964, and it retains its usefulness today (Grayhack et al. 1964). A unilateral shunt may be sufficient because of venous cross-communication between the corpora (Figure 2). One theoretical disadvantage of this procedure is the loss of the saphenous vein, which is used so frequently in vascular reconstruction in elderly patients. In the procedure, a 1 cm incision in Buck's fascia and the tunica albuginea is made into the substance of the corpora on its dorsolateral aspect close to the base of the penis. After irrigation of the corpora and removal of clots, and after the establishment of brisk bleeding, the saphenous vein is ligated and divided about 10 cm from its junction from the femoral vein. The vein is brought subcutaneously to the opening in the corpora cavernosa and anasto-

mosed to it using a continuous vascular nonabsorbable suture. A urologist undertaking this procedure for the first time should review Grayhack's original article.

The second shunting procedure presently in use was first described in 1964 (Quackles 1964). This is the spongiocavernosum shunt (Figure 3). In this procedure, the spongiosum and corpora cavernosa are anastomosed to each other on each side in the perineum. The anastomoses are 1.5 to 2 cm in length. Caution is necessary in incising the spongiosum to avoid penetrating the urethra because the spongiosum is very thin. A number of urethrocutaneous fistulae have been created during this procedure. As in the saphenocavernosum shunt, brisk bleeding after evacuation of clots must be obtained prior to creating the shunt. Some authors recommend

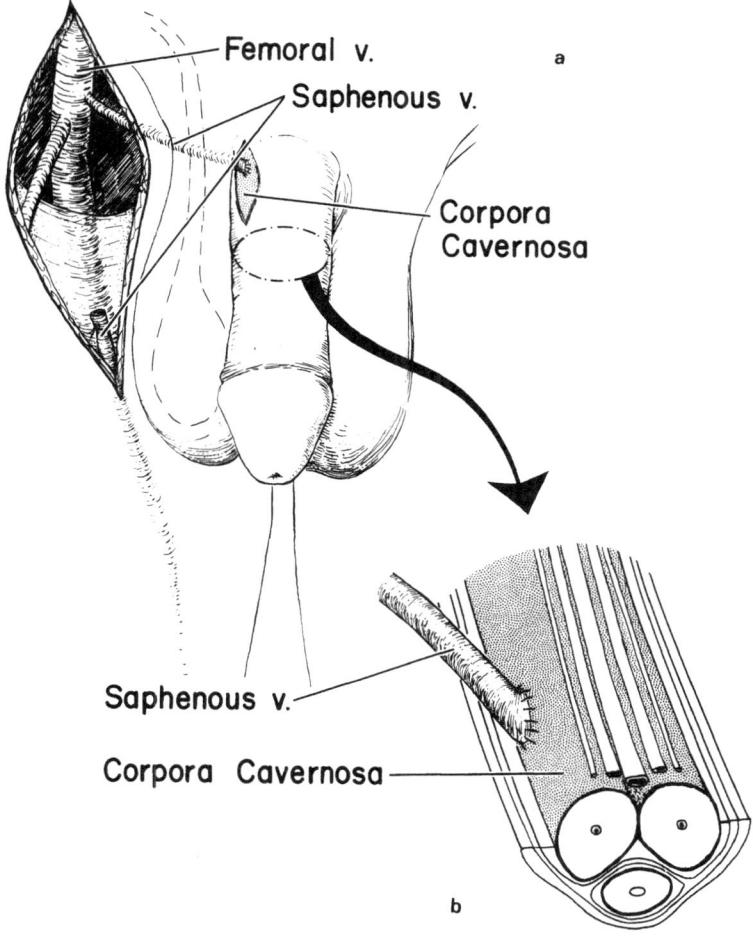

Figure 2. Saphenous-corpora cavernosa shunt. a. Showing saphenous vein anastomosis with corpus cavernosum at base of penis. b. Magnified view of completed anastomosis.

postoperative heparinization. With either of these methods, one can expect that the majority of patients will lose their erections, and potency will be retained by about 50 percent. The use of the deep and the superficial dorsal penile veins to create shunts with the corpora cavernosa was reported in 1976. We have not used this shunt, and there are only two successful cases reported in the literature (Barry 1976) (Figure 4 and 5). The principles involved, however, are the same as for the sapheno-cavernosum shunt. In 1976, the use of a new and simple technique for creating a shunt between the corpora cavernosa and the spongiosum was reported (Winter 1976, 1978). This involves the use of a biopsy needle to remove a core of tissue from the septum between the glans penis and the corpora cavernosa. We have used this technique successfully. This method is quick, simple and may be followed by more formal procedures if unsuccessful

(Figure 6). It may be performed under local anesthesia if necessary.

Another method of shunting blood away from the corpora cavernosa has been described using extracorporeal shunting from the corpora cavernosa to a vein in the arm by means of dialysis equipment and a roller pump (Douglas 1976). In 8 patients, detumescence was achieved after varying periods of time, with potency retained by 4 patients. Recently, attempts have been made to attack the problem of priapism from the arterial inflow side by using autologous clot to obstruct the internal pudendal artery (Wear et al. 1977). This author noted that ligation of the internal pudendal artery might lead to permanent impotence, and therefore autologous clot seemed to offer a temporary method of occluding this vessel. Two patients were thus successfully treated.

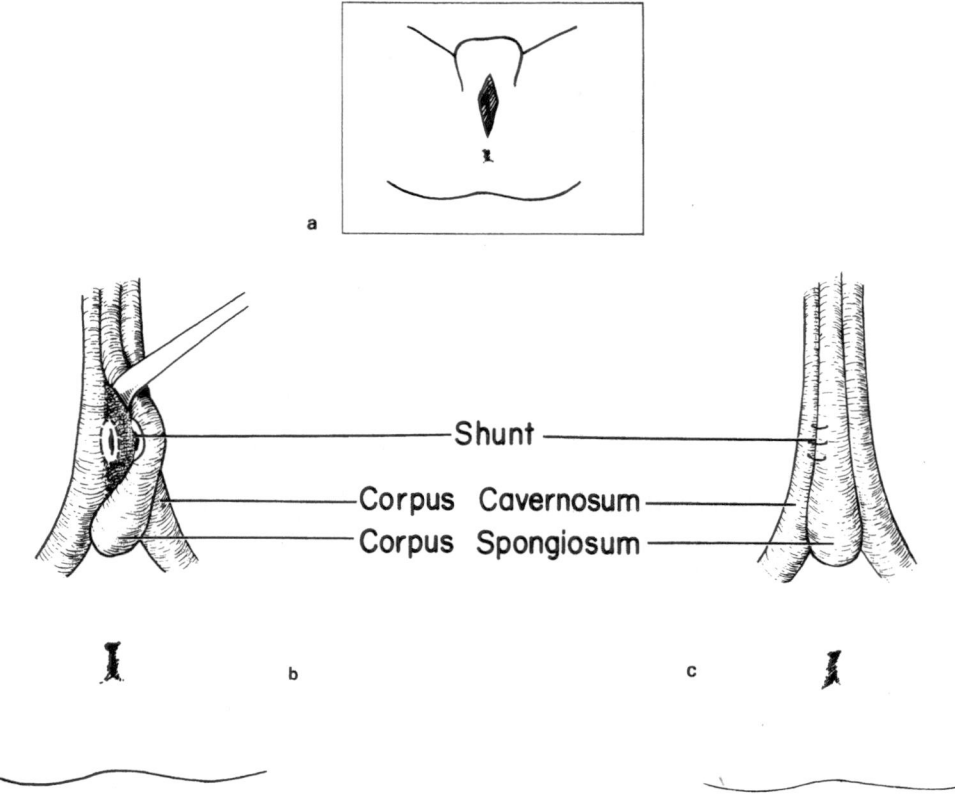

Figure 3. a. Perineal incision. b. Site of corpus cavernosum-corpus spongiosum shunt. c. Completed shunt.

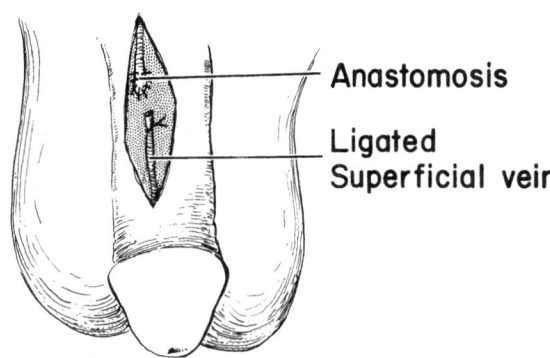

Figure 4. Shunt created using superficial dorsal vein of penis and corpus cavernosum.

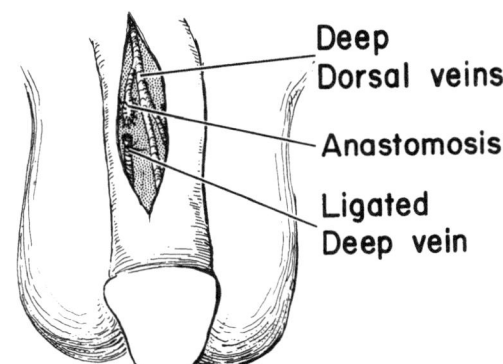

Figure 5. Shunt created using deep dorsal vein of penis and corpus cavernosum.

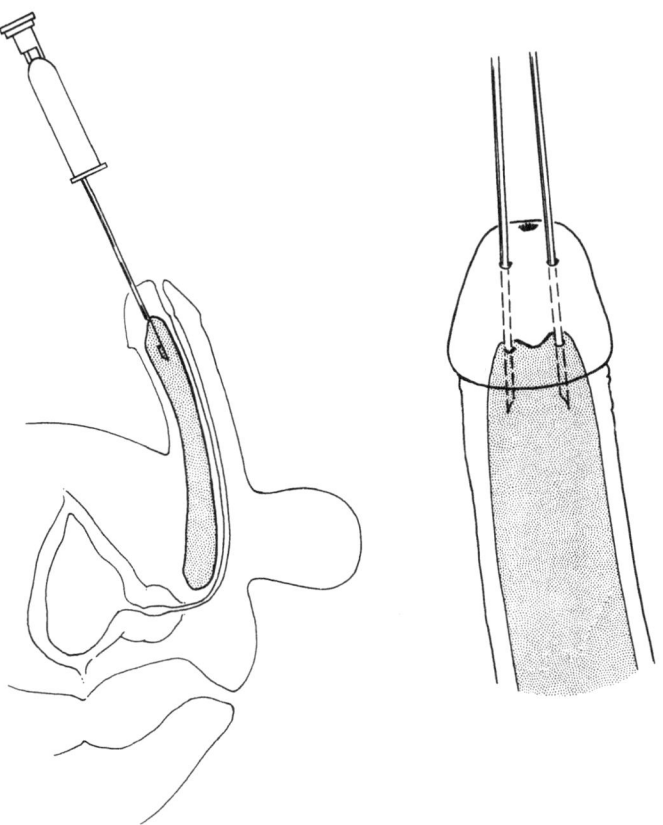

Figure 6. Winter's simplified method of creating a shunt from the corpus cavernosum to the corpus spongiosum using a disposable biopsy needle.

REFERENCES

Appell RA: Thorazine-induced Priapism. Brit J Urol 49: 160, 1977.

Austin, G: The spinal cord: basic aspects and surgical considerations. 2nd ed. Charles C Thomas, 1972.

Baron M and Leiter E: Management of Priapism in sickle cell anemia. J Urol 119: 610, 1978.

Barry JM: Priapism: Treatment with corpus cavernosum to dorsal vein of penis shunts. J Urol 116: 754, 1976.

Becker LE and Michell AD: Priapism. Surgical clinics of North America, p 1523-34. 1965.

Carter RG, Thomas CE and Tomsky GC: Cavernospongiosum shunts in treatment of priapism. Urology 3(3): 292, 1976.

Darwish ME, Atassi B and Clark SS: Priapism: Evaluation of treatment regimens. J Urol 112: 92, 1974.

Dorman B: Association of priapism in phenothiazine therapy. J Urol 116: 51, 1976.

Douglas LL: Extracorporeal circulatory management of priapism. Urology 7(2): 198, 1976.

Duggan M: Heparin: A cause of priapism. Sou Med J 63: 1131, 1970.

Goulding F: Priapism caused by glucose phosphate isomerase deficiency. J Urol 116: 819, 1976.

Grayhack JT, McCullough W, O'Connor WJ Jr and Trippel O: Venous bypass to control priapism. Invest Urol 1: 509, 1964.

Haar H, Shanbrom E and Miller S: The treatment of leukemic priapism with A-139. J Urol 83: 429, 1960.

Harlow B: Simple technique for treating priapism. J Urol 101: 71, 1969.

Hasen HB and Raines SL: Priapism associated with sickle cell disease. J Urol 88: 71, 1962.

Hinman F Jr: Priapism: reasons for failure of therapy. J Urol 83, 420, 1960.

Kandel GL, Bender LI and Grove JS: Pulmonary embolism: A complication of corpus-saphenous shunt for priapism. J Urol 99: 196, 1968.

Karayalcin G, Imran M and Rosner F: Priapism in sickle cell disease. Am J Med Sci 264(4): 289, 1972.

Kraus EM and Tessler AN: Gangrene of the penis following bilateral corpus-saphenous shunts for idiopathic priapism. J Urol 109: 1021, 1973.

Larocque M and Cosgrove M: Priapism: A review of 46 cases. J Urol 112: 770, 1974.

Maloney PJ, Elliott GB and Johnson HW: Experiences with priapism. J Urol 114: 72, 1975.

Narayana AS, Kelly DG and Duff FA: Malignant priapism. Brit J Urol 49: 326, 1977.

Nelson JH and Winter CC: Priapism: Evolution of management in 48 patients in a 22-year series. J Urol 117: 455, 1977.

Port FK, Hecking E, Fiegel P and Kohler H: Priapism during regular dialysis: Lancet Nov: 1287, 1974.

Quackles R: Cure of a patient suffering from priapism by cavernospongiosa anastomosis. Acta Urol Belg 32: 5, 1964.

Resnick MI, Holland JM, King LR and Grayhack JT: Management with cavernosaphenous shunt. Urology 5(4): 492, 1975.

Rosenbaum EH, Thompson HE and Glassberg AB: Priapism and multiple myeloma. Urology 12(2): 201, 1978.

Rubin SO: Priapism as a probable sequel to medication. Scand J Urol Nephrol. 2: 81, 1968.

Schreibman S, Gee TS and Grabstald H: Management of priapism in patients with chronic granulocytic leukemia. J Urol 111: 786, 1974.

Seeler RA: Intensive transfusion therapy for priapism in boys with sickle cell anemia. J Urol 110: 360, 1973.

Seeler RA: Priapism in children with sickle cell anemia. Clin Ped 10(7): 418, 1971.

Snyder GB and Wilson CA: Surgical management of priapism and its sequelae in sickle cell disease. So Med Jour 59: 1893, 1966.

Stein J and Martin D: Priapism. Urology 3(1): 8, 1974.

Tarasuk AP and Schneider IM: Management of priapism by cavernoglandular shunt. Urology 3(2): 141, 1976.

Wear JB Jr, Crummy A B and Munson BO: A new approach to treatment of priapism. J Urol 117: 252, 1977.

Weisman EB, Hardison JE and Burns JB: Priapism as the initial manifestation of renal carcinoma. Arch Intern Med 123: 58, 1969.

Weiss JM and Ferguson D: Priapism: The danger of treatment with compression. J Urol 112: 616, 1974.

Wilson S, Klionsky L and Rhamy R: A new etiology of priapism: Fabry's disease. J Urol 109: 646, 1973.

Winter CC: Priapism cured by creation of fistulas between glans penis and corpora cavernosa. J Urol 119: 227, 1978.

Winter CC: Cure of idiopathic priapism. New procedure for creating fistula between glans penis and corpora cavernosa. Urology 3(4): 389, 1976.

13. VASECTOMY

J.E. DAVIS

Vasectomy, or more exactly, vas sectioning and occlusion, has become a popular elective procedure for permanent male contraception in the United States, Asia, and parts of Europe. Though cultural barriers to its acceptance currently exist in other parts of the world, vasectomy has been introduced into Africa, Latin America, and the Middle East. In spite of dire predictions that men will not accept the procedure for fear of lost masculinity or castration, reports indicate that when properly presented, men in all societies will welcome the procedure when their concern for limitation of family size and economic and educational advancement outweigh desire for more children; and where concern for risks of maternal morbidity and female contraceptive method failure are overriding considerations.

As with many other contraceptive methods for which popularity and acceptance preceded thorough scientific understanding of effects and sequelae, so the effects of vasectomy upon the proximal genital tract have only come under scrutiny by serious investigators in the past ten years. Immunologic response, effects on lipid metabolism, effects on spermatogenesis and epididymal function are under scrutiny. Such studies are necessary. Though millions of men have undergone uncomplicated vasectomies, and prospective studies of vasectomized and nonvasectomized matched controls have not as yet revealed significant differences in chemical or endocrine parameters, one cannot doubt that some changes, probably subclinical, do occur and that some men with as yet undefined diseases may be at greater risk if they undergo the operation. Intensive study of the effects of vasectomy may lead to discriminants which assist the physician and family planning counselor in helping the individual decide on the most appropriate contraceptive technique.

The risk-benefit ratio of vasectomy, as with other contraceptive methods, will be better understood as a result of current studies.

Although the techniques for female sterilization have become increasingly simpler and safer, vasectomy has been extremely popular in the United States since 1965. It is estimated that more than 250,000 men have the operation yearly. Over three million men in the United States have had the operation.

As the demand for voluntary male and female sterilization has grown, governments have begun to remove the remaining legal restrictions. In 1972, U.S. courts struck down the last state law prohibiting sterilization. Since then, the poor have been able to obtain free or inexpensive operations through Medicaid or state health funds. The only restriction on the use of government money for sterilization is that the person involved must give informed consent, be 21, and be legally competent.

In the industrialized world, sterilization is legal or unregulated except Italy, France, Turkey, and some provinces of Canada. Sterilization is a government-sponsored family planning method in Thailand and the Philippines. The only nations where sterilizations are still prohibited or difficult to obtain are in sub-Sahara Africa and the Arab world.

The clinical development of the vasectomy procedure is historically linked with the course of experimental investigation. The first experiment in tying of the vas was reported as early as 1785, but it was not until the 1800s that several investigations into the effects of vasectomy were undertaken. Cooper is generally credited with initiating the first systematic experimental work in 1830 when he demonstrated that closing the ducts of the testes (the vas) had no effect on the production of sperm by the testes for as long as six years after the operation.

Gosselin in 1847 and Simmonds in 1921 noted that even in cases in which the vas deferens had been occluded for many years, there was no apparent injury to the sperm producing functions of the testicles.

In the late 1890s, the clinical uses of vasectomy were begun by surgeons in conjunction with operations on the prostate. Ochsner performed such operations in 1897 and reported in the Journal of the American Medical Association, April 22, 1899, that no change whatever had been noted in the sex lives of his patients following successful vasectomies. Although the operation gained in popularity over the years, it was the consensus among physicians that a vasectomy, once done, was irreversible. However, an accidental vasectomy during a hernia repair led to the first attempt to rejoin the vas in 1945. Following this attempt, other surgeons reported cases of vasovasostomy with complete recovery even when the vasectomy had been performed several years earlier. The popularity of vasectomy for contraception has increased sharply in the past decades. The Association for Voluntary Sterilization estimates that 75 percent of all voluntary sterilizations performed in the U.S. during 1970 were vasectomies, which represented a considerable upward trend in male sterilization from 10 years earlier when 60 percent of all voluntary sterilizations were performed on the female.

Most men requesting vasectomies are over 30 and have two or three children. Most couples seeking vasectomy have utilized other forms of contraception. Some have found them inconvenient and others have suffered ill effects such as hormonal or blood disturbances related to oral contraceptives, or pelvic infections due to intrauterine devices. Other males suffer the consequences of contraceptive failure, necessitating abortions or continued unplanned pregnancies.

Whereas failure rates of temporary methods of contraception are additive year by year, the 0.1 percent chance of recanalization decreases after the first year of vasectomy to virtually zero, making it, along with closure of the female tubes, the most effective method of contraception.

I. BIOLOGY OF THE VAS

A. Anatomy

The vas deferens is easily palpable in the scrotum as a portion of the spermatic cord. It is 35 cm in length and extends from the tail of the epididymis to the prostate, where it forms the ejaculatory duct together with the duct of the seminal vesicle.

The vas deferens is composed of three layers of smooth muscle: the outer and inner longitudinal and middle circular layers. It is capable of powerful peristaltic motion. The lumen of the vas, like the tubules of the epididymis, is lined with epithelium lying on a basement membrane arranged with submucosa and longitudinal folds. There is a thick sheet of connective tissue exterior to the muscle layer. The vas deferens may be divided into five portions: (1) the sheathless epididymal portion contained within the tunica vaginalis, (2) the scrotal portion, (3) the inguinal division, (4) the retroperitoneal or pelvic division, and (5) the ampulla. The portion of the vas of clinical interest for vasectomy is generally in the midscrotal portion.

The blood supply of the vas deferens is from the deferential artery, a branch of the inferior vesicle artery and an important collateral circulation mechanism for the testicle. It is also an important artery in terms of possible hemorrhage following vasectomy if it is not carefully separated from the sheath of the vas or suitably ligated or coagulated. The sheath of the vas in the scrotal portion contains pain nerves. Careful infiltration of the sheath with long-acting local anesthetic agents is valuable in limiting pain.

B. Histology

The human vas deferens is a firm, tubular structure about 3-4 mm in diameter. It is composed of epithelial mucosa, surrounded by a thick, muscular wall and adventitia. Collagen fibers are found interspersed in the muscle layers. The epididymis has two concentric smooth muscle layers that turn into three at the junction of the vas deferens. The middle layer of the three muscle layers gradually thickens as it approaches the urethra, whereas the innermost layer thins and disappears at the ampulla. In turn, these muscle layers are surrounded by adventitia, which contains small branches of the inferior spermatic nerve and blood vessels.

The epithelium and lamina propria of the vas deferens are folded into 8 to 12 longitudinal ridges. The epithelium, which is pseudostratified, is composed predominantly of tall, thin principal cells extending from the base to the lumen and small, round pyramidal basal cells. The principal cells have long stereocilia on their luminal surfaces. Scanning microscopy has revealed that the vas mucosa is carpeted with microvilli, which appear particularly tortuous in man. Surface blebbing of the epithelial cells is a further indication of secretory or absorptive processes.

C. Innervation and Theories of Sperm Transport

Innervation of the vas consists of short adrenergic post-ganglionic neurons (Baumgarten et al. 1975). The nerves of the testis, i.e., the superior spermatic nerves, arise from the renal plexus and inter-mesenteric nerves and travel in association with the testicular arteries, whereas the inferior spermatic nerves arise from the hypogastric plexus and course around and along the vas deferens to innervate the epididymides. In man, the middle spermatic nerves arise from the hypogastric ganglia, whereas innervation to the testis is generally by classical long neurons. At the junction of the epididymis and vas deferens, the amount of adrenergic innervation increases. Histological and pharmacological studies indicate both adrenergic and cholinergic components. Adrenergic fibers, revealed by histochemical fluorescence methods for catecholamines and by electron microscopy, are found in both longitudinal and circular muscles; these fibers are most likely the motor supply of the vas muscle.

Physiological studies and structural studies have been conducted on the vas deferens. Generally, the vasa from most species respond similarly. Stimulation of the hypogastric nerve causes the isolated duct to contract longitudinally. If the vas is bathed in noradrenaline, the intensity of contraction increases (Ventura et al. 1973). If the tissue has been previously exposed to reserpine, the contractions diminish unless the nerve is again exposed to noradrenaline. Phentolamine blocks contractions. Exposure to guanethidine or bethanidine, which especially damage the short adrenergic neurons,

greatly reduces or abolishes contractions. Thus, the pharmacologic evidence as well as the histochemical studies support adrenergic innervation (Batra and Lardner 1976).

The mechanism of sperm transport through the vas deferens is still not totally understood. The heavy, smooth muscle layers equip the vas deferens for vigorous peristalsis. Several hypotheses have been advanced. It is hypothesized that spermatic fluid could be transported by: (1) pressure exerted by the epididymis, (2) peristalsis of the walls of the vas deferens, and (3) active contraction at ejaculation of the wall of the vas deferens constricting the lumen. A combination of these propulsion mechanisms is probable.

Though there are different theories currently under consideration, the sequence of events in sperm transport probably include: (1) continuous movement of spermatozoa through the cauda epididymis and vas deferens due to peristalsis caused by contractions of smooth muscle, (2) emission that involves a coordinated contractile wave from the epididymis to the urethra, (3) strong adrenergically caused contractions of the wall that push the majority of the sperm of each ejaculate through the vas deferens, and (4) propulsion of the sperm to the ampulla and urethra by short, powerful, adrenergically mediated contractions of possibly the cauda epididymis and certainly the vas deferens.

II. CONTRAINDICATIONS TO VASECTOMY

Although vasectomy is a simple operation which can be performed almost anywhere, the more removed the setting is from medical back-up, the more important it is to screen out men who are likely to develop complications.

The major physical contraindications to vasectomy are local infections and systemic blood disorders. Local infections, which can prevent normal healing, are easily recognized and should be treated and cleared up before the operation is performed. Other local conditions which make vasectomy more difficult to perform include: inguinal hernia or previous surgery for hernia or orchiopexy, hydrocele, varicocele, pre-existing scrotal lesions, or a thick, tough scrotum.

Systemic blood disorders which call for special

precautions would include any disease (e.g., hemophilia) that interferes with normal blood clotting. In such cases, the technique used should minimize tissue trauma and emergency equipment should be available. The therapeutic use of anticoagulants may require the same precautions. Other systemic diseases such as diabetes or hypertension are not contraindications to vasectomy but hospitalization may be advisable in case emergencies arise.

There is no physiological basis for an adverse psychological response to vasectomy. Although there is a paucity of reliable information on the subject, available literature suggests that a normal, sexually well-adjusted male will experience no significant psychological changes following elective sterilization if he understands what he can expect during and after the procedure, and if he is given an opportunity to express his fears and have his questions answered in advance (Freund and Davis 1973). When psychological problems do occur postoperatively, they usually stem from preoperative attitudes and conditions.

For the man with serious neuroses or sexual maladjustments, vasectomy may not be advisable. If professional counseling is available, vasectomy candidates with suspected psychological problems should be interviewed and evaluated individually. Tests measuring psychological adjustment indicate that postoperative problems can usually be traced to preoperative ones (Ziegler et al. 1969).

III. PREOPERATIVE COUNSELING AND PREPARATION

A patient's request for vasectomy must be made voluntarily and must be accompanied by written, educated and informed consent. The operative permission must include statements that the man seeking sterilization was given: (1) a fair explanation of the surgical procedure, (2) a description of the attendant discomforts and risks, (3) a description of the benefits to be expected, (4) an explanation concerning appropriate alternative methods of family planning, and the effect and impact of the proposed sterilization, including the fact that it must be considered to be an irreversible procedure, (5) an offer to answer any inquiries concerning the procedure, and (6) information that the individual is free to withhold or withdraw consent to the

procedure at any time prior to the sterilization.

In the counseling process, special attention must be paid to the fact that sterility is not guaranteed, to the immediate physical effects of the procedure, and to the possible long-range psychological reactions. Counseling may be done by a trained non-physician; however, a physician must assume the responsibility for the content of the material provided by the counselor to the patient, for ascertaining that such counseling has been done prior to performance of the procedure, for seeing that all the patient's questions have been satisfactorily answered, and for assuring that informed consent has been obtained.

Consent of the spouse is not required by law, but inclusion of the spouse in the counseling and decision-making process is recommended when feasible. While there should be no rigid guidelines regarding the waiting period between the interview and the performance of the procedure, the physician should use his judgment based upon evaluation of the patient (preferably the couple) as to a reasonable period in which the patient can reflect upon his decision. In general a two to three week period is adequate, but this should be determined individually. The interview should include a general history, system review, attention to previous genital surgery, and any adverse reactions to drugs. Ideally, the patient should receive a complete physical examination following the interview. Attention to genital anomalies, individual characteristics such as associated hydrocele, undescended or retractile testes, scars, or thick scrotum should be noted, so that the surgeon may be prepared to manage them intraoperatively. In some instances the procedure may best be performed in the hospital under anesthesia. The patient should be instructed about the area to be shaved. The hair from the base of the penis extending onto the scrotum should be shaved prior to surgery. Blood count, bleeding and clotting time, urinalysis and semen analysis determinations may be useful.

Preoperative sedation is not advised if the procedure is being performed on an outpatient basis. The outpatient facility should have available emergency equipment, including oxygen, epinephrine, steroids, and other agents, consistent with local standards of ambulatory surgery and local statutory and health code requirements.

IV. TECHNIQUE

Several general statements should be made about vasectomy techniques. Palpation and isolation of the vas from the spermatic cord is the first step in the performance of vasectomy – usually the vas can be identified as a firm cord, approximately 1-2 cm in diameter, unlike other structures of the spermatic cord. Relaxation of the scrotal wall can assist in this maneuver. A warm room and a relaxed patient are essential. The patient is usually apprehensive and appreciates reassurance and a friendly, relaxed attitude on the part of the surgeon. Downward displacement of the testicle assists the surgeon in localizing the vas. Occasionally, a thick, tough scrotum is encountered and vas isolation is difficult and indeed painful. In such instances, the procedure may more appropriately be performed in a hospital setting under general anesthesia.

Though reversibility should not be in the mind of the patient, it should be in the mind of the surgeon. Vasocclusion by simple interruption of vas continuity, closure of the proximal (testicular) end by fulguration of the mucosal surface (Schmidt 1966), or compression by tantulum clip or suture (Leader et al. 1974; Moss 1972) followed by fascial interposition describes the technique considered most acceptable today. The danger of damaging the vital sympathetic innervation of the vas by removing a segment of the vas and accompanying nerves exists. An intact nerve supply may be vital to the transport of sperm from the epididymis at the time of ejaculation, should reanastomosis be performed (Freund and Ventura 1974).

Other technical considerations which may improve chances of restoration of fertility include sectioning of the vas as high as possible away from the convoluted portion, careful preservation of the vas sheath, and preservation of the artery to the vas. Silber (1977) has suggested that fulguration of the distal end of the cut vas be performed rather than of the proximal end, so as to allow sperm leakage to occur. He feels that this will promote sperm leakage and sperm granuloma formation, thereby reducing intravasal and epididymal tubular pressure so as to prevent epididymal rupture. Although an increasing number of surgeons favor the Schmidt technique of mucosal fulguration described above, there is no conclusive evidence that external compression, particularly with inert tantulum clips with fascial interposition, is in any way less effective or more apt to result in sperm granuloma or failure.

Routine resection of the vas for pathologic study is not essential or recommended. The presence of two vas specimens does not substitute for determining the end point of azoospermia. Since the same vas might have been sectioned twice, or a double vas may be present, the patient may still be fertile despite the fact that two separate specimens have been sent to the laboratory. Conversely, if the laboratory cannot confirm the presence of vasa on microscopic examination, the patient may still have had a successful procedure, since tissue can be distorted in removal or lost in transit to the laboratory. All patients must be followed carefully until fully healed and demonstrated to be azoospermic, regardless of the pathology report.

Moreover, removal of a segment is no assurance that spontaneous recanalization cannot occur. This unfortunate complication, though rare (three to four per thousand in large series), is more apt to be prevented by interposition of fascia between the cut ends of the vas and avoidance of the use of catgut suture material. There is also evidence that removing portions of the vas may damage its sympathetic innervation, making subsequent efforts to reestablish fertility less successful, even though continuity of the ends is achieved.

The vas is grasped and fixed between thumb and middle fingers while injecting approximately 3-5 cc of 1 percent procaine into the scrotal skin, scrotal layers and perivasal tissues in the upper scrotal portion of the vas (Figure 1). Anesthetic effect is almost immediate.

An incision is made with the fingers still grasping and fixing the vas (Figure 2). A transverse incision is an acceptable alternative. The incision should be carried into the perivasal tissues.

It is important to clamp and ligate (or coagulate) subcutaneous bleeding points (Figure 3). Attention to this operative detail will prevent hematomas, which can complicate the postoperative course.

The vas is grasped in its sheath with an Allis clamp (Figure 4). With experience, the operator will learn how deep to make the initial incision, with the vas in a fixed position, so that the Allis clamp will grasp the vas in its sheath with a minimal amount of overlying and surrounding tissues.

A vertical incision is made into the vas sheath (Figure 5). Since the vas sheath will serve to provide tissue for a fascial barrier, care should be taken to define and separate the sheath from the vas itself. The definitive occluding procedure should not include the sheath, but should be performed upon the isolated vas. Once the sheath is opened, the vas can be readily mobilized as illustrated in Figure 6, using

a second Allis clamp. It may be advisable to place stay sutures in the vas sheath for future identification.

Two tantalum clips are applied to both the proximal and distal parts between which vas sectioning will be performed (Figure 7a, b). The author prefers tantalum clips since they seem to cause less

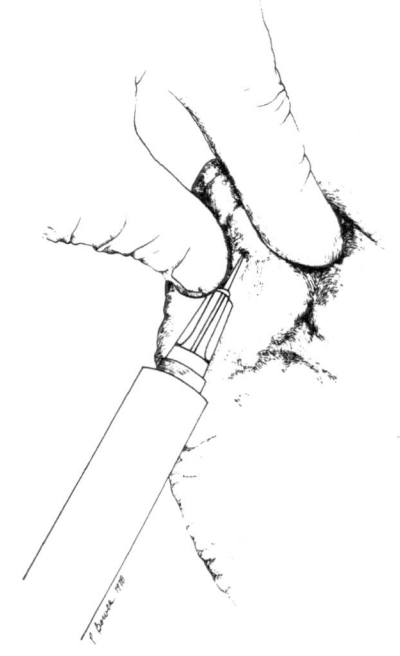

Figure 1.

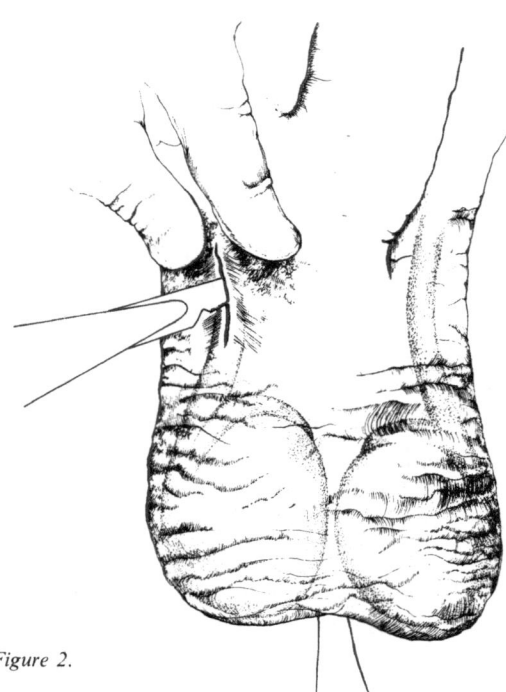

Figure 2.

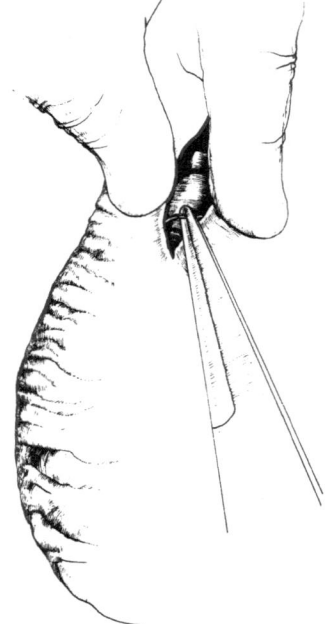

Figure 3.

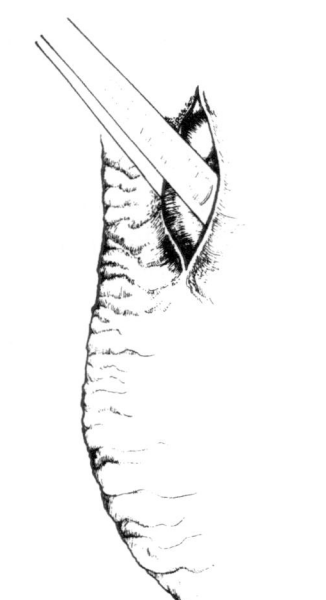

Figure 4.

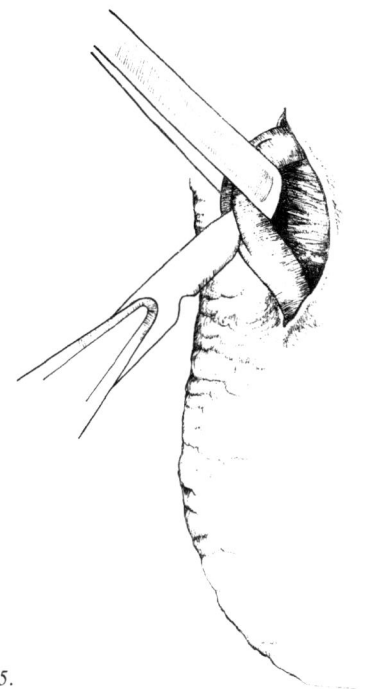

Figure 5.

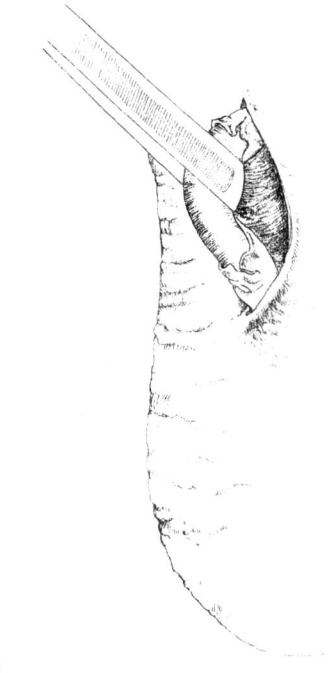

Figure 6.

postoperative reaction and pain, and they are easy to apply.

Previous animal studies (Jhaver et al. 1971) suggested that clip migration could occur, when a clip was applied to the vas in continuity. However, in over 1,000 reported vasectomies using this technique, there has been no evidence of this in the sectioned vas.

The vas sheath is then drawn over the distal end of the vas for fascial interposition (Figure 7c) This maneuver is aided by the tendency of the distal vas (once clipped) to retract distally, and is also assisted by drawing the proximal end forward which further allows for ease in suturing over the distal end. A triple 0 chromic catgut or triple 0 black silk suture is used for connective tissue interposition.

In the vas flush technique, blunt tipped No. 23 gauge needle or attached polyethylene tubing can, with some practice, be inserted into the distal vas lumen (Figure 8). One of several agents (the author has utilized 0.1 percent nitrofurazone solution) can be injected. Approximately 3-4 cc of the solution fills the vas to the ejaculatory duct. The patient usually feels a desire to void, due to stimulation of the ejaculatory duct at the level of the posterior urethra. The purpose of this technique is to shorten the end point of azoospermia. Albert (1974) used

the nitrofurazone solution to flush the distal vas at the time of vasectomy so that in the first ejaculation following the operation there were at most only a few immotile sperm. Following vas flushing, hematospermia has been observed in some cases. This may indicate irritation of the distal tract. Further evaluation of flushing techniques and appropriate agents are required, but they hold the promise of further simplifying vasectomy procedures and reducing the time period to render the patient sterile.

Schmidt (1966) has described an excellent alternative technique (Figure 9). Utilizing coagulating current, fulguration of the proximal vas lumen for a distance of several millimeters is performed. This damages the vas mucosa and allows for the formation of a scar, thereby 'perfecting' vas occlusion by an intraluminal technique, rather than depending upon external compression of the vas wall. It is Schmidt's observation that external compression, particularly with suture material, may result in pressure necrosis and gangrene of the devitalized tissue, allowing the proximal vas to open, followed by sperm leakage and sperm granuloma formation. In some instances the sperm granuloma may present postoperatively as a painful nodule which may be so annoying to the patient as to require excision. Furthermore, recanalization between the proximal and distal ends may develop through the medium of

Figure 7.

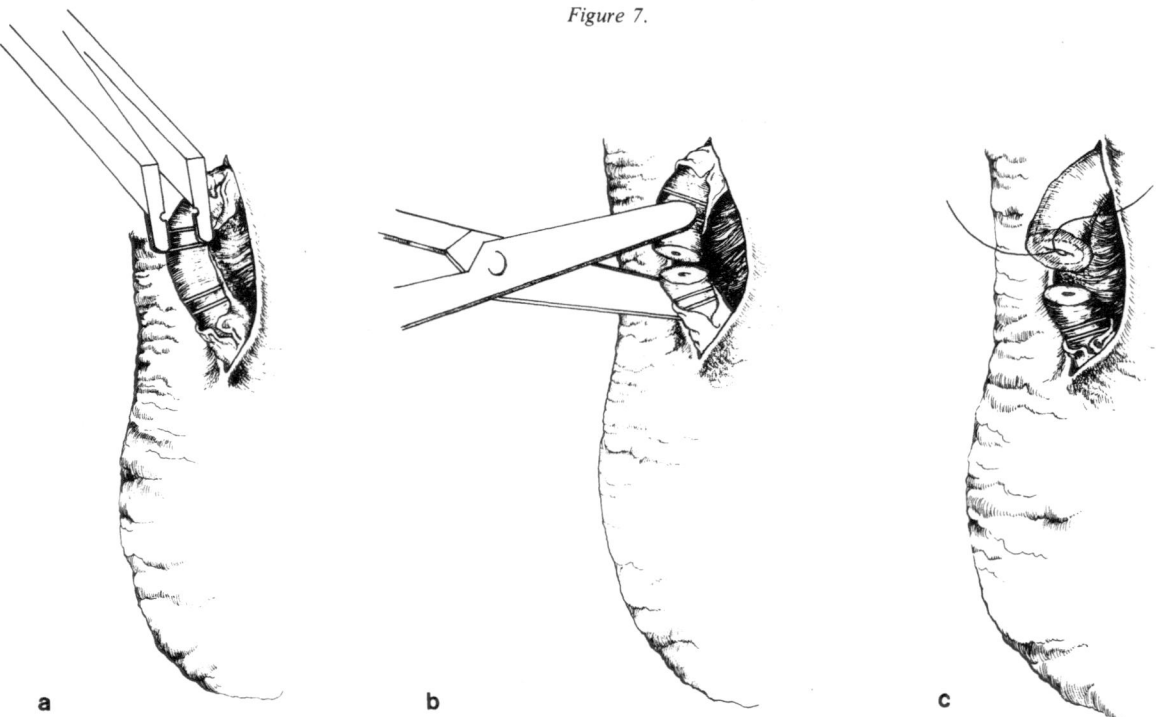

a   b   c

the sperm granuloma. After mucosal fulguration, fascial interposition over the proximal end is usually performed (Figure 9b).

Silber (1978) has recently taken exception to proximal vas occlusion of any type, theorizing that sperm extravasation and granuloma formation may prevent elevated vasal and epididymal pressures. This in turn could prevent intratubular rupture and occlusion in the proximal tract, making the success of vasectomy reversal more likely.

The author utilizes an absorbable suture for skin closure (Figure 10). The patient is told that these sutures will dissolve in one to two weeks, leaving a temporary gap in the skin, which requires a daily dressing until healing is complete. Some surgeons prefer to use nonabsorbable sutures, which require removal after one week. This provides an opportunity to inspect the wound and observe any possible complications.

A percutaneous injection technique for vasocclusion, utilizing a 4 percent formalin solution originally described by Coffey and Freeman (1975) is currently under study by the author. Utilizing a No. 25 gauge needle, 0.5 ml of the agent is injected into the vas through the locally anesthetized scrotal skin. No attempt is made to find the vas lumen, but simply to inject the agent into the vas wall. Very preliminary observations suggest that sperm transport can be affected by this technique, though several injections may be necessary to obtain azoospermia. Long term followup of semen analyses is required.

V. EFFECTS AND SEQUELAE OF VASECTOMY

A. Disappearance of Sperm

Research into vasectomy and its sequelae and effects has resulted in better understanding of the

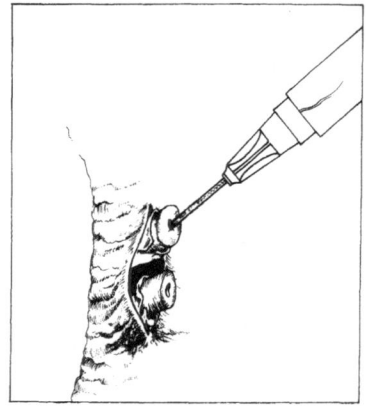

Figure 8.

mechanism of sperm transport during ejaculation. Formerly, urologists had advised a period of from six weeks to several months of contraception following bilateral vasectomy, or until two semen specimens without sperm had been produced. Freund and Davis (1969) determined the exact end point in terms of the number of ejaculations post-vasectomy required to render a patient's semen aspermic. Preoperative and consecutive postoperative semen specimens were studied. Approximately 60 to 70 percent of the sperm found in the normal ejaculate from an intact (i.e., unoperated) man come from that part of the vas proximal to the point of vasectomy and from the epididymis, since the first specimen after vasectomy consistently contained about 30 to 40 percent of sperm found in the preoperative specimen. A constant percentage decrease in sperm output with successive specimens after vasectomy suggested that ejaculation is a true biologic emptying phenomenon, and that at ejaculation approximately 65 percent of the sperm distal to the point of vasectomy are expelled from the vasa. In over 100 patients studied, absence of sperm was noted after six to ten ejaculations following vasectomy. By virtue of this technique, the urologist and the patient, with the cooperation of the laboratory performing the sperm counts, can determine

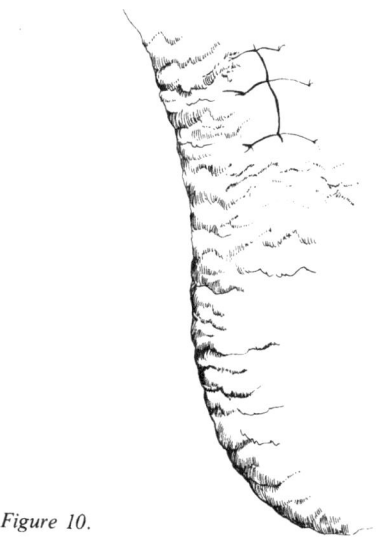

Figure 10.

within a relatively short period of time after the operation that aspermia has been produced, and that the procedure has been successful.

Jouannet and David (1978) repeated and confirmed these findings. They also observed that motile sperm were not observed in freshly ejaculated semen specimens 15 days after successful vasectomy. The reappearance of any number of mobile sperm postvasectomy after 15 days strongly suggested failure or recanalization.

B. Effects of Vasocclusion

Although prospective endocrine studies suggest that there is an increase in mean plasma levels of testosterone and luteinizing hormone and estradiol when compared with mean hormone levels measured prior to vasectomy, the changes were not found to be outside the normal range in adults (Smith et al. 1975). An ongoing prospective study by the National Institute of Health, studying all clinically significant parameters in vasectomized men, matched with comparable nonvasectomized men, has failed to show any abnormality.

Morphologic effects of vasocclusion vary significantly from one species to another (Alexander 1976). For example, sperm granulomata form rapidly in the rat vas and epididymis (Kwart and Coffey 1973). In biopsies of epididymal epithelium from the rhesus monkey (Alexander 1975), similarity of cellular organelles before and after vasectomy indicates that many functions of the epidi-

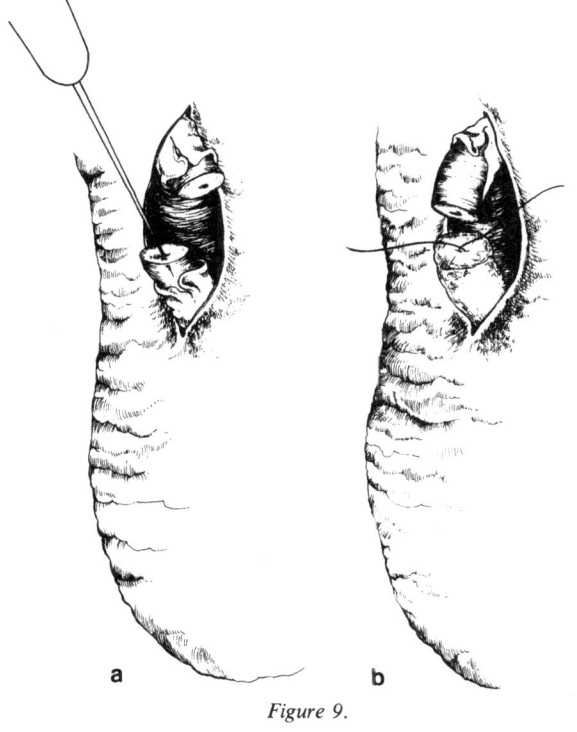

a   b

Figure 9.

dymis, including secretion and resorption, continue and are probably not changed to any great extent. The epithelial cells appear to remain metabolically active.

Kiviat et al. (1978) studied vas specimens obtained during vasovasostomy by scanning and transmission electron microscopy and compared them with vas specimens obtained during vasectomy. Atrophy of microvilli was found in the vasovasostomy specimens on both the proximal and distal sides of the occluded vasa, suggesting that the changes were not due to increased pressure, but to a deprivational state of these cells in which androgenic steroids or some other trophic substance functioning to maintain the height of the epithelial microvilli and normally secreted into the ductal system are decreased or absent.

In men undergoing vasovasostomy, it has become possible to do ultrastructural studies of the testis and to study the long term effects of vasocclusion upon human spermatogenesis (Hagedoorn and Davis 1974). To study the morphologic effects of vasectomy, testicular biopsy specimens from three to seven years postvasectomy were fixed, embedded, and stained for light and electronmicroscopic examination. Sections of the seminiferous tubules showed: (1) the blood supply to the tubules was intact, (2) the lumen of each tubule examined was patent, (3) the Sertoli cells appeared to be intact, with elongated cell outlines, radially oriented, dense cytoplasm, prominent endoplasmic reticulum, lipid droplets, subsurface cisternae adjacent to Sertoli cell junction, and nuclei with characteristic clefts and large tripartite nucleolus. However, a large number of lysosomes were present in the area between the nucleus and basement membrane as intact dense bodies and as membrane coated electron-lucent formation, and (4) the germinal epithelium was present and showed normal stages of spermatogenesis, suggesting that vasectomy does not inhibit sperm formation. Spermatids were seen in the usual clusters of four to five. However, spermatozoa were not observed in their typical location close to the lumen, enwrapped by digitations of Sertoli cells, but rather appeared abutting the basal portion of Sertoli cells, often close to the basement membrane of the tubules. This peculiar location might indicate that these Sertoli cells were acting to absorb or eliminate the

sperm. These ultrastructural findings suggest that the human testicle may actually deal with the sperm which are not ejaculated and which do not pass through the vas deferens. This is a deviation from the current concept of sperm absorption occurring in the epididymis. These studies are in progress, and they will be complemented by studies in animals of a prospective nature to determine ultrastructural and histochemical effects of vasectomy.

The question of immunologic consequences following vasectomy is of great interest today. No systemic diseases of an immunologic nature have been proven to be due to vasectomy, but Zappi et al. (1970) and Ansbacher (1971) have shown that in over 50 percent of men in the first year following vasectomy, there are factors in the serum which cause agglutination of donor sperm. Normally, spermatozoa are sequestered behind a barrier limiting both their potential to immunize the male and their vulnerability to immune damage. Disturbances of this barrier might occur after vasectomy when massive sperm absorption may take place somewhere in the genital tract, or as a result of testicular biopsy through a transient release of an immunizing dose of spermatozoa. This immunity usually is not a high titer response, and it may decline with time. The immunity following vasectomy or biopsy need not be deleterious. When the testis barrier is breached, however, a further possibility arises, namely, autoallergic orchitis. Clinically, the incidence of orchitis following vasectomy is extremely low. Ansbacher (1973) has shown that the titers of humoral antibodies decrease two to three years following vasectomy. The mechanism of the humoral response is not yet known. It should be noted that the standard Kibrick test measures only IgG, while the sperm immobilization test measures both IgG and IgA. The origin of the immune response that may take place after vasectomy in man has not been demonstrated. Although antibodies have been reported in the blood of a certain percentage of men after vasectomy, the antigenic stimulus for antibody production has not been localized. Since the presence of such antibodies in only about one-half the vasectomy patients can be demonstrated, it is difficult to propose a unifying hypothesis. If the immune response is a classic pathophysiologic response in the epididymis to the presence of excess numbers of sperm that takes place weeks, or even months after vasectomy, it should occur in all immunologically competent men. The verification of such a classic immune response requires the experimental demonstration of the steps involved, including the primary reticuloendothelial system response with the presence of IGS-containing lymphocytes, the secondary response in the epididymis which involves macrophage activation with the stimulation of the large lymphocytes to produce the characteristic small lymphocytes, and the migration of the small lymphocytes to the testis. The experimental verification of such an immune response has not as yet been provided, and the need for such research work is urgent.

It is also necessary to characterize the specific immunoglobulins involved in the immune response. The basic research in immunology should have a high priority since it is essential to understand the underlying phenomena involved in view of the anecdotal, unsubstantiated and damaging reports in the lay media on the long term sequelae of vasectomy that are attributed to the immune response.

Undoubtedly pressure changes may occur in the human epididymis following vasocclusion resulting in epididymal blockage due to sperm extravasation, granuloma formation and scarring. Yet clinically, epididymal enlargement and epididymal congestion or inflammation are unusual postoperatively.

C. Other Studies

Reports implying that vasectomy causes such damage as thrombophlebitis, hyperinsulinism, and recurrent infections are anecdotal, but have stimulated wide ranging studies.

Kisker and Alexander (1978) studied vasectomized rhesus monkeys for changes in coagulation factors that might reflect an increased incidence of thrombosis. The results of these tests were compared with nonvasectomized animals, and there were no significant differences between the groups.

Perera (1978) found spermatogenesis to be qualitatively and quantitatively affected after vasectomy with associated epididymal changes, including development of spermatoceles, granulomas, as well as disturbances in the process of sperm maturation.

Wilson et al. (1977) found reduced cell-mediated immunity in vasectomized rhesus monkeys. In this

study, the longer an animal had been vasectomized, the more likely it was to have reduced mitogenic activity. These animals, however, did not manifest a higher incidence of infection or malignancy.

In summary, there does not appear to be any reason to limit vasectomy in men because of its occlusive effects on the testis or epididymis, at this time. The reasonable (and improving) success rates of reanastomosis suggest that in many instances, at least in the human, the vasocclusive effects are reversible.

As yet there is little knowledge as to the effects of vasectomy upon the function of the human epididymis. Jones' (1973) studies in vasectomized rabbits suggested that the procedure does not seriously impair the capacity of the cauda epididymidis to maintain a stable milieu in the lumen of the duct, and it seemed unlikely that the normal maturation and survival of spermatozoa would be effected. He emphasized that if spermatocele formation occurred (due to epididymal rupture), then a different situation might arise and the function of the epididymis might then be impaired. Flickinger (1975) found species variation in the ability of the proximal vas and epididymis to distend following vasectomy. Despite the distention, the epithelium of the epididymis and vas deferens of vasectomized rabbits remained columnar. The epithelium also continued to be functionally active as indicated by the persistence of the characteristic complement of cellular organelles, including vacuoles and lysosomes thought to be involved in secretion. Though the rabbit duct is more distensible and undergoes expansion for months, ultimately the epididymis may rupture and sperm may escape. Thus, regardless of species, sperm may reach the outside of the duct system at some point in time and be phagocytosed by macrophages in connective tissue. Johnson and Howards (1975) measured intratubular hydrostatic pressure in the testis, caput epididymis and cauda epididymis of the golden hamster. Postvasectomy pressures in the cauda were significantly greater than the controls and reflected the accumulation of sperm and fluid. The high incidence of spermatic granuloma formation and/or rupture of the epididymis observed after vasectomy emphasized that in this species there are definite limits to both distensibility and reabsorptive capacity. No similar experimental studies are available in humans, but clinical observation of thousands of vasectomized males over ten years has rarely revealed postvasectomy epididymal lesions, spermatoceles or enlargement of the epididymis. Clinical epididymitis is rare. The mechanism whereby sperm can be accommodated in the epdididymis is still not known, but at least clinicopathologically does not resemble the events which occur in the rabbit, rat and hamster.

VI. COMPLICATIONS

Surgical complications are technique-related, except where anomalous conditions or anatomic variations exist. The physician must pay particular attention to hemostasis and cannot hope for subcutaneous bleeding points to stop by themselves, since the complex scrotal fascial layers do not readily tamponade bleeding. Sterile technique is required. The occurrence of epididymitis, though rare, may be related to infection or may be a result of back pressure from the occluded vas. That this does not occur very often and that gross distension or pain from the epididymis is not noted clinically are indicative of some as yet unknown homeostatic mechanism in the human male, not seen in other animals.

Sperm granuloma is an inflammatory response to the leakage of sperm from the vas or epididymis into surrounding tissues. It has been reported in 0.1 to 3.0 percent of vasectomy cases. Most granulomas are small and harmless, however, and would go unnoticed except in cases of later surgery. Thus, it is estimated that the true incidence may be as high as 20 percent in the vas and 15 percent in the epididymis. Some have been discovered only a few weeks after the procedure, others as long as 25 years later. Although generally asymptomatic, sperm granulomas can be troublesome if they become infected, create vasocutaneous fistulae, cause recanalization of the vas through ducts formed within the granuloma, or if they prevent later surgical reanastomosis. In theory at least, an immune response may result from absorption of sperm from the granuloma.

A diagnosis of sperm granuloma should be considered if the patient complains of pain and swelling at the site of vasectomy one or two weeks postoperatively. Specifically, if the patient has been asymptomatic for some time after the operation, a sudden onset of pain suggests a granuloma; but because their symptoms are similar, cancer, tuberculosis and neoplasms should first be ruled out. On gross examination, granulomas begin as an inflammatory response surrounding creamy-white, thick, seminal fluid. The initial lesion is usually pea-sized. If the lesion becomes large and cystic, its contents may become tinged with blood. As the inflammation subsides, the lesion becomes yellowish-brown, and the walls become fibrous and sometimes calcified.

A sperm granuloma should be considered a complication, not a necessary sequela of vasectomy. Sperm extravasation and resultant granuloma formation may be preventable by the fulguration technique of Schmidt or by techniques of compression by inert instruments such as tantalum clips. Sutures, especially catgut, which cause pressure necrosis are more apt to be a setting for sperm leakage. As stated above, Silber feels that sperm granuloma should be allowed to occur to reduce proximal intravasal and epididymal pressure, anticipating the need for reversal. However, recanalization is more apt to occur in an area of sperm granuloma, according to Schmidt.

Although vasectomy is not completely foolproof, it is the most effective male method of fertility control now available, and it is becoming more effective as practitioners gain greater skill and experience. Studies conducted in the late 1960s reported failure rates up to four per 100 procedures performed. Recent studies show failure rates of less than one per 100 procedures (Hackett and Waterhouse 1973). This decline probably reflects increased experience and the use of more effective and less traumatizing operative techniques. Nevertheless, a vasectomy candidate should understand that a small possibility of failure exists.

Failure may or may not result in pregnancy in the female partner. Failure is usually discovered when semen examinations indicate the presence of sperm more than three months after the operation or after 10 to 12 ejaculations, when there are motile sperm in the semen after a period of azoospermia, or when pregnancy takes place in the female partner. Although the female partner may be impregnated by another male, pregnancy in the partner accompanied by the appearance of even a few motile sperm in a patient's semen is generally conclusive.

The likelihood of recanalization may be influenced by the vasectomy technique employed. For example, crushing and tying the vas, particularly with absorbable sutures, a widely used procedure, can lead to recanalization. Members of the workshop on clinical aspects of male sterilization at the 1973 Geneva conference on voluntary sterilization agreed that separating the treated vas ends with a barrier of fascia is an effective means of preventing vasectomy failure (Schima et al. 1974).

The likelihood of operative failure is reduced if the surgeon has performed the procedure frequently. The importance of frequent practice was emphasized by Sobrero et al. (1973) of the Margaret Sanger Research Bureau, New York. They reported six failures in 236 procedures performed during the first year of the vasectomy service at the Bureau. Four of these procedures were performed by physicians-in-training and two by general surgeons with little experience in the operation. Failure also results from inadequate occlusion of the vas ends. If ligatures or clips are applied too loosely, sperm continue to pass through the vas; if they are applied

too tightly, they may cut through the vas wall and permit the sperm to exit.

VII. CONCLUSIONS

Vasectomy (vas sectioning and occlusion) is a short, outpatient surgical procedure which has a demonstrable end point of azoospermia after ten to fifteen ejaculations (or shorter, using one of several vas flushing methods now available). As a contraceptive method, it is not coitally related, appears in prospective studies to cause no hormonal, biochemical or other changes in the human male, and with appropriate screening and counseling it should result in no psychological problems. Refinements and improvements in technique, especially sectioning without resecting vas to preserve blood and nerve supply, and emphasis on high sectioning of the vas away from the convoluted portion appear to result in even less postoperative discomfort and morbidity; and, as an added benefit, refinements may offer a better chance should a reversal be desired.

REFERENCES

Albert PS, Mininberg DT and Davis JE: Nitrofurans: Sperm immobilizing agents. Urology 4: 307, 1974.

Alexander NJ: Immunologic and morphologic effects of vasectomy in the rhesus monkey. Federation proceedings 34: 1692, 1975.

Alexander NJ: Vasectomy: Morphological and immunological effects. In: Human semen and fertility regulation in men, Hafez (ed), Chapter 28, St. Louis, CV Mosby, 1976.

Ansbacher R: Sperm agglutinating and sperm-immobilizing antibodies in vasectomized men. Fertility and Sterility 22: 629, 1971.

Ansbacher R: Vasectomy, sperm antibodies. Fertility and Sterility 24: 788, 1973.

Batra SK and Lardner TJ: Sperm transport in the vas deferens. In: Human semen and fertility regulation in men. Hafez (ed), Chapter 10, St. Louis, CV Mosby, 1976.

Baumgarten HG, Owman C and Sjoberg NO: Neural mechanisms in male fertility. In: Control of male fertility, Sciarra, Markland, Spiedel (eds), Chapter (26-40), Hagerstown, MD, Harper and Row, 1975.

Coffey DS and Freeman C: Vas injection: a new, non-surgical procedure to induce sterility in human males. In: Control of male fertility. Sciarra JJ, Markland C and Speidel J (eds). Hagerstown, Ind, Harper and Row, 1975.

Craft I and McQueen J: Effect of irrigation of the vas on post-vasectomy semen counts. Lancet 1: 515, 1972.

Flickinger CJ: Fine structure of rabbit epididymis and vas deferens after vasectomy. Biology of Reproduction 13: 50, 1975.

Freund M and Davis JE: Disappearance rate of spermatozoa from the ejaculate following vasectomy. Fertility and Sterility 20: 163, 1969.

Freund M and Davis JE: A follow-up study of the effects of vasectomy on sexual behavior. The Journal of Sex Research 9 (3): 241-268, 1973.

Freund M and Ventura W: Male sterilization – basic science aspects. In: Advances in voluntary sterilization (Proceedings of the Second International Conference, Geneva, Feb. 25-Mar. 1, 1973). Schima ME, Lubell I, Davis JE and Connel E (eds), American Elsevier Publishing Co, Inc, 1974, p 338-345.

Hackett RE and Waterhouse K: Vasectomy – reviewed. Amer J Obstetrics and Gynecology 116 (3): 438, 1973.

Hagedoorn JP and Davis JE: Fine structure of the seminiferous tubules after vasectomy in man. Physiologist 17: 236, 1974.

Hulka JF and Davis JE: Sterilization of men. In: Human reproduction – conception and contraception. Hafez and Evans (eds), Chapter 19, Hagerstown, Md, Harper and Row, 1973.

Jhaver PS, Davis JE, Lee H, Hulka JF and Leight G: Reversibility of sterilization produced by vas occlusion clip. Fertility and Sterility 22: 263, 1971.

Johnson AL and Howards SS: Intratubular hydrostatic pressure in testis and epididymis before and after vasectomy. Amer J Physiology 228: 586, 1975.

Jones R: Epididymal function in the vasectomized rabbit. J Reprod Fert 36: 199, 1973.

Jouannet P and David G: Evolution of the properties of semen immediately following vasectomy. Fertility and Sterility 29: 435, 1978.

Kisker CT and Alexander NJ: Coagulation changes following vasectomy: A study in primates. Fertility and Sterility 29 (5); 543, 1978.

Kiviat MD, Eddy EM and Chapman WH: Changes induced in the epithelial surface of the vas deferens by vasectomy of long standing. Surg Gyn & Ob 147: 328, 1978.

Kwart AM and Coffey DS: Sperm granulomas: Adverse effects of vasectomy. Journal of Urology 110: 416, 1973.

Leader AJ, Axelrod SD, Frankowski R, Mumford SD: Complications of 2,711 vasectomies. Journal of Urology 111 (3): 365-339, 1974.

Moss WM: A sutureless technique for bilateral partial vasectomy. Fertility and Sterility 23: 33, 1972.

Perera BM and Oswin A: Changes in the structure and function of the testes and epididymides in vasectomized rams. Fertility and Sterility 29 (3): 354, 1978.

Schima M, Lubell I, Davis JE, Connell E (eds): Advances in voluntary sterilization, p 232. Excerpta Medica American Elsevier Publishing Co, 1974.

Schmidt SS: Technics and complications of elective vasectomy: the role of spermatic granuloma in spontaneous recanaliza-tion. Fertility and Sterility 17: 467, 1966.

Silber SJ: Microscopic vasectomy reversal. Fertility and Sterility 28 (11): 1191, 1977.

Silber SJ: Vasectomy and vasectomy reversal. Fertility and Sterility 29 (2): 125, 1978.

Smith KD, Chowdhury M, Teholakian RK: Endocrine effects of vasectomy in humans. In: Control of male fertility, Sciarra JJ, Markland C and Spiedel J (eds), Hagerstown, Md, Harper and Row, 1975, p 169.

Sobrero AJ, Kohli KL, Edey H, Davis JE and Karp R: A vasectomy service in a free-standing family planning center: One year's experience. Social Biology 20 (3): 303, 1973.

Ventura WP, Freund M and Davis JE: Influence of norepine-phrine on the motility of human vas deferens. Fertility and Sterility 24: 68, 1973.

Wilson BJ, Alexander NJ, Porter G and Fulgham D: Cell mediated immunity in vasectomized rhesus monkeys. Fertility and Sterility 28 (12): 1349, 1978.

Zappi E, Ahmed U, Davis J, Shulman D: Immunologic conse-quences of vasectomy. Federation Proceedings 29: 728, 1970.

Ziegler FJ, Rodgers DA and Prentiss RJ: Psychosocial response to vasectomy. Archives of General Psychiatry 21: 46-54, 1969.

Ziegler FJ: Vasectomy and adverse psychological reaction. Annals of Internal Medicine 73: 853, 1970.

14. VASOVASOSTOMY

S.S. SCHMIDT

Almost one-half of American couples between the ages of 30 and 44 have resorted to sterilization as a means of birth control (Ford 1978). Single men and women who have undergone sterilizing surgery are in equal numbers. The statement that vasectomy is the operation most frequently performed upon adult males is thus supported. Not surprisingly, some of these men wish or are convinced that they wish to have their fertility restored: once one in 400 patients, they are now one in 300 in my practice.

I. RESTORATION OF FERTILITY: THE FACTS

Before a vasectomy, I inform all candidates that a reversal is often successful. Unfortunately, many physicians still tell their patients that it is impossible to rejoin the vas, thus preventing some men from seeking it. An information booklet displays bureaucratic stupidity by stating, 'Can vasectomy be undone? No!' (California State Department of Health 1977). A vasectomy should always be done so that a spontaneous reanastomosis is prevented, but a deliberate surgical anastomosis is later possible. Every surgeon has a duty to tell his patients that a vas anastomosis may be attempted in the future – but that it does not always succeed. Happily, successes are becoming more common as the problems of vasovasostomy are better understood and as familiarity with the surgical procedure increases (Schmidt 1975; Silber 1977; Middleton and Henderson 1978).

Who seeks restoration of fertility, and why? Almost all men undergoing sterilization by vasectomy fully intend it to be permanent. Indeed, any man who has a vasectomy with the intent of a later reversal shows great imprudence, since various circumstances may cause reversals to fail, regardless of who performs the operation.

Happily, the most feared event – death of a child or of an entire family – is the reason given least frequently by candidates for vasovasostomy. Usually, the vasectomized man has remarried, often to a younger woman who either has never had children of her own or who wishes to have a child by this husband 'to make the marriage more secure'. The husband's mind is thus influenced. In these circumstances, it is usually the wife who inquires about the operation, who is delighted to hear that surgical reversal of the vasectomy is possible and who makes the appointment for her husband. In such cases, followup appointments are frequently difficult to secure. The husband feels that one operative attempt is sufficient and fears that a demonstrated failure will cause his wife to insist that he undergo a second anastomosis. Therefore, he avoids testing. When it is the man himself who wishes to have his fertility restored, he is likely to be a fully cooperative patient.

Most patients undergoing vasovasostomy have had children previously, thus have proved their fertility. However, there are men who are sterilized without knowing whether they are fertile. Most of them, although not all, prove to have been fertile originally. Occasionally, it is necessary to later correct a varicocele or to assist the patient in some other way to increase his fertility after the vasovasostomy. Sometimes one encounters patients (and their wives) who keep changing their minds. I have one patient upon whom I have performed two vasectomies, and two vasovasostomies, all successful.

II. OPERATION: GENERAL CONSIDERATIONS

Many of the surgical principles governing a vaso-vasostomy are peculiar to this operation and differ from those for surgery of other ducts in other parts of the body.

Before discussing these points, it must be emphasized that an overriding factor is that the surgeon has usually had no control over the original vasectomy and must work with the results of an operation done by someone else. Many different techniques are used for performing vasectomies, and some of them are difficult to follow (Figure 1). Frequently, the vas is divided in its convoluted portion, sometimes even at its origin from the epididymis. In an attempt to guarantee a successful vasectomy, different lengths of vas may be excised unnecessarily, even to the entire scrotal vas from the epididymis to the external inguinal ring. Occasionally, one must follow another surgeon's unsuccessful vasovasostomy. Recently, I encountered a vaso-vasostomy done by a technique in which absorbable sutures had been used. There was a minimum of reaction at the site of vas junction, patency of anastomosis had been secured on one side, and there was an obstruction of the epididymis on that side. As one can imagine, inspection and palpation of that vas failed to disclose the point of previous anastomosis, and probing revealed only patency of the vas. Fortunately, most often the site of vasectomy is detectable by palpating either as a thickening or as a defect in the vas.

III. PRINCIPLES OF VASOVASOSTOMY

It is easier to perform anastomosis in the straight portion of the vas and when there is little or no defect in the vas length. Sometimes, however, it may be necessary to elevate the cauda of the epididymis or to invade the inguinal canal in order to secure enough length to approximate the vas ends.

The vas is thick walled, with a lumen that has a mean diameter of 1.0 mm (third to half of the total diameter of the vas) (Brueschke et al. 1974). This is in marked contrast to the thin walls of the ureter or of blood vessels. Therefore, a somewhat different management in doing the anastomosis is necessary.

The lumen of the testicular side of the vas dilates after obstruction, at the expense of the muscular wall (Figure 2). In the straight vas, this increases the mean diameter of the lumen by 70 percent, the outside diameter remaining unchanged (Schmidt and Brueschke 1976). This dilatation begins after vasectomy and appears to reach a maximum at about six months, after which it is apparently permanent. If this dilatation is not found, one should suspect a more proximal obstruction either in the epididymis or in the vas, reminiscent of the obstructions that can follow a gonorrheal or tubercular vasitis (there are surgeons who obstruct the vas in two places when performing a vasectomy). If both testicular and urethral sides are dilated, a distal obstruction is usually present, either in the vas or in the ejaculatory duct. When the usual one-sided dilatation is found, *one must anastomose lumens of different diameters.*

Spermatic granuloma of the vas lessens the luminal dilatation of the testicular end and keeps spermatozoa flowing through the vas to the granuloma, where they are digested (Silber 1977). These factors make the likelihood of a successful anastomosis more favorable when such a granuloma is found. *However, one should never perform a vasectomy in such a way that a granuloma will result.* Granulomas are abscesses and when they involve the spermatic nerve, the resulting pain may be extreme (Schmidt 1979).

End-to-end anastomoses are more successful. Because the walls of the vas are thick, spatulated, oblique and side-to-side anastomoses are less practical (Figure 3). This thickness of walls makes the completed anastomosis rigid, so that kinking cannot occur. Stents are unnecessary to align and support the anastomosis and may even cause its obstruction or obstruction at the point of emergence of the stent.

The anastomosis must be watertight and sperm-tight. Should sperm leak through the suture line, a spermatic granuloma may follow, with concomitant obstruction, pain or both (Schmidt 1959). Within the vas, the mucosa must be accurately approximated so that there is no raw area between its margins. The muscular wall of the vas should be compressed against the other side to seal and strengthen the anastomosis (Figure 4). A mucosal defect, when exposed to sperm, may lead to a fibrous contracture and occlusion of the lumen, just

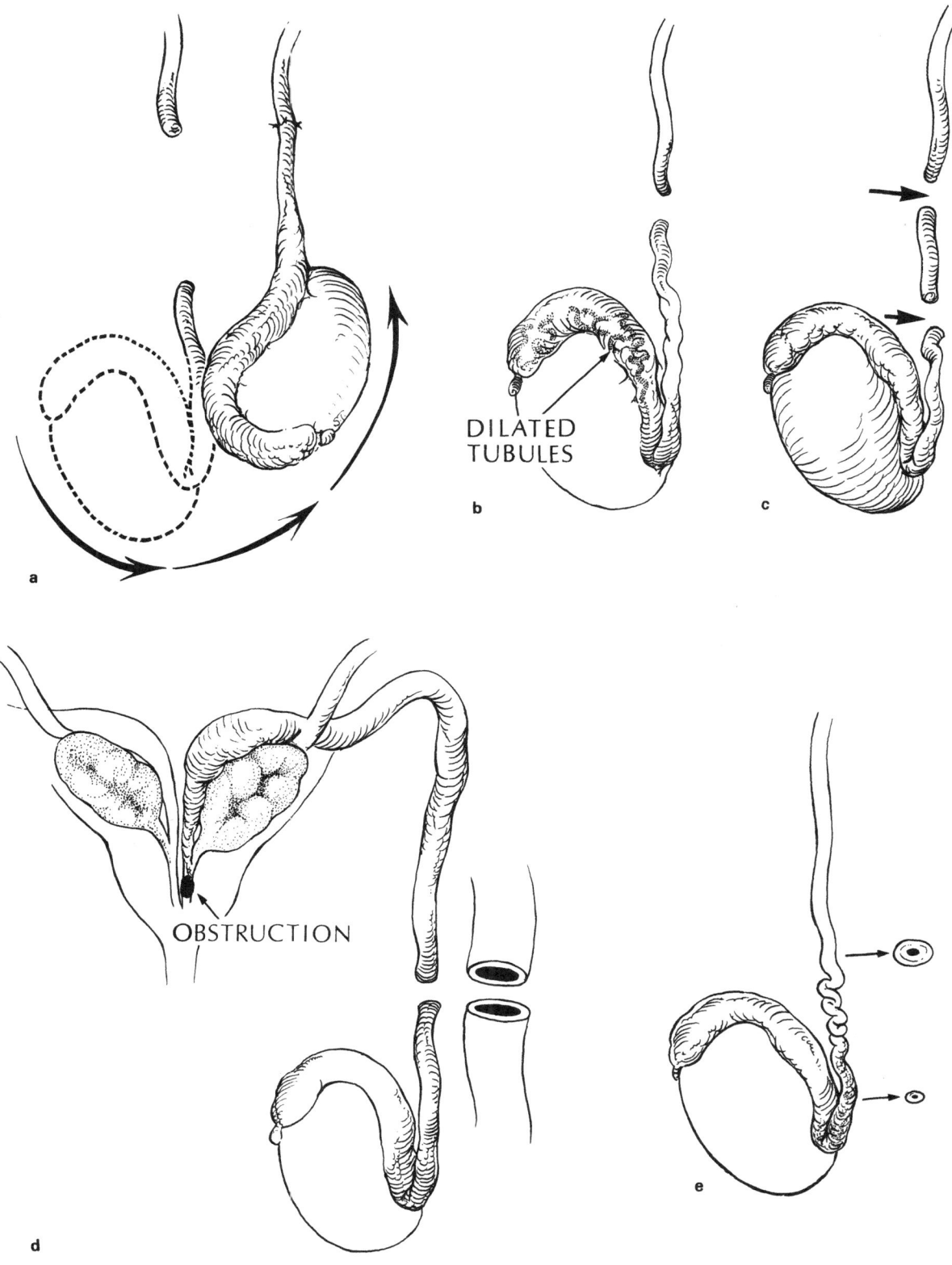

Figure 1. Possible problems created by previous vasectomy: a. Large defect in vas – which necessitates inverting testis in order to join vas ends. b. Obstruction in lower third of epididymis, with concomitant absence of spermatozoa in vas fluid. c. Vas interrupted in two places. d. Obstruction in ejaculatory duct (distal to point of vasectomy) with urethral side of vas dilated. e. In convoluted vas note · smaller diameter near epididymis.

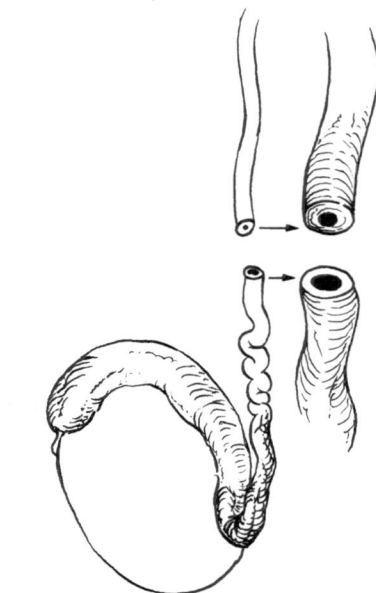

Figure 2. Cross sections of vas showing dilatation of lumen on testicular side.

as an area of raw skin, ungrafted, may lead to a contracture (Hagan and Coffey 1977). When the muscle has been accurately sutured, the fine film of blood clot between the muscular faces of the anastomosis will act as nature's own tissue cement to make the anastomosis even more watertight. In the absence of proper suturing, however, it may not prevent leakage of sperm.

Fine, nonreactive, monofilament sutures should be used. Braided sutures may act as a conduit for

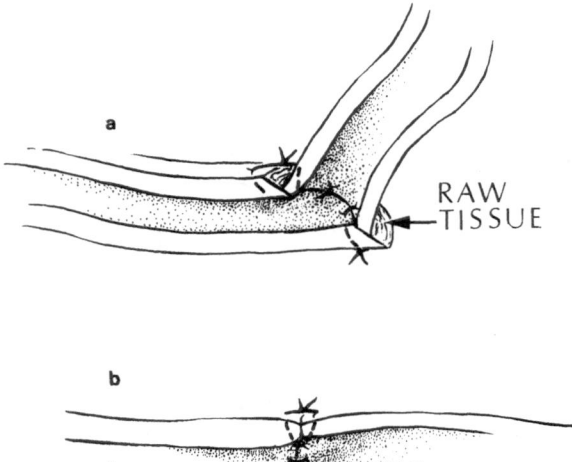

Figure 3. Oblique (a) versus straight (b) anastomosis.

sperm to leak from the lumen and reactive sutures add additional inflammation to an area where healing with a minimum of inflammation is desired. Nylon and polypropylene, in sizes 7-0, 9-0 and 10-0 (which is 1/3 to 1/5 the diameter of pubic hair [DeHaan, unpublished study]) are most commonly used (Figure 5). Tissue sections fail to show reaction around these sutures, even when the latter enter the lumen of the vas. They should be tied firmly without cutting through the tissue.

Unless a gross defect in the vas exists, *reinforcing fascial sutures is unnecessary to support the anastomosis,* since an anastomosis made with even 10-0 nylon has surprising strength.

Optical aids and special instruments should be used in performing the operation. The naked eye is simply not capable of accurate placement of suture as fine as 10-0 at the cut mucosal edge. Magnification helps the physician to perform the task more easily and with greater precision. Additionally, microsurgical instruments have been designed for operation on minute structures: with practice, the surgeon is better able to handle tissues gently, to guide tiny needles properly, to place them accurately, and to tie the sutures without breaking them. I use a visor (magnification $2\frac{1}{2} \times 8$ inch focal distance) to dissect out the vas ends and an operating microscope ($6 \times$ magnification for tying knots; $10 \times$, $16 \times$ and $25 \times$ for placing sutures). However, it is not sufficient to merely possess the microscope and the microsurgical instruments; courses in microsurgery are available and the surgeon should secure instruction in these techniques before attempting to use them upon his patients (Owen 1976). Similarly, the surgeon who does a vasovasostomy only occasionally will not be as accurate as the surgeon who performs the operation frequently. The once-a-year vas anastomosis should be referred to a specialist.

Occasionally, the vas is obstructed above the scrotum on the side possessing a good testis, and open on the side of an atrophic testis or a testis with a scarred epididymis: in such a case, *a crossover* (right to left, or vice versa) *vasovasostomy can be carried out with full anticipation of success* (Figure 6).

In most cases, *if the operation does not succeed on the first try, it may be repeated* with good expectation. Since both sides of the vas are usually anastomosed, and since one patent side is sufficient to

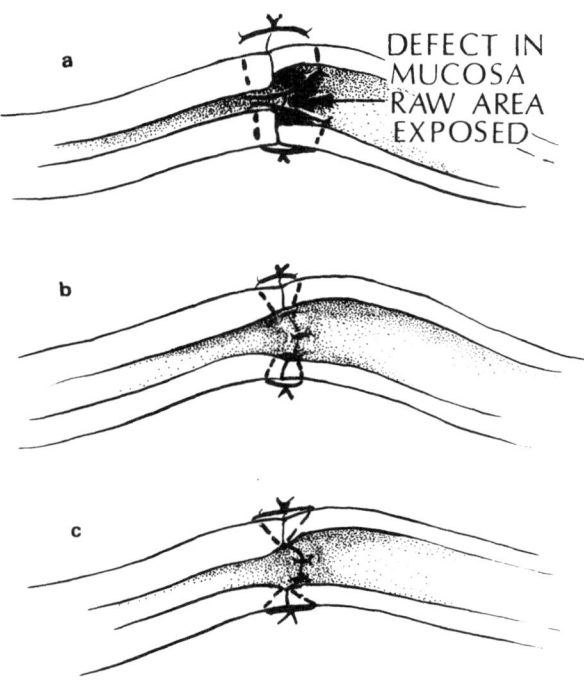

Figure 4. Types of full thickness sutures: square (a), narrow triangle (b), and *broadbases triangle* (c) (best).

bring about a pregnancy, the odds are favorable.

The operation can be performed – in a manner comfortable for both patient and surgeon – as an outpatient procedure under local anesthesia. For years, I felt that the patient should be hospitalized and that he should be operated upon while under general anesthesia: I now wonder why it took so long for me to change that opinion. My last 150 or more patients have been under local anesthesia (both during vasovasostomies and epididymovaso-

stomies), and I do not intend to return to utilization of general anesthesia. Complete anesthesia of the scrotal contents is easy to attain. The site of operation is immobilized with a suspensory that permits undisturbed healing. Administration of codeine seems adequate to control discomfort. In short, hospitalization and general anesthesia involve additional expense and discomfort for the patient without offering any advantages.

IV. REQUIREMENTS FOR OPTIMAL SURGICAL RESULTS

A. The setting

What, then, is required to perform the operation in an easy, successful manner? First, a sterile operating area, suitably equipped, is needed. This may be found in a hospital, but is increasingly available in the surgeon's office. When only local anesthesia is employed, the requirements for such an area are simplified. Adequate operating lights may be portable, as long as they procure a six-inch spot of light. I employ an excellent portable light

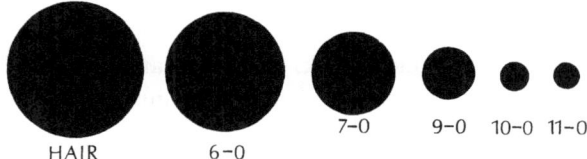

Figure 5. Comparative sizes of sutures and of pubic hair in cross-section.

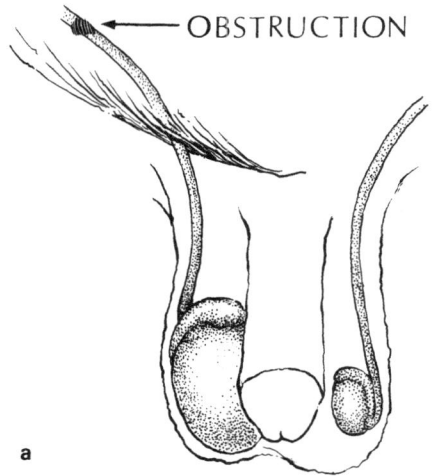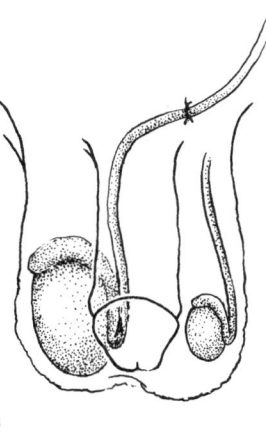

Figure 6. a. Vas obstructed from good testis. Vas open from atrophic testis. b. Successful crossover anastomosis.

which uses only a 60 watt bulb. A trained assistant accelerates and facilitates the operation, and provides support for the surgeon. If necessary, however, a vasovasostomy can be performed without assistance.

B. The instruments

An electrosurgical unit, which provides a coagulating circuit, is needed for hemostasis and is used with a needle electrode for pinpoint coagulation of fine vessels. Disposable sterile packs of paper gowns and drapes are readily available. A small dissecting set, containing scalpel, forceps (regular and Adson, toothed and serrated) and hemostats (straight and curved mosquito clamps, possibly including several Jacobson mosquito clamps) will serve as a basic set of tools.

Additional instruments for either vasovasostomy or epididymovasostomy include: Pediatric Allis clamps to grasp and hold the vas – they fit around it without crushing or otherwise harming its tissues; a basic set for microsurgical surgery (Barranquer needle holders, Pierse Corneal forceps with either 0.3 mm or 0.1 mm teeth; No. 5 straight and No. 7 curved jeweler's forceps; tying forceps; and Castroviejo type scissors, Edward Weck and Co. Inc.. Research Triangle Park, N.C.). Many types of clamps are available for vas approximation, but I find most of them awkward to use. Syringes are needed for both anesthesia and irrigation. I prefer to use a No $27 \times {}^5/_8$ hypodermic needle for anesthesia and a blunt tipped No. 23 needle for irrigation and for testing the urethral vas for patency. I use 9-0 and 10-0 double armed nylon sutures in the vas, whereas I prefer a 3-0 plain catgut with a swaged needle for stay sutures and to close the skin. For probing the vas, No. 0 or No. 00 nylon works well.

C. Optical aids

For optical assistance, I use an OptiVISOR model E with $2\frac{1}{2} \times$ lenses. By merely tilting one's head, normal vision is changed to magnified vision. This does not interfere with vision through the operating microscope. I use the Zeiss OPMI 1 operating microscope, changing magnification manually as needed. Finer, more expensive microscopes are available, some of which permit both surgeon and assistant to view the operative field, to focus and magnify by motor, etc. These instruments are superb, but I can work comfortably with the simpler models.

D. The operation proper: Importance of anesthesia

The best local anesthesia is that administered to a confident, relaxed person (one only has to think of the frightened dental patient, whose jaw is completely anesthetized, but who becomes rigid at the approach of the drill). Friendly conversation is a reliable and simple method of relaxation.

Since many of my vasovasostomy patients come from rather distant areas, the patients are met and examined the day before surgery. They are asked about the date of their vasectomy, postvasectomy complications, general health, sensitivity to drugs and whether they have had children. They are informed about local hotels and restaurants. The patients are instructed to shave their genitalia and to have a light breakfast the next morning – with only one cup of liquid to avoid the possibility of a full bladder during operation.

They receive an intramuscular injection (100 to 125 mg of meperidine hydrochloride) of a sedative *after* they are on the operating table, so that the effect will be rapid and will last the duration of the operation. The scrotum is examined for location of vasectomy, possible presence of spermatic granuloma of the vas, defect in the vas, testicular size and consistency, and for any possible pathologic conditions of the epididymis. When possible, urinalysis is done to rule out infection or presence of sugar. Everything is done in a reassuring manner, with the intent of relaxing the patient and gaining his confidence.

To avoid delay and nervousness on the morning of the operation, the preadmission paperwork is usually carried out the afternoon before at the hospital. On that morning, the patient is dressed in an operating room gown and shaving of the genitalia is completed when necessary. The skin is prepared with antibacterial solutions (never mercurials) and draped. An area overlying the vasectomy site is selected, and the skin and subcutaneous tissues are infiltrated between cutaneous vessels for a distance of 5 cm with 1 percent lidocaine, containing 1:100,000 epinephrine. This area is the only one to receive this type of anesthesia.

The skin is then incised and the subcutaneous tissue is spread apart for the length of the incision. At this point the patient often asks whether the incision has been made yet, or if the operation has begun – which indicates a successful anesthesia. The vas is next grasped with the fingers and the perivasal tissues are filled with 1 percent lidocaine *without* epinephrine. At this point it is important to remember that the sheath of the vas is composed of many layers, derived from the abdominal fascia. Nerve filaments run in these layers, particularly the innermost one. Thus, these layers should be filled with lidocaine, and especially that next to the vas. The arteries to the testis communicate with each other and course with the vas, making testicular ischemia likely if epinephrine were part of the anesthetic mixture – not to mention the possibility of delayed bleeding.

The vas is then grasped gently with an Allis clamp, so that additional anesthetic may be injected more exactly into the perivasal tissues toward the urethra. Only then, and cautiously, is this clamp locked around the vas. At this time testicular anesthesia is usually complete.

E. Site of vasectomy

The sheath of the vas is incised longitudinally down to the vas itself and opened to the point of previous vasectomy: this area is usually marked by scarring, a defect in the vas or nonabsorbable suture material, but locating it may be a tedious and slow task. Frequently (one case in three), a spermatic granuloma of the testicular end of the vas is visible as a cluster of creamy yellow or golden yellow nodules. Often, the lumen on the testicular side is filled with cream colored spermatic fluid – a favorable prognostic sign. Yet, occasionally none of these signs are found and the site of vasectomy is undetectable.

While scarring of the sheath may indicate the location of vasectomy, it is sometimes necessary to partially transect the vas so that a probing nylon suture or blunt hypodermic needle may enter the lumen and saline solution be injected to prove patency to the urethra. An outflow of spermatic fluid at this point will indicate that the vasotomy is on the testicular side of the obstruction, while an undilated lumen will suggest that the obstruction is toward the testis. In the latter case, one may need to open the tunica vaginalis and inspect the epididymis, looking for dilated tubules. These dilated tubules often extend only to the middle or lower portion, and empty tubules in the cauda epididymidis indicate the location of the obstruction. Whatever the findings, this vasotomy is easily closed with several full thickness sutures of fine nylon. Saline solution may be injected through a fine needle passed obliquely through the vas wall into the lumen; however this method does not permit as accurate probing as a vasotomy.

F. Vas transection and dissection

When the point of vasectomy is obvious, the vas is transected on either side to expose the lumen and to conserve vas length. It is not desirable to resect the vasectomy scarred tissue or a granuloma (lest blood and nerve supply be impaired); thus, this tissue is simply pushed to the side. I dissect the fascia free from the vas for a distance of only 5 mm so that it will not be caught in the anastomosis and trauma to the tissues will be minimal. Other surgeons deliver the testis out of the scrotum and dissect the vas away from its sheath for several centimeters on each side, finding it easier to use approximating clamps. They claim that this procedure does not produce ischemia of the vas. I prefer to leave the testis in the scrotum and to mobilize only the vas ends.

The testicular end of the vas usually emits spermatic fluid, either clear or creamy white. This fluid is examined microscopically for presence of spermatozoa. Sometimes motile spermatozoa are seen, sometimes spermatozoa heads without tails, and sometimes merely amorphous debris (Figure 7). If spermatozoa are not seen initially, a continued flow of spermatic fluid may eventually show them. For this reason, repeated examinations are in order. It is safe to strip the vas to secure fluid (or to empty it of fluid so that it will not flood the anastomotic site), but one should not squeeze the more easily traumatized epididymis. When no fluid is present in the vas, the epididymis should be inspected. Patency of the urethral side is proved by injecting saline solution up the vas.

I next place a stay suture in the sheath to

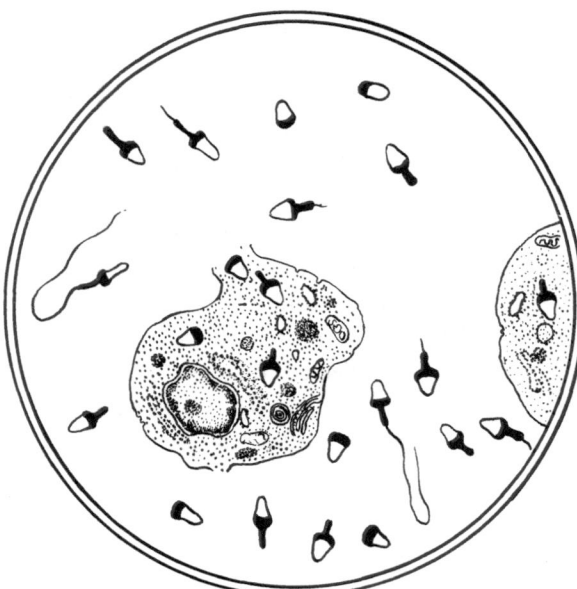

Figure 7. Spermatic fluid from vas containing phagocytes with ingested spermatozoa heads and free spermatozoa heads.

approximate the vas ends until they almost touch, and bring these ends up out of the scrotum (Figure 8). From there on to the completion of the procedure, I work with the help of the microscope.

G. Mucosa to mucosa approximation and Sutures

Inasmuch as the lumens of the vas ends will differ in diameter, it is a challenge to approximate mucosa to mucosa, without raw tissue at the suture line. The mucosa is attached somewhat loosely to the muscularis, thus the urethral side of the lumen can be dilated with the help of special forceps (modified No. 7 jeweler's forceps, Norris Graham, Louisville, Kentucky) until it has the same diameter as the testicular end; the sutures can then be placed. Since the sutures are commonly made with needles swaged on both ends, the posterior suture is placed first, from lumen side out (Figure 9). The needles enter the wall of the vas just at the cut edge of the mucosa and emerge from the muscular wall about 3 mm from the vas end, so that a triangular suture is made, with the apex of the triangle bringing mucosa and emerge from the muscular wall about 3 outside the vas bringing the muscular walls snugly together. A 7-0 suture is strong enough to permit one to rotate the vas for suturing but a 9-0 suture may be used throughout the anastomosis; $^3/_8$ curve needles on a 9-0 nylon are easier to employ for full

thickness sutures, whereas $\frac{1}{2}$ curve needles are easier to handle for mucosal sutures.

I place the successive sutures (now single-armed) around the vas, again bringing mucosal edge to mucosal edge, but starting outside the vas and passing the needle toward the lumen. When the anastomosis is completed, I inspect it for gaps in the suturing. If any exist, they are closed by sutures placed in the muscle but not entering the lumen. While placing these sutures, I remove any outpouring of spermatic fluid by sponging and irrigation. The mucosa is usually easy to distinguish from the muscle under magnification. In case of difficulty, a free floating stent of plain catgut may make it easier to see the lumen.

A two-layer anastomosis may also be constructed, suturing the mucosa as a row and the muscle as a row. Because of the thick wall of the vas, one may even use a circumferential full thickness running suture without fear of crimping the lumen, although this method makes it difficult to maintain uniform tension.

The skin is then closed with subcutaneous and cutaneous sutures of plain catgut, and the procedure is repeated on the other vas. A suspensory is applied, which must be worn for the next two weeks. Bandages are discarded after three days, and bathing is then permitted. Sexual activity must be avoided for the first seven postoperative days.

H. Postoperative testing for spermatozoa

Testing for the presence of spermatozoa is done one month postoperatively, and a full semen analysis is obtained after an additional two months. It is common for the number and motility of spermatozoa to improve during the first six months and

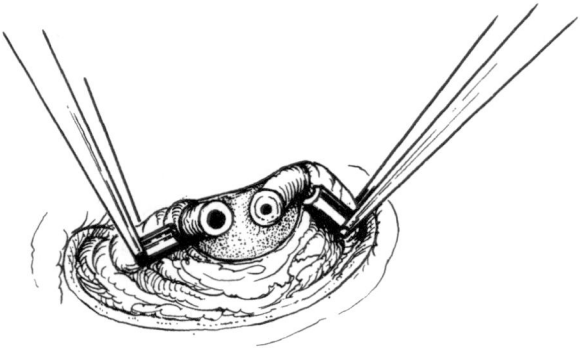

Figure 8. Vas ends delivered out of scrotum, ready for suture.

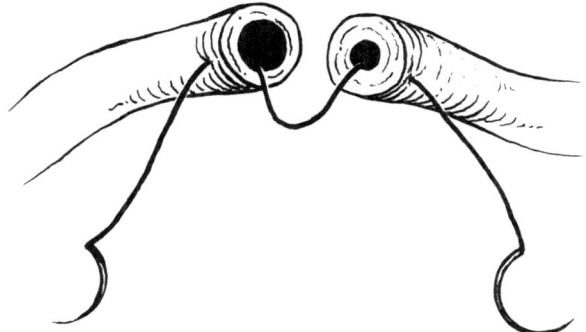

Figure 9. Placement of initial, posterior suture, using suture with two needles.

occasionally after that period of time. A good spermatozoa count may become much lower. Spermatozoa may even disappear from the ejaculate, which indicates that an initially patent anastomosis has scarred shut and should be repeated. Probing of the anastomosis is useless in the hope of reopening it. It is better to excise the scarred anastomosis and to reconstruct a new one.

I. Microsurgery

Practice in microsurgical techniques is essential to perform this operation comfortably and accurately. One must be familiar with instruments, microscope and anatomy of the vas deferens. Tremor can be minimized by resting the forearms and wrists on the table and by holding instruments with thumb and index finger, the other fingers resting against those of the opposite hand. The technique of Belker and his associates is recommended for this anastomosis. It has the superb advantage that one may make an anastomosis upon preserved segments of vas deferens and then open the vas longitudinally, thus being able to inspect the anastomosis from inside, where precision is crucial.

J. Repeat anastomosis

Failures do occur, and reoperation often brings success. Examination of these failures is the means by which we learn to improve our skills. Occasionally, one will find a spermatic granuloma at the site of anastomosis, although this is uncommon in my experience. Sometimes the anastomosis has been performed in spite of an obstruction in either the epididymis or the ejaculatory ducts, so that it may prove patent but fails to produce fertility. Most commonly, fibrous occlusion of the anastomosis has occurred and has followed the butt-together type of anastomosis, where the muscle has been approximated without attempting to bring the mucosal edges together inside the anastomosis. When raw tissue is exposed to spermatozoa, inflammation ensues, which leads to contracture.

As more sophisticated surgical techniques are developed, success in restoring fertility, leading to pregnancy, is becoming more common and fully justifies all the efforts involved.

REFERENCES

Belker AM et al: Microsurgical two layer vasovasostomy: Laboratory use of vasectomized segments. Fertil Steril 29: 48, 1978.

Brueschke EE et al: Development of a reversible vas deferens occlusive device: I. Anatomical size of the human and dog vas deferens. Fertil Steril 25: 659, 1974.

California State Department of Health, Office of Family Planning: What about vasectomy? 1977.

DeHaan John D: Human scalp and pubic hair: A comparison of physical properties. Unpublished Study. California Department of Justice, Sacramento, Ca 95813.

Ford K: Contraceptive utilization in the United States: 1973 and 1976. Advance data. USPHS National Center for Health Statistics, August 18, 1978.

Hagan KF and Coffey DS: The adverse effects of sperm during vasovasostomy. J Urol 118: 269, 1977.

Middleton RG and Henderson D: Vas deferens reanastomosis without splints and without magnification. J Urol 119: 763, 1978.

Owen, Earl: The operating microscope isn't everything – A warning and a prediction. Editorial, J Bone Joint Surg (BR) 58-B: 397, 1976.

Schmidt SS: Anastomosis of the vas deferens: An experimental study. II. Successes and failures in experimental anastomosis. J Urol 81: 203, 1959.

Schmidt SS: Vas anastomosis: A return to simplicity. Br J Urol 47: 309, 1975.

Schmidt SS and Brueschke EE: Anatomical sizes of the human vas deferens after vasectomy. Fertil Steril 27: 371, 1976.

Schmidt SS: Spermatic granuloma: An often painful lesion. Fertil Steril 31: 178, 1979.

Silber SJ: Microscopic vasectomy reversal. Fertil Steril 28: 1191, 1977.

IV. GENDER REASSIGNMENT

15. ORCHIECTOMY, PENECTOMY, VAGINOPLASTY FOR THE MALE TRANSSEXUAL

L.I. LIPSHULTZ

Although the first technical description of male to female sex reassignment surgery appeared in the German literature in 1931, it was not until 1953 that similar operations were reported with any frequency from other centers (Abraham 1931; Hamburger et al. 1953). Individuals seeking this gender conversion were defined as 'transsexuals' by Caldwell in 1949, but it is Money's description of these patients that has persisted, i.e., '(those with a) . . . disturbance of gender identity in which the person manifests with constant and persistent conviction, the desire to live as a member of the opposite sex and progressively takes steps to live in the opposite sex role on a full time basis' (Money 1970). Utilizing statistics from both the United States and abroad, it would appear that male transsexuals (biologic males requesting surgical creation of external female genitalia) outnumber female transsexuals in approximately a 4:1 ratio (Montague 1973). This article is about this group of biologic males and describes our surgical technique of sex reassignment.

Using a modification of the technique described by Pandya in 1973 and Granato in 1974, surgery is directed primarily at creating the external genitalia of the normal biologic female. The operation should produce adequate vaginal depth for intercourse, retain erectile tissue for increased sensation during sexual arousal, and provide a normally located female urethral meatus that permits micturition to occur in the sitting position (Lipshultz and Corriere 1978). During the procedure, the normal male tissues serve as homologues to create the external neogenital organs of a female (Table 1).

The homologous retainment of the male tissue is shown graphically in Figure 1. As illustrated here, the scrotal skin is used to form the new labia. The erectile tissue representing the remnants of the corpora cavernosa are fashioned into a clitoral-like organ, while the bulbous urethra becomes the female perineal urethra. The penile skin is transformed into the lining of the vagina by creating a penile skin tube, the apex of which, the glans penis, becomes a pseudo-cervix.

I. SURGICAL TECHNIQUE

The operation is performed under general anesthesia with the patient in the exaggerated dorsal lithotomy position. Having prepped and draped the perineum as is standard for any perineal procedure, a midline incision is made from below the base of the penis to approximately one to two centimeters above the anal verge (Figure 2). As seen here, the testes have already been removed via a routine high scrotal orchiectomy. This then leaves the corporal bodies isolated within the perineum, i.e., the corpus spongiosum located most ventrally and surrounding the bulbous urethra with the erectile tissue of the paired corpora cavernosa located dorsolaterally. The corporal bodies have been isolated using a Penrose drain which is located at the upper limit of the wound.

Using blunt and sharp section (Figure 3), a plane is established between the corporal bodies and the surrounding perineal tissue. With gentle traction,

Table 1. Operative homologues.

Male	Transsexual
Scrotum	Labia
Corpora cavernosa	Clitoris
Bulbous urethra	Perineal urethra
Penile skin	Vagina
Glans penis	Cervix

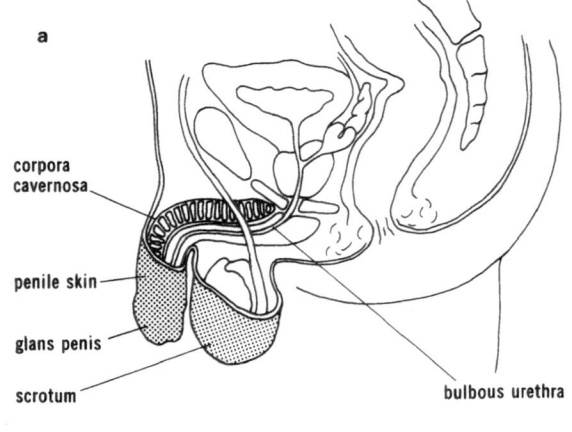

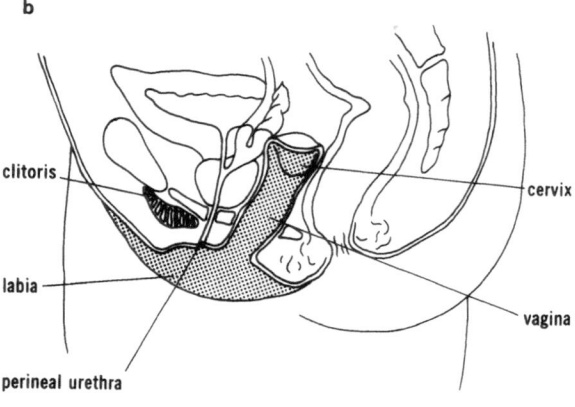

Figure 1.

the corporal bodies are then freed from the penile skin. The operating surgeon's finger, as well as the Penrose drain, is placed beneath the corporal bodies and the penile skin is pushed cephalad until the skin is inverted up to the corona. A Foley catheter helps to identify the urethra at all times and allows urinary drainage during the procedure.

After the corporal bodies have been completely separated from the surrounding penile skin, they are sharply transsected at the level of the corona (Figure 4). Prior to transsecting the corpora, a Kocher clamp must be carefully placed at the lower limit of the proposed incision site on the corpora cavernosa and the incision made cephalad to the clamp. This significantly reduces the amount of bleeding from the hypervascular corpora cavernosa, which can be quite brisk. In addition, the original Foley catheter must be removed and repositioned within the urethra which has now been transsected. In this figure, one sees the inverted base of the glans penis and the newly sectioned portion of the corporal bodies which subsequently must be

shortened to form the erectile tissue of the clitoris and the neo-urethra.

The urethra and corpus spongiosum are now freed from the corpora cavernosa as depicted in Figure 5. Dissection of the urethra is carried down to the deep portion of the bulbous urethra. At this point, the corpora cavernosa decussate and the suspensory ligament of the penis must be incised for better mobilization of the erectile tissue. Also seen in Figure 5 is the 'penile skin tube' everted here in its original position to demonstrate, once again, that it has remained intact.

The corpora cavernosa must now be shortened and refashioned into a clitoris-like organ. This is done by mobilizing the corpora cavernosa after freeing the suspensory ligament of the penis, cross-clamping the erectile tissue at a level that will allow the tissue to rest easily against the superior part of the symphysis pubis, and excising and discarding the excess tissue. Kocher clamps are placed at the appropriate level and the hollow penile skin tube is reinverted to prevent desiccation (Figure 6). The Foley catheter drains the urethra, which has been separated completely from the erectile tissue.

As demonstrated in Figure 7, the excess corporal tissue has been removed, leaving two stumps of these erectile bodies. Held by Kocher clamps, the free edges of the corpora have already been oversewn with two layers of continuous zero chromic suture. The two remaining free ends of this running layer of chromic suture are then used to secure the stumps of the corpora cavernosa to a comfortable position on the symphysis. Interrupted 3-0 chromic sutures are used to further attach the erectile tissue to the pubis, creating a smooth edge between

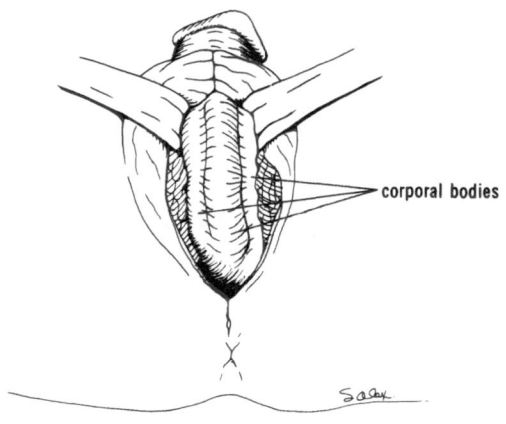

Figure 2.

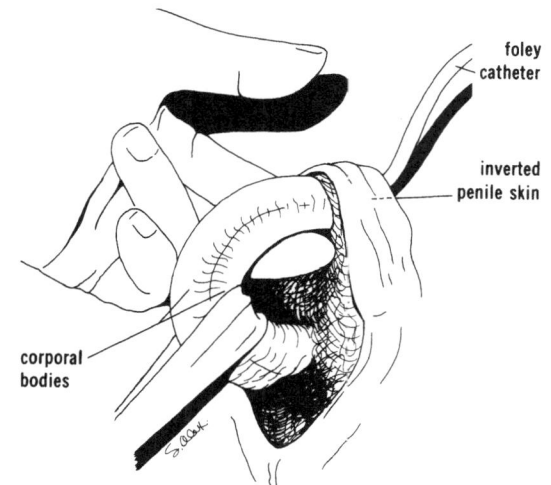

Figure 3.

erectile tissue and bone and insuring complete hemostasis. The final chromic stitch is being tied in Figure 7. Note the decussation of the corporal bodies and the ventral course of the urethra with the indwelling Foley. The pubic symphysis lies beneath the sutured corporal tissue. This newly positioned vascular tissue will have the necessary tactile sensitivity and erectile potential that corresponds to the normal female clitoris.

Our attention is now turned to the creation of the neovagina. In Figure 8, a cavity for the neovagina has been surgically created by dissecting a deep plane between the rectum and the urethra, pushing Donovillier's fascia cephalad. As seen in the diagram, long deep Deavers have been placed in the cavity to allow better dissection and demonstrate a depth of approximately 10 cm. The urethra is pointing upwards with a Foley catheter still in place.

The scrotum and penile skin tube must now be brought down towards the rectum in order to permit easy inversion of the penile skin into this

newly formed cavity. To accomplish this, the inverted penile skin and scrotum are elevated and the lower abdominal skin freed from its attachment to the underlying abdominal fascia half-way to the umbilicus, as seen in Figure 9. This permits the entire skin of the scrotum and penis to be mobilized and moved ventrally. Care must be taken to insure hemostasis under the freed abdominal skin, for a hematoma forming in this dissected area may cause impeded perfusion of the skin tube and subsequent tissue loss.

The penile skin tube is then inserted into the neovagina. In Figure 10, a deeper Deaver has been placed inferiorly and a Parker retractor laterally to enable better visualization of the new introitus. The depth of the cavity varies from 10 to 15 cm, depending on the available skin from the penile skin

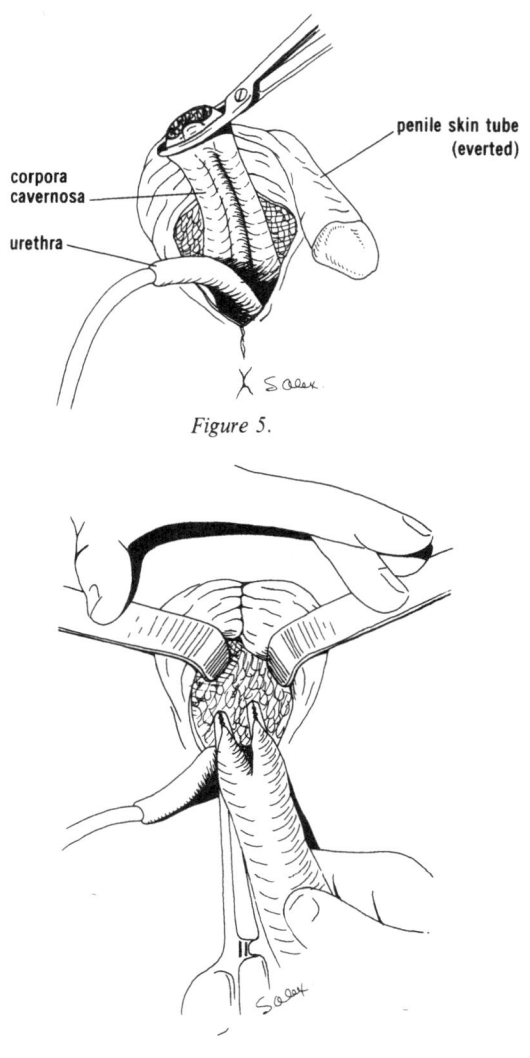

Figure 5.

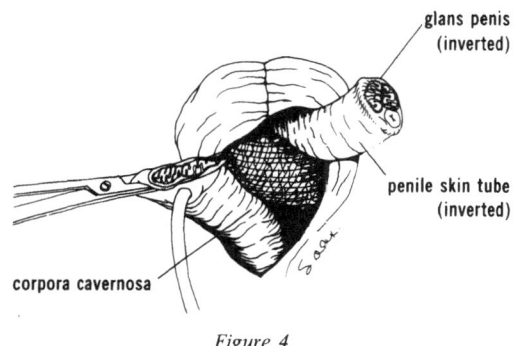

Figure 4.

Figure 6.

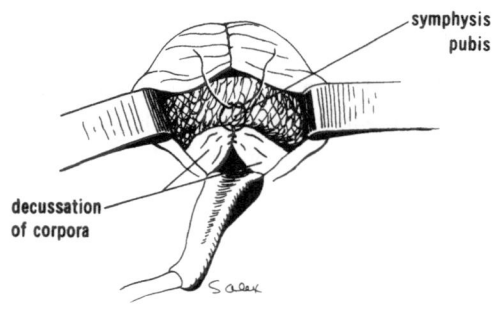

Figure 7.

tube and the depth of the newly created perineal cavity. The urethra must be brought through a new meatus located superior to the neovagina and inferior to the erectile tissue of the corpora cavernosa, previously fashioned into the clitoris. The excess tissue of the urethra has already been transsected at the skin level and the edges of the urethral mucosa sutured to the new meatus with interrupted 3-0 chromic.

The procedure is then completed by forming the external genitalia (Figure 11). The redundant tissue of the scrotum has already been excised and the free edges sutured with 3-0 interrupted polyglycolic acid suture to the edges of the original wound, thus forming the labia. The inverted penile skin tube must be held firmly against the walls of the neovaginal cavity to insure firm attachment and prevent hematoma formation. This is done by placing a vaginal stent in the inverted skin tube and leaving it in place for 48 hours. A pressure dressing is firmly applied to prevent swelling of the labia as well as to insure proper positioning of the vaginal stent. The patient is confined to bed rest during the first two days, after which the pressure dressing is

removed and the patient is instructed to remove and replace the vaginal stent three times daily during a sitz bath. Twenty-four hours after removal of the pressure dressing, the Foley catheter is discontinued. If the patient is then able to manage dressing changes as well as to void without difficulty for at least 24 hours, she is discharged. The vaginal stent must be worn until complete healing of the vaginal cavity has occurred. This takes four to six weeks, after which the vaginal stent can be worn only as needed. It is usually completely discontinued by four to six months after surgery.

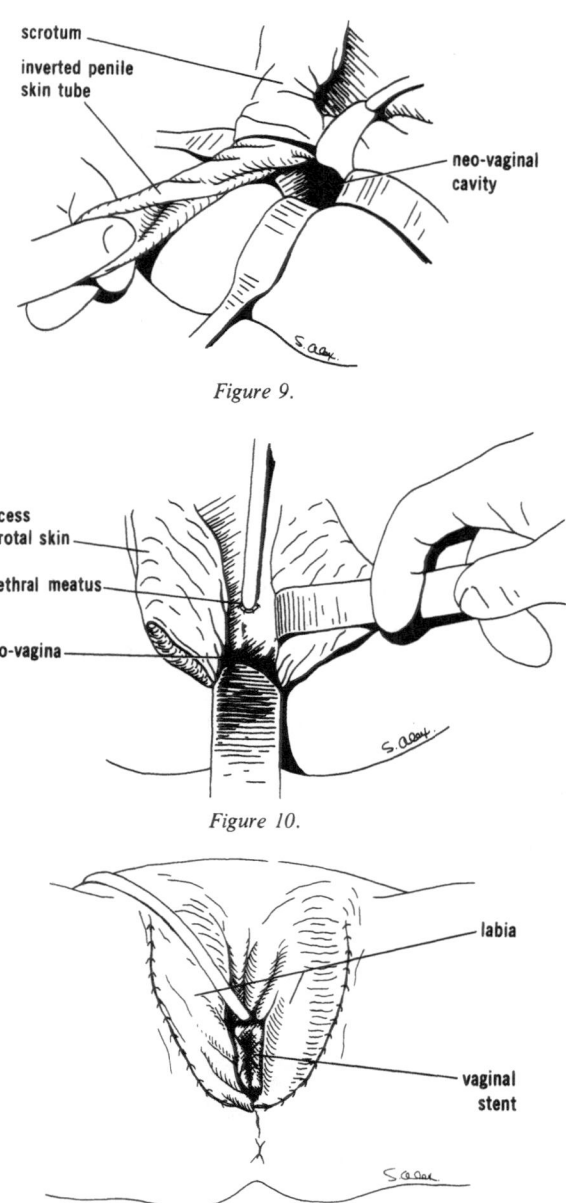

Figure 9.

Figure 10.

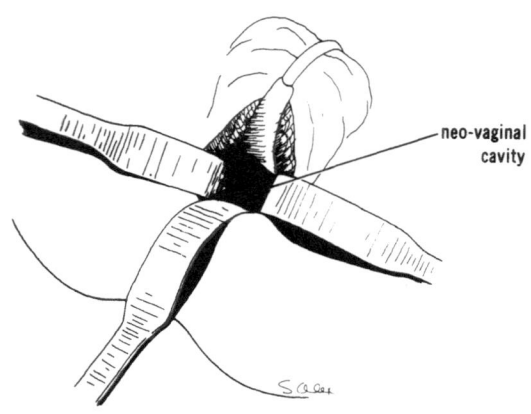

Figure 8.

Figure 11.

II. COMPLICATIONS AND RESULTS

Limiting our transsexual surgery to approximately one operative procedure per month, 40 patients have undergone male to female sex reassignment surgery from 1975 to 1978. Statistics on these patients are seen in Table 2. The ages have ranged from 20 to 54, with a mean age of 26. Of these 40 patients, 30 have had no complications whatsoever. Six have had minor complications and four have had major complications, all of which are listed in Table 2.

The significant part of successful sex reassignment surgery, however, is not the operative technique itself, but more importantly, the method of correct and careful patient selection. All patients under our care must undergo initial in-depth psychiatric and endocrinological evaluation as well as a predetermined, *minimum* one-year waiting period prior to any type of surgical intervention. It is during this time that both psychiatric analysis and endocrinological evaluation are concluded. As noted in our description, surgery can be effective

Table 2. Review of transsexual surgery. University of Texas Medical School at Houston: 1975-1978 (N = 40).

Age: 20-54 years	
Average 26 years	
Complications:	
None:	30
Minor:	Urethral stenosis – 2
	Urethrovaginal fistula – 1
	Loss of vaginal depth (< 2 cm) – 1
	Labial abscess – 1
	Redundant labial skin – 1
Major:	Severe introital stenosis – 1
	Significant loss of vaginal depth (> 2 cm) – 1
	Slough of penile skin tube – 1
	Recto-vaginal fistula – 1

in accomplishing the desired result of successful female gender reassignment in a one stage procedure with a minimum of operative complication. To be considered successful, the operative technique must result in the formation of normal appearing external female genitalia, adequate vaginal depth for intercourse, and a normally located female urethral meatus that permits micturition to occur in the female sitting position.

REFERENCES

Abraham F: Genitalwandlung an zwei maennlichen Transvestiten. Z Sexualwiss 18: 223, 1931.

Caldwell DO: Psychiatric aspects of transsexual surgery management. J Nerv Ment Dis 147: 525, 1968.

Granato RC: Surgical approach to male transsexualism. Urology III (6): 792, 1974; 26: 277, 1973.

Hamburger C, Stump GK and Dahl-Iversen E: Transvestism: Hormonal, psychiatric and surgical treatment. JAMA 152: 391, 1953.

Lipshultz LI, Corriere JN Jr: Construction of a neovagina in male transsexuals. In: The human vagina, Hafez ESE and Evans TN (eds), Elsevier Biomedical Press, 1978.

Money J: Sex reassignment. Int J Psychiatry 9: 249, 1970-71.

Montague DK: Transsexualism. Urology II (1): 1, 1973.

Pandya NJ, Stuteville OH: A one-stage technique for constructing female external genitalia in male transsexuals. Brit J Plas Surg 26: 277, 1973.

V. BENIGN DISORDERS OF THE MALE ACCESSORY GLANDS

16. PROSTATECTOMY FOR BENIGN PROSTATIC HYPERPLASIA

S.G. MULHOLLAND and J.R. DALTON

I. HISTORICAL BACKGROUND OF PROSTATECTOMY

Prostatectomy has evolved into a well-defined procedure which may be performed in many ways, according to the urologist's preference. It has been observed (Weyrauch 1959) that prostatic surgery provides the romance of Urology. All urologists have enjoyed the satisfaction of performing uncomplicated prostatectomies with excellent post-operative results. The unexpected complication or failure, however, continually reminds us of the need to search for even better techniques.

The critical anatomical position of the prostate itself makes this operation challenging. Inaccessibility, relationship to continence and potency, rich blood supply, proximity of ureters and rectum, infection, and myriad of associated medical problems further compound the challenge. It is difficult to assess the number of men who may need this operation. One study (Lytton et al. 1968) showed that just under two percent of patients under 60 years of age required prostatectomy. The incidence gradually increased in patients up to the age of 70 of whom ten percent required treatment.

Benign enlargement of the prostate undoubtedly had a similar incidence prior to our modern surgical era. The cause of bladder obstruction was not known until the middle of the 16th century when a Venetian physician, Niccolo Ulassa, recognized the prostate gland as the cause. The first efforts at relieving obstruction were by catheterization, followed by tunneling through the gland. Very little in the way of recognizable surgical procedures was done until the middle of the 18th century when surgical procedures were instituted for removal of bladder stones. Cystotomy was practiced for centuries prior to the development of the surgical procedure, prostatectomy. The major route to the bladder was perineal, and, on occasion, fragments of prostatic tissue were removed. In 1556, Pierre Franco first attempted a suprapubic cystotomy. In 1639, a perineal prostatectomy was performed by Couvillard. Throughout the remainder of the 18th and 19th century, a number of other surgeons reported performing perineal prostatectomy. In the 1800s, the operation matured through the efforts of many others including Ferguson (1848), Billroth (1867), Goodfellow (1891), Young (1903). The eight routes to the prostate originated with the following (Weyrauch 1959):

Suprapubic	– Amusset	1834
Retropubic	– Von Stockum	1909
Transpubic	– Billroth	1867
Infrapubic	– Langenbuch	?
Transurethral	– Guthrie	1834
Transrectal	– Demarquay	1873
Ischiorectal	– Dittel	1890
Sacral	– Boeckel	1908

Well-known urologic surgeons have developed and refined these techniques in the 20th century.

II. DEVELOPMENT OF BENIGN PROSTATIC HYPERTROPHY

At about the twelfth week of fetal development, five groups of epithelial buds appear in the prostatic urethra (Table 1). By the fourth month, branched tubules appear and the groups of tubules from the five primitive buds develop into lobes. Two accessory groups may develop which occasionally are recognized clinically:

Subcervical group of Albarran – Subcervical lobe
(Lowsley 1912)
Subtrigonal glands of Home   – Subtrigonal lobe

Table 1.

Bud	Location	Lobe
One middle	Floor of urethra proximal to Wolffian ducts	Middle
Two lateral	Posterolaterally	Lateral
One posterior	Floor of urethra distal to Wolffian ducts	Posterior
One ventral	Anterior proximal prostatic urethra	Anterior

A. Pathology

In a patient's early adult life, the prostate consists of sets of acini and ducts which grow out radially from the prostatic urethra. The bulk of ducts are located in the middle and lateral lobes. The ducts are surrounded by smooth muscle. The detrusor muscle fibers pass down through the gland with a condensation of these fibers at the periphery of the gland merging with the capsule, but the majority pass down between the acini and ducts to insert into the urethra just distal to the entry of the ejaculatory ducts (Blancy 1976). With aging, the arrangement of these muscle fibers changes. The vertically running fibers begin to collect as a septum, forming an inner and outer zone of acini (Semple 1963). In this inner periurethral zone, nodular hyperplasia begins.

There has been, in the reports, a great deal of confusion concerning the exact pathology and correct nomenclature. The pathology reveals a benign enlargement of the gland due to hyperplasia of glandular, or fibromuscular tissue, or both. Benign prostatic hypertrophy; prostatic adenoma, adenomatous hypertrophy; benign enlargement; glandular and stromal hyperplasia; hyperglandular and stromal hyperplasia; fibro-glandular hyperplasia; nodular hyperplasia have all been used as attempts at clinico-pathological nomenclature (Mostofi and Price 1973).

Areas of nodular hyperplasia begin along the urethra in the middle and two lateral lobes. These areas grow and coalesce, pushing the urethra inwards and compressing the normal prostatic tissue outwards. The muscle fibers are pushed out and form a septum. This septum clearly divides a nodular hyperplastic area from an outer layer of normal prostatic tissue. Microscopically hyperplasia glands show considerable variation (Mostofi and Price 1973). The hyperplasia may be fibrous, fibrovascular, fibromuscular, muscular, fibroadenomatous, fibromyoadenomatous, and purely adenomatous.

The enlargement of the prostate due to nodular hyperplasia can occur in various gross anatomical combinations (Weyrauch 1959). The classic enlargement, well known to the urologist, is referred to as trilobar hypertrophy or nodular hyperplastic enlargement of the middle and lateral lobes. Certainly more unusual involvements of the other lobes may occur. The relationship of prostatic enlargement to obstruction is not absolute. There can be a massive enlargement and virtually no obstruction and vice versa.

B. Incidence of nodular hyperplasia

Nodular hyperplasia begins in the fifth decade and thereafter its incidence rises markedly (Moore 1944). By the ninth decade, 75 percent of human prostate glands demonstrate benign prostatic hyperplasia (BPH) which is the most common cause of prostatic obstruction (Grayhack et al. 1975). Fifty percent of men past fifty years and 75 percent past eighty demonstrate pathologic changes in the gland (Randall 1931; Weyrauch 1959). Another study (Franks 1954) showed BPH in 73 percent of cases in the seventh decade at autopsy, but yet another report (Robinson 1964) showed only 37 percent. This difference is probably the result of different histologic criteria.

In Africa, BPH has been reported (Dodge 1963) as uncommon in Uganda but common in Bantus (Lisoos 1973). Many studies indicate that the incidence is lower in the black race when compared to the white race (Walker 1922; Rodman 1919; Day 1921; Hirsch 1932; Smith and Jaffe 1932; D'Aunoy et al. 1939; Burns 1940). Other recent studies have shown the incidence and operative procedures more equal in both races (Whitfield 1950; Hunt 1928; Lytton et al. 1968).

An increasing incidence has been reported (Walker 1922) in Mongolian, Indian, Arabic, Semitic, and Caucasian races. The Chinese have been reported to have a lower incidence than the

Caucasians (6.6-47.2 percent) at age 41 years (Chang and Char 1936). BHP has been thought to be low in Koreans, Japanese and other Asiatics, but recent studies demonstrated the incidence to be much higher than previously thought (Oomura et al. 1965; Ahluwalia and Tandon 1965; Tan 1961). In Wales, men of Welsh origin have a higher incidence than those of English origin (Ashley 1966). BPH was found (Lytton et al. 1968) to be three times more common in Jews than in Catholics or Protestants, but the majority of Jews were foreign born. It could not be determined whether geographical or religious origin was responsible for the difference. Differences in incidence by anthropological, geographical, social, or national classification is not clear cut.

Mortality rates appear higher in more sophisticated European countries, where records are more reliable (Iceland, Austria, Scandinavia and The Netherlands). The lowest mortality appears in oriental areas (Japan, Hong Kong, China, Philippines, Ceylon· and Singapore).

C. Natural History, Sequelae and Symptoms of BPH

The natural history of BPH is not well known. Variables in the progression of the disease make it difficult to predict the course in a single patient at any given time. The urologic surgeon should strive to have an adequate knowledge of the natural history, in order to prognosticate accurately and to determine the need for surgery.

Benign enlargement of the prostate in the human is a common occurrence, but the reason is not known. Experimentally, growth and secretion of the prostate can be prevented by castration. Estrogen suppresses and androgen stimulates specific areas of the prostate. Unfortunately no animal has a prostate identical to man embryologically, histologically, or pathologically. Animal studies, therefore, are of limited value in answering these questions. Studies of experimental work concerning development of BPH are discussed in depth elsewhere in this text.

Benign prostatic hypertrophy does progress over the years and can be measured objectively. However, worsening of symptoms correlates very poorly with this increase in size. In some patients prolonged periods of regression of symptoms occur in spite of increasing size of the gland. Furthermore, the size of the gland bears no relationship to the degree of obstruction measured objectively or to the patient's symptoms.

As obstruction at the bladder neck develops, hypertrophy of the bladder wall gradually ensues and voiding intravesical pressure rises. If the hypertrophy progresses, saccules then diverticula or herniation of urothelium occur through hypertrophied bladder muscle. Some individuals develop very thick-walled bladders with many diverticula while others develop gradual distention of the bladder with increasing residual urine volumes.

As hypertrophy of the bladder wall develops, the upper tracts usually begin to show obstructive changes, at first with dilation of the lower ureter, then gradual hydro-ureteronephrosis ensues. The hydronephrosis may be a result of: (1) increased intravesical pressure being transferred back to the ureter, (2) obstruction from hypertrophied bladder muscle at the ureterovesical junction, or (3) reflux. Further development of obstruction may result in renal damage.

Although the pathological changes of obstruction progress as described, the patient's symptoms do not follow a routine pattern. Roughly speaking, however, the following symptoms are commonly seen singly or in combination. With bladder hypertrophy irritability of the bladder muscle occurs and the patient complains of frequency and urgency. With obstruction and distortion of the urethra, straining and difficulty in starting the stream, poor stream, intermittence and terminal dribbling occur. With decompensation of the bladder muscle, frequent voiding of small quantities with incomplete emptying occurs and culminates often in complete retention. These symptoms may wax and wane from week to week or may never appear so that the patient may present with uremia and polyuria, the so-called silent prostatism. At any stage, infection may occur to give a marked increase in frequency with cystitis, and pyelonephritis and epididymitis may also occur.

Acute retention may precipitate hospitalization and there is not always a natural progression of symptoms toward retention. Acute retention may be brought about suddenly by increased fluid load (e.g., alcohol), drugs (e.g. common cold remedies containing anticholinergics and sympathomimetics), or sudden prostatic enlargement from infection or infarction. Hematuria may develop secondary to infection, stone, or BPH itself, but other causes (e.g. malignancy) should be ruled out by intravenous pyelogram and cystoscopy.

III. INDICATIONS FOR PROSTATECTOMY

A. *Absolute*

1. Chronic obstruction with azotemia.
2. Acute exacerbation on chronic obstruction.
3. Bladder calculi plus chronic obstruction.
4. Damage to the bladder and upper tract from obstruction.
5. Recurrent urinary infection from obstruction.
6. Hemorrhage from benign hypertrophy.

B. *Relative*

1. Acute retention.
2. Urinary frequency interfering with sleep or work.
3. Early obstructive changes in the bladder or upper tracts.
4. Residual urine.
5. Bladder stones.
6. Recurrent prostatitis.

There is little controversy about the absolute indications for prostatectomy because in this group the obstructing disease will not remit spontaneously and secondary life-threatening changes may have begun to appear. With increasing sophisticated testing, fewer patients within this classification are admitted to the hospital.

The patients with relative indications are now the major group for a number of reasons. The risks of prostatic surgery are minimal (Singh et al. 1973; Valk 1975). Referring doctors are now aware that delay in seeking advice until acute retention occurs increases the operative mortality (Salvaris 1960). Furthermore, with increasing use of annual physical examinations, physicians are referring more men to urologists for presymptomatic evaluation of the enlarged prostate.

In one study (Anikwe 1978), it has been shown that 80 percent of patients will be assessed purely by clinical methods and the remaining 20 percent will need specialized urodynamic tests.

In the presence of a normal intravenous urogram, normal BUN, creatinine and sterile urine, minimal symptoms such as voiding twice per night and slight tailing off of the stream can be ignored. However, in the absence of a stricture, bi-annual urinalyses and maximum urinary flow rate either by the trained eye or the simple uroflowmeter of Drake (Grewe Plastics, Newark, N.J.; Drake 1948) is a simple, convenient and inexpensive followup. The residual urine can be assessed by catheterization or on an intravenous urogram if the post-void film is taken immediately. While cystograms and voiding cysto-urethrograms are suggested (Culp 1975) as aids in decision making, with the moderately symptomatic patient most urologists rely more heavily on pan-endoscopy with observation of the prostatic urethra from the external sphincter with the water flowing in and out as well as the presence of trabeculation of the bladder. For patients with minimal symptoms, one should first exclude low-grade prostatitis as the cause of symptoms. Post-rectal examination or post-prostatic massage, urine, commonly called V.B. 3 (Meares and Stamey 1968), will show many white blood cells on microscopic examination if prostatitis exists. This condition should be treated appropriately before a final assessment is made. At this time, an inexpensive simple objective test is needed to avoid premature 'prophylactic' surgery and too late surgery where increased mortality and morbidity is added to the operation. A recent study (Anikwe 1978), using mean urinary flow rate, mean maximum intravesical pressure, mean maximum intrinsic bladder pressure, mean minimum urethral resistance and mean micturation wall tension and the mean mean residual urine, showed the pattern of the urethral resistance to be the single most valuable parameter. A computer instrument named The Resistanceometer was designed to make the necessary calculations from urethral flow and pressure. However, the authors of this article do not use such an expensive, invasive method of assessment, but rely upon the uroflowmeter, the urogram (Susset et al. 1973) and urinalysis together with the patient's symptoms.

In spite of all the sophisticated aids of urodynamics, there will still be cases where other factors lead to an earlier operation than objective signs indicate, for example, the patient with recurrent low-grade prostatitis and prostatic calculi. Seventy-two percent of patients with prostatitis were reported cured by transurethral resection (Smart and Jenkins 1973). The authors observed that resection must be as complete as possible to remove all of the infected tissue. The patient with complicated medical problems, e.g., severe respiratory disease needing adrenergic drugs plus a mildly obstructing prostate, may need an early prostatectomy. Severe cardiac disease and straining to void often can be relieved by transurethral resection. Chronic renal disease with some added obstructive element can be improved by TURP. Prior catheterization and review of serial BUN and creatinine studies will show improvement, confirming the possible value of TURP in this group of patients. Finally, the elderly man with recent onset of hernia, with a poorly emptying bladder as the only precipitating cause for his hernia, needs prostatectomy before hernia repair.

IV. PREOPERATIVE EVALUATION

Most patients undergoing prostatic surgery are in the older age group and may need some preoperative treatment to bring them to optimal condition for surgery. The great improvement in mortality and morbidity over the last 20 years has been to a large extent the result of better selection of operative procedure and preoperative treatment of cardiorespiratory problems and control of bacterial infection.

A. Work-up

1. Complete history and physical examination.
2. Rectal examination.
3. Urinalysis with culture and sensitivity.
4. Complete blood count: *SMA-12* (total protein, albumin, calcium, phosphorus, cholesterol, glucose, uric acid, creatinine, total bilirubin, alkaline phosphatase, LDH, SGOT); *SMA-6* (sodium, potassium, chloride, CO_2, sugar, BUN); *Serum acid phosphatase*; prothrombin time, partial thrombo-plastin time.
5. Intravenous urogram.
6. Chest x-ray.
7. Electrocardiogram.
8. Cystometrogram when urgency or urge incontinence may suggest an uninhibited neurogenic bladder.
9. Panendoscopy.

An intravenous urogram is an essential investigative procedure. Not only does it show the presence of obstructive changes in the bladder and upper tracts, but it may also show significant renal and ureteric lesions which demand more urgent treatment (Hodges and Barry 1975). Any unexplained anemia should be investigated before preoperative transfusion is given. Similarly, diabetic patients should be stabilized before operation and, while not all urologists are agreed that a coagulation survey is essential, prothrombin time and partial thromboplastin time are two adequate screening tests.

From time to time, patients are seen whose urinary problems consist more of urgency than of frequent voiding. A cystometrogram is advisable in these patients if unpleasant postoperative complications of incontinence from an unstable bladder or neuropathic disease and poor sphincter control are to be avoided. All patients should be cystoscoped before prostatectomy. Many surgeons combine this with the operative procedure so that bladder stones, cancer and diverticula can be diagnosed and the operative plan changed accordingly.

B. Use of Antibiotics: Sterile urine and uncatheterized cases

Although there are series of cases that show that antibiotics are unnecessary following prostatectomy, most surgeons use a urinary antiseptic while catheters are indwelling and for a short period after the patient is discharged from the hospital (Wear and Haley 1973).

C. Infected or catheterized patients

Virtually all are agreed that appropriate preoperative, intra- and postoperative antibiotics are necessary in the presence of infected urine and in the patient catheterized for five days or more (Herr 1973).

V. DETERMINATION OF OPERATIVE TECHNIQUE

The standard methods of prostatectomy are:

1. Transurethral resection.
2. Retropubic enucleation.
3. Transvesical suprapubic enucleation.
4. Perineal enucleation.

Ninety-five percent of patients with prostatic obstruction are advised of transurethral resection of the prostate as the operation of choice (Valk 1975). A number of factors are responsible for this figure: most patients present with prostatic obstruction and small glands, more adequate control of blood loss and hemostasis by the transurethral method, and the increasing number of urologists and other surgeons who have expertise in this particular method of prostatectomy. Since the retropubic technique was first described (Millin 1945), more and more surgeons perform enucleation prostatectomy by this approach. The exposure of the prostatic fossa and control of bleeding is more easily accomplished with the wider view of the prostate obtained with this method. Transvesical prostatectomy has the great advantage since large stones and diverticula can be treated at the same time as the enucleation of the prostate gland, but hemostasis is more difficult than with the retropubic approach. The vertical vesico-capsular approach (Ward 1948) incising both the bladder and the prostatic capsule has been described as giving the best of both worlds. The retropubic operation was said to have a high incidence of osteitis pubis. However, with increased use of antibiotics to clear up preoperative infection in the bladder and prostate, a study was reported in which there were no cases of osteitis pubis in 761 retropubic prostatectomies (Marshall 1967).

Perineal prostatectomy is the least used method at the present time. Of all the open methods of prostatectomy, however, the perineal approach gives the most comfortable postoperative course for the patient. If there is a question of a malignant nodule in an otherwise benign gland, open perineal biopsy and frozen section can be performed before the gland is treated perineally. Elderly (poor risk) patients with chronic obstructive airway disease have difficulty in breathing out and the head-down position aids the expiratory movement (Melchior et al. 1974).

VI. RETROPUBIC PROSTATECTOMY

The retropubic approach to the prostate gland is the most satisfactory in the patient who has a large (50 grams or more) gland. Abdominal obesity is no particular problem to the surgeon using this approach, because the head-down position helps in exposure of the prostatic capsule and incidentally takes some of the abdominal fat upwards towards the head. Furthermore, in the patient with an abdominal apron, the tissue for two to five centimeters above the pubis is less infiltrated with fat than that which falls down over the pubis and it is in this region that the transverse incision of the Pfannenstiel exposure is made.

Satisfactory anesthesia for this operation can be obtained by using low spinal technique with or without local infiltration or a general anesthetic. Where there is any question, it is generally left to the personal preference of the anesthetist.

While vasectomy was a mandatory part of open prostatectomy for a good many years, most surgeons nowadays select the patient on the basis of number of days of catheter drainage before surgery and the presence or absence of infection. However, some urologists (Brooks et al. 1971) perform routine vasectomy in open cases with or without prior catheterization as a good prophylaxis against postoperative epididymitis.

Before the operating session, cystoscopy is performed and a catheter should be inserted to empty the bladder completely.

Either a Pfannenstiel or a midline incision is made to expose the prostate. By remaining close to the posterior aspect of the pubis, the surgeon can easily find the prostate and bleeding from anterior prostatic veins is minimized. The anterior aspect of the prostate and bladder is exposed and a self-retaining retractor, such as that designed by Millin, is inserted into the wound. The bladder is then depressed in the wound either with the Millin third blade or a malleable strip of copper over a folded laparotomy pad (see Figure 1). This will expose the capsule effectively so that the anterior prostatic veins may be under-run and ligated against the anterior capsule one to two centimeters below the prostatovesical junction. Having inserted two such sutures, the prostatic capsule is opened transversely by a three-to-four centimeter incision. The white shiny surface of the adenoma is seen marking the plane of cleavage. The adenoma can be dissected distally either with scissors or with a finger and the urethra cut across under direct vision just above the external sphincter. Alternatively, the adenoma can be dissected proximally to enter the bladder. A finger is inserted through the bladder, down the prostatic urethra to break through the mucosa proximal to the external sphincter. It is particularly important during this part of the operation that the external sphincter be left intact and that no urethral mucosa be pulled from the sphincter region lest the patient be rendered incontinent postoperatively. Having broken through

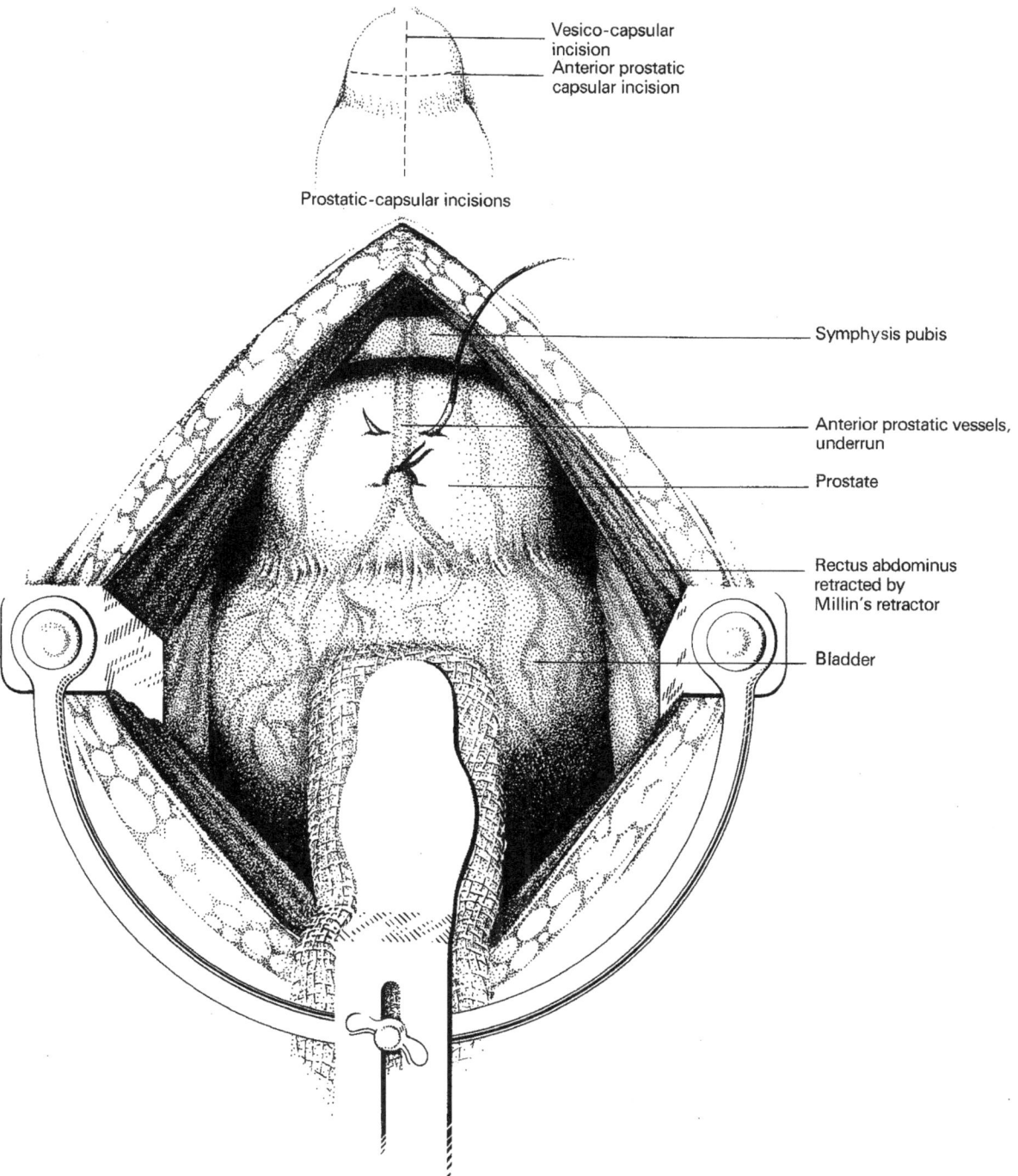

Figure 1. Vesico-prostatic area exposed by Millin's retractor.

the plane of cleavage, at the apex, the urologist can enucleate both lateral lobes until the gland is merely attached at the bladder neck and trigone. If the gland is small, it can be withdrawn whole through the prostatotomy. Using the bladder neck spreader, the surgeon can incise the bladder neck and remove a wedge of tissue at the bladder neck as the gland is removed (see Figure 2). If the gland is large, it can be broken up within the prostatic fossa and removed as two lobes rather than tearing the capsule laterally and risking brisk hemorrhage to pull out the complete enucleated adenoma. After the adenoma has been removed, the fossa can be packed firmly with vaginal packing for two to three minutes. This usually stops small bleeders. After the packing is removed inspection of the prostatic fossa will show most of the bleeding arising from the vessels at the five and seven o'clock positions. These can be under-run with 000 catgut for hemostasis. Smaller vessels can be coagulated with elec-

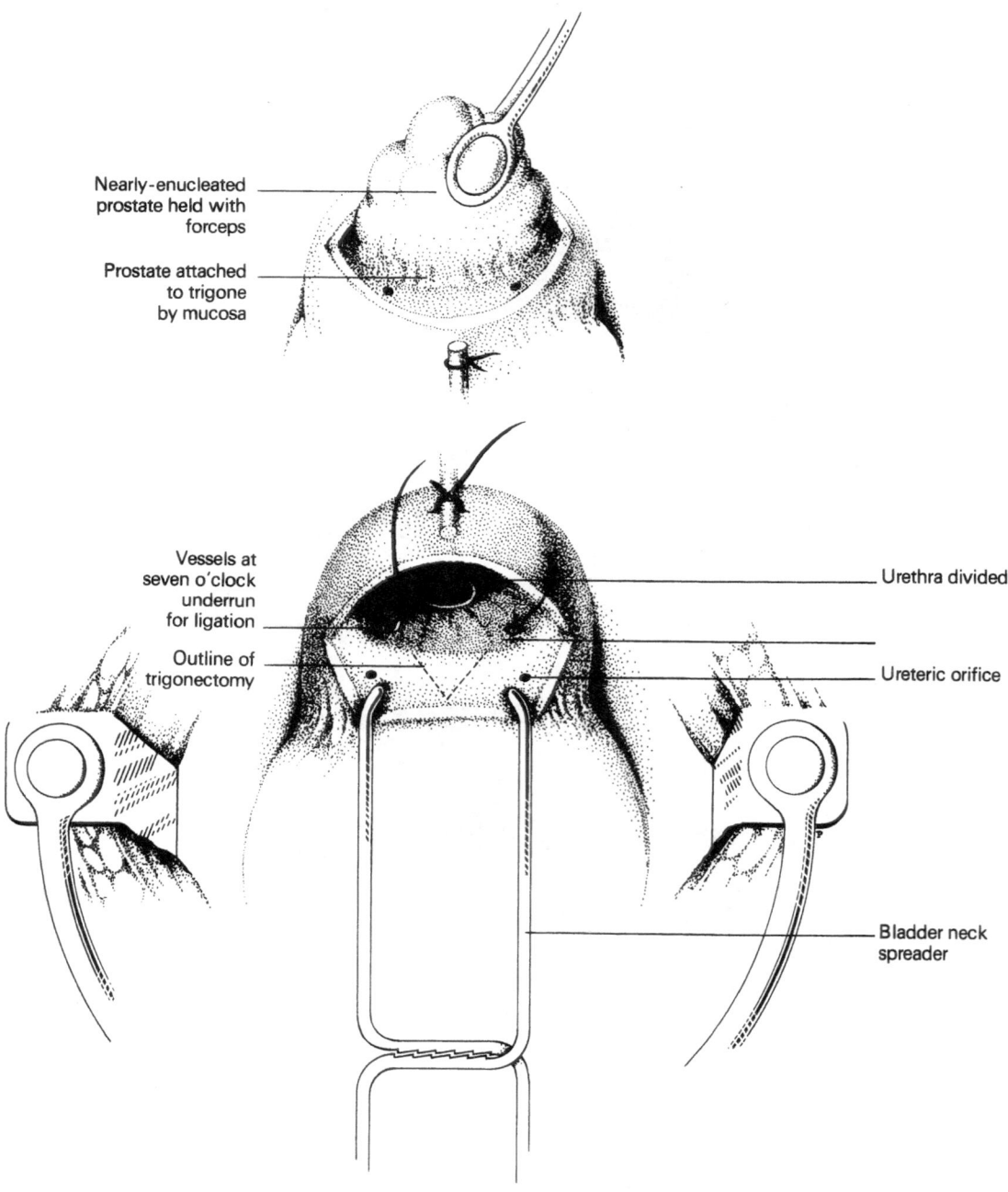

Figure 2. Prostatic fossa exposed for haemostasis.

trocoagulation. Time is usually well spent at this particular part of the operation to secure hemostasis and avoid postoperative troubles. Having secured hemostasis, a Foley catheter is inserted and the capsule closed. If there is a persistent ooze from the prostatic fossa, traction on an inflated Foley catheter will usually tamponade the bleeding source. If this fails (which it rarely does) and the patient bleeds persistently without control, sutures can be run around the prostatic capsule, the catheter inserted and the sutures tied compressing the prostate against the catheter for hemostasis. Twenty-four to thirty-six hours later, the sutures can be cut and the catheter left indwelling. Postoperatively the Foley catheter is left in place for five to seven days. Drains placed in the retropubic space are advanced when dry.

The retropubic approach as described by Millin (1945) used an anterior transverse prostatotomy to expose the adenoma (Figure 1). However, other surgeons using this approach to the retropubic space have described a number of variations, such as the low transverse incision into the bladder (Harvard and White 1960). This incision is made a centimeter above the vesico-prostatic junction. Using the cutting electrode, the enlarged prostate can be circumcised from within the bladder and the prostate enucleated. If necessary, a finger can be inserted into the rectum to elevate the prostate to the enucleating finger and aid in the definition of the correct plane of cleavage.

A further modification (Ward 1948) of this approach used a vertical vesico-capsular incision (Figure 1). In this procedure, the capsule and junction of the bladder neck and prostate are cleaned of fat by blunt dissection and the dorsal veins are under-run as low down as possible. A further holding suture is placed through all coats of the bladder vertically above the lower-most suture and two to three centimeters above the prostato-vesical junction. The lowest suture is inserted deeply through the capsule and serves the purpose of a marker for later repair, but also acts as a stay suture to prevent or minimize the possibility of the incision splitting further distally through the external sphincter mechanism and rendering the patient incontinent. Two further stay sutures of catgut are inserted at the region of the bladder neck which, when elevated, allow an incision to be made

easily into the prostatic capsule and bladder neck. The adenoma is seen as the capsular incision is made and, using curved scissors, hugging the lowermost margin of the apex, the urethra is transsected without avulsing the mucosa within the membranous urethra. The mucosa over the prostate can be circumcised via the bladder part of the incision with a cautery to limit the amount of mucosal bleeding before enucleation. Also, the bladder can be inspected for other pathological processes, although these should have been seen by the preoperative cystoscopy. Having enucleated the gland, the urologist can secure hemostasis in very much the same way as in the retropubic operation. The vesico-capsular incision is usually closed with a running suture of 00 chromic catgut with the middle stay sutures tied over the repair for added support. However, if at the end of the enucleation the bladder neck appears to be narrow, then the vertical incision can be closed in a transverse direction by drawing the lateral sutures of the bladder neck laterally and the inferior and superior stay sutures of the prostate and vesical incision together.

A similar principle for widening the bladder neck has been used. Instead of making a horizontal incision into the prostatic capsule, a 'Y' shaped incision is made and repaired as a 'V' by bringing the apex of the 'V' to the bottom of the 'Y' thus performing a large 'Y-V' plasty.

An early fistula sometimes occurs if there has been faulty closure of the prostatic capsule or where enucleation of the prostate has resulted in a tear in the posterior part of the capsule. It can occur as the result of, rather than, overenthusiastic coagulation of capsular bleeders immediately after the capsule is opened. In the majority of cases, spontaneous closure occurs. However, if there is a persistent leak, a Foley catheter which has a hole specially cut in the urine lead just below the Foley bag as it rests on the bladder neck will usually result in closure. The point of drainage will then be distal or below the level of the fistula, whereas the usual drainage point of a Foley catheter with the balloon inflated is two to three centimeters above the fistula site. Osteitis pubis and pelvic cellulitis occurred in some of the earlier cases but none in recent years (Marshall 1967). However, it is important that adequate retropubic drainage should be established for the first four to five days following operation.

VII. TRANSVESICAL (SUPRAPUBIC) PROSTATECTOMY

This is the procedure by which the enlarged prostate is removed through the cavity of the bladder. The approach to the bladder can be through the Pfannenstiel incision already described for retropubic prostatectomy or by a midline vertical incision through the skin and the anterior sheath with a rectus muscle separation. Where cystoscopy has been performed before the prostatectomy, the bladder is filled before the scope is removed or alternatively a catheter is used to fill up the bladder. By this maneuver, the peritoneum is displaced upwards leaving a part of the anterior wall of the bladder easily exposed. Where previous cystotomy has been performed to allow preoperative drainage, the skin cystotomy wound can be circumcised and the tract followed down to open the bladder. Through the cystotomy, two narrow Deaver retractors can be inserted and the bladder inspected. The obstructing prostate can be inspected with a bladder retractor and the mucosa overlying it circumcised with a cautery to reduce mucosal bleeding. When the retractors are removed, and an index finger can be inserted through the bladder into the prostatic urethra, the anterior commissure is split for the start of the enucleation by pressing anteriorly towards the pubis (Figure 3). The finger is inserted as far as the apex of the prostate and, by

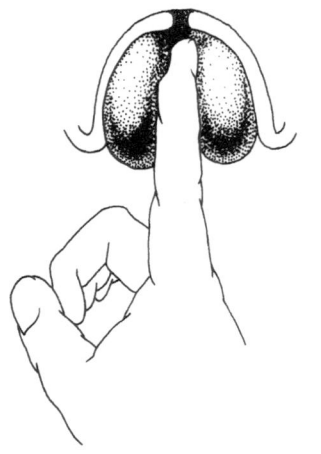

Prostate broken through anteriorly

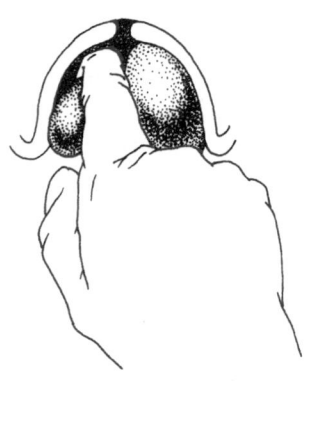

Left lateral lobe enucleation

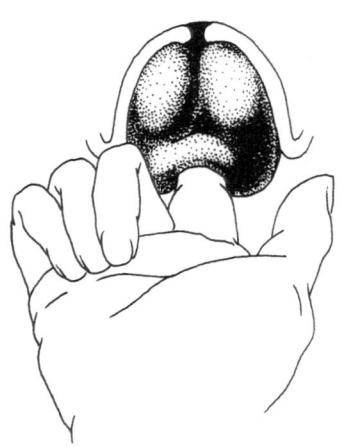

Lateral and median lobes, gland enucleated

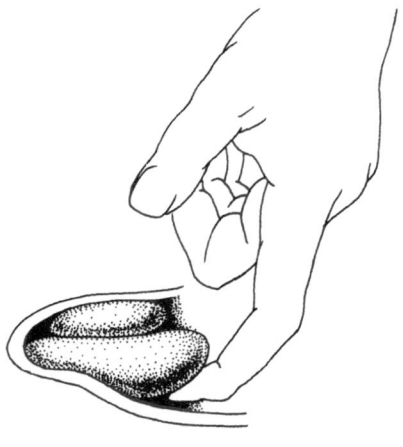

Middle lobe enucleation

Figure 3. Digital enucleation of prostate, transvesical approach.

flexing the distal phalanx laterally with a scratching maneuver, the mucosa over the apex of the gland can be breached without avulsing the membranous urethra. The adenoma is then enucleated. If difficulty is encountered with enucleation, a finger can be inserted into the rectum and, with upward pressure, will bring a large prostate well within the reach of the average finger and also aid in definition of the plane of dissection. It is sometimes useful to run a layer of 000 plain catgut around the mucosal edge, closing this to the prostatic fossa to secure hemostasis. Bleeding vessels at five and seven o'clock at the bladder neck may be under-run with catgut for hemostasis, but this is more difficult to perform with the transvesical operation than in the retropubic exposure. Having performed enucleation, most urologists insert a cystotomy tube as well as a urethral catheter to allow the facility of through and through irrigation if necessary in the immediate postoperative phase. A DePezzer, Foley, or Malecot catheter is used, depending upon the preference of the surgeon. After the suprapubic tube is inserted, the prostatic area is again inspected and if hemostasis is secured, the bladder is closed.

The immediate postoperative care is concerned with prevention of clotting in the catheters. Many methods have been described by staunch and vocal advocates of their own particular systems. However, as a general principle, the method the surgeon prefers is the method that should be used because he is comfortable with it and knows its advantages and limitations. A selection of these methods includes a continuous drip of saline through the supra-pubic catheter or through a urethra catheter and out through a cystotomy tube. The older tidal drainage system which was in vogue in the early 1950s has been replaced by an intermittent method of irrigation using a reservoir and an agitator in the input line so that 50 ml of saline can be washed in and out of the bladder with a closed system. This system is called The Bristol Irrigating System in England and the cysto pump unit in the United States. This system has the advantage of irrigating the bladder as necessary without breaking the sterile tubing from the bladder to the drainage bag. Being a semi-automatic system, it also has the advantage that a nurse or other personnel sees the patient at half or three-quarter hourly intervals depending upon the amount of bleeding throughout the patient's early

postoperative course. This encourages close observation and attention to the patient's vital signs. Finally, there are surgeons who merely connect the catheter to a drainage bag and irrigate the catheter manually whenever there is a question of clotting. This has the disadvantage of breaking the sterile arrangements for manual irrigation. Blood loss is difficult to assess in open prostatectomy because first the bladder is sucked clean of urine, then the bladder is irrigated of clots immediately after it has been closed and much blood and fluid is taken up in the drapes around the wound. However, in most institutions, the anesthetist has a fairly accurate assessment of blood loss from the general condition of the patient and the number of dressings soaked with blood. Following the operation, hematocrit and hemoglobin levels will indicate the need for further transfusion.

VIII. PERINEAL PROSTATECTOMY

This is essentially a North American operation. 'British surgeons have never understood why this difficult operation was ever as popular as it once was in some centers in North America. Even those of us who have been privileged to watch it being done, remain puzzled as to why anyone should want to make an easy operation so difficult' (Blandy 1976). There is no doubt that this once popular technique is now fourth on the popularity poll and many surgeons have never seen the operation, let alone receive training in it. However, it still remains a useful operation in the urologist's repertoire. Of all the open techniques of prostatectomy, it is the most comfortable for the patient and least likely to have complications. To those who are horrified by the position of the patient on the operating table, amazement is added the next morning by seeing just how well the patient looks for the first postoperative day.

A. Indications for perineal prostatectomy

1. The patient who has a questionable nodule in an otherwise moderately enlarged benign gland. A perineal biopsy can be taken for frozen section and if this is benign, the gland can then be enucleated without change of position of the patient.

2. The patient who has had a recent lower abdominal operation or hernia repair and a large obstructing gland can be treated by perineal prostatectomy without disturbing the recent abdominal incision.

3. Patients with chronic obstructive airway disease have difficulty in exhaling and the inverted position necessary for perineal prostatectomy aids the patient's expiratory movements. Respiratory depression is avoided since the operation is performed under a spinal anesthetic (Giesecki et al. 1968). The operation has been performed in patients undergoing abdominoperineal resection for malignant rectal disease, but one author of this article (Dalton) has been loath to perform this operation for fear of opening 'another system' and risking possible spread of malignant seedlings to the urinary tract.

The main contraindication to perineal prostatectomy is the young patient in whom sexual performance is extremely important, as this form of prostatectomy probably interferes with potency more than any other technique.

B. Preoperative Preparation

The ideal patient for this surgical approach is one in whom the perineum is thin and the pelvis is wide. Because of the proximity of the prostate to the rectum, preoperative preparation includes enemas and washouts to clear the bowel before operation, plus a low residue diet and neomycin sulphate forty-eight hours before operation. The operation is usually performed under spinal anesthesia. While there are still old models of the specialized perineal table designed by Hugh Young, most modern-day operating tables with leg supports and a wedge under the sacrum will give excellent exposure of the perineum. An important detail is that the sacrum and buttocks are raised so that the perineum is placed horizontally. The weight of the patient plus skin traction usually prevents the patient sliding head-down the table, but shoulder rests should be inserted to avoid this complication. To avoid traction injury to the brachial plexus, one should be able to move a finger between the shoulder rests and the shoulder so that the rest is a guard against slipping and not a constant pressure support over the period of the operation. While a number of specialized surgical instruments have been designed for the performance of the perineal prostatectomy, the operation can be performed with the usual urologist's armamentarium plus a urethral sound and a Foley catheter in place of the Lowsley or Young prostatic tractor. Again while it is more rapidly performed with two or three assistants plus a scrub nurse, in fact the operation can be performed with a surgeon, his assistant and a scrub nurse. This operation has been described and illustrated so well that any further description of the operation itself would be quite redundant (Hudson 1970). A number of practical details, however, can be added. It is extremely important to protect the rectum with gauze under a finger or retractor so that injury does not occur. In the event of rectal injury early in the operation, the procedure of prostatectomy should be abandoned and the rent repaired in two layers with 000 chromic catgut: one layer for the mucosa and the other for the muscle. A further layer approximating the levator ani muscle as it attaches to the rectum acts as a tension-relieving suture. A perineal drain is inserted and the wound closed. Dilatation of the anus to six fingers slowly, as in Lord's treatment for anal fissure will result in some temporary paralysis of the anal sphincter and prevent gaseous distention within the rectum. Either a catheter is inserted into the bladder and left to continuous catheter drainage or alternatively another method of prostatectomy may be used considering that the patient is already anesthetized. If the rectal tear is found at the end of the surgical procedure, then the rectal injury is repaired as described and the anal sphincter stretched. The preoperative neomycin sulphate medication is continued into the postoperative period for five to seven days. Intravenous therapy is continued for two to three days longer than the usual period and oral feeding is delayed for two to three days. The perineal drain should be left for a total of a week and the catheter, instead of being removed on the seventh or eighth postoperative day in the uncomplicated case, is left for a full two weeks, providing there is no evidence of fecal leak through the skin.

In spite of suturing the urethral catheter to the penis, the catheter can still be inadvertently removed. Where the urethra has been drawn down to the bladder neck during the operation, a waiting policy can be followed as the patient is likely to pass urine with no problem. If the prostatic capsule has merely been closed, reinsertion will be necessary, unless the catheter has been inadvertently removed on or later than the third or fourth postoperative day. Now that the Coudé's Foley catheter is available, it is possible to pass this catheter intact along the anterior wall of the urethra and into the bladder. Sometimes a finger in the rectum is necessary to avoid posterior capsule and rectal tear. If a Coudé catheter is not available, a Foley catheter on a stilette is passed along the urethra, 'hugging' the anterior wall of the urethra and prostatic cavity so that the catheter will slide safely into the bladder rather than run under the posterior lip into the rectum or sub-trigonal space. If there is any question about the position of the catheter after insertion, 5 to 10 ml of Urographin and a lateral x-ray film will usually show the position of the catheter. If there is any difficulty in reinsertion, the preferable course is to allow the bladder to fill to above the pubis and to insert a No. 12 or 14 cystocath for drainage. This can subsequently be clamped and the patient tested for ability to void spontaneously.

C. Urinary Extravasation

Urinary extravasation for the first 48 hours or so after removal of the perineal tube can be expected; this usually stops spontaneously. If it reappears following removal of the urethral catheter, the catheter is reinserted and left indwelling until the perineum has been dry for seven days.

As in other forms of prostatectomy, following removal of the catheter, the patient has a period of uncertainty about his urinary control, but in the vast majority of cases by the first postoperative day control is practically normal and will remain so merely with the suggestion that the patient perform perineal exercises of a stop, start, stop, start variety during voiding for a month.

IX. TRANSURETHRAL RESECTION: PROSTATECTOMY

Transurethral resection of the prostate (TURP) is now the most popular method of prostatectomy in the United States and is rapidly becoming more accepted throughout the world as surgeons learn the technique. Approximately 95 percent of the prostatectomies in our institution and in other similar institutions are done transurethrally (Valk 1975). Most residency training programs are now designed to offer the resident as much experience as possible. Although this procedure is initially difficult and sometimes dangerous, TURP is adequately learned after the first 100 cases. Then the surgeon gradually acquires expertise and skill and with years of experience, he learns his limitations. Many expert resectionists will resect 100 grams or more of tissue. We prefer to resect no more than 80 grams to avoid excessive resection time, over-instrumentation, and fluid absorption overload. Most surgeons should be able to resect about a gram per minute and the operation rarely takes more than one hour.

The size of the gland is generally the first consideration of the surgeon. If he feels he can comfortably resect the gland, there are really very few specific contraindications to the transurethral procedure. A careful medical evaluation, especially of the cardiopulmonary status of the patient, is absolutely essential. If heart failure is present, or impending heart failure, great care must be taken with the patient. Amazingly large amounts of irrigating fluid can be absorbed into the venous system in a relatively short period of time. Fluid overload and congestive heart failure can occur quite rapidly so continuous electrocardiographic monitoring and a central venous pressure catheter should be used intraoperatively in the severe cardiac patient. Urethral pathology is a relative contraindication. If strictures are present, often they can be slowly dilated preoperatively with a soft silastic catheter of increasing size, or it is possible to bypass the stricture by operating through a perineal urethrotomy. Wide caliber strictures may be gently dilated just prior to introducing the resectoscope. A urethrotomy prior to surgery has been advocated by some (Emmett et al. 1963), but we have had unwanted morbidity with this procedure.

All patients should have sterile urine prior to a transurethral resection. If the patient has a urinary tract infection or if a catheter has been placed for bladder drainage, suitable antimicrobials should be instituted prior to surgery. Routine use of antimicrobials during or after surgery in patients with sterile urine is currently a point of argument. Our patients do better postoperatively with oral antimicrobials for three to four weeks.

Proper positioning of the patient, meticulous care and organization of the instruments, and a comfortable working position for the surgeon are absolutely necessary. Many instruments and modifications are available. We prefer the Iglesias resectoscope and certainly fiber optic lighting. Low spinal anesthesia is preferable so that it is possible to monitor and communicate with the patient in order to recognize possible complications early (cardiac heart failure, fluid overload, electrolyte imbalance, or fluid extravasation). Isotonic irrigating solutions should be used to obviate hemolysis, renal tubular damage, or both. Smaller size sheaths (25 French) can now be used routinely especially with a continuous flow apparatus to allow the surgeon to resect without pausing to empty the patient's bladder.

The surgeon should check out his own instruments to assure proper working order. Careful cystoscopy and panendoscopy should be carried out first. If the transurethral resection procedure is elected, the sheath should be introduced gently with copious lubricant. Meatotomy is wise if any suggestion of narrowing is present. Gentle dilation of strictures is advisable so that the sheath slides freely. The surgeon should first identify his landmarks well: The bladder neck – most proximal extent of his resection; area of the verumontanum – most distal extent of his resection; bladder; trigone; and ureteral orifices (Figures 4a, b). We have found the classical resection technique to be best (Nesbit 1970). First, the area of the vesical neck is resected down to fibers. These fibers serve as a good landmark for the surgeon to follow as the procedure progresses. Next the bulk of the adenoma is resected from the bladder neck to the verumontanum. We begin in the roof (Figure 4c), resect down to fibers, then follow this depth of resection out laterally, resecting first the left lateral lobe (Figure 4d), then the right lateral lobe (Figure 4e) and finally the median lobe. Major bleeders are coagulated as the operation progresses. Minor ones can be ignored till the end of the procedure. The apical area is resected last (Figure 4f). In this area, the surgeon must take great care not to overresect. Usually he can withdraw the scope just distal to the verumontanum and see the distal parts of the lateral lobes which can be resected. The median

lobe, if large, may have to be resected first, to allow free passage of the resectoscope. Resection of adenomatous tissue in the prostatic floor can be facilitated by elevating the prostate with a finger in the rectum (via an O'Connor sheath). At the end of the procedure, all arterial bleeders should be coagulated with care. Venous bleeders will stop as the capsule contracts. Prostatic chips can be best removed with an Ellik evacuator and a No. 24 Foley catheter inserted into the bladder with 50 cc placed in the bag. With gentle irrigation, the bleeding stops in two to four minutes. If not, gentle traction on the catheter for 10-15 minutes should clear the irrigant. The catheter should be removed as soon as the urine clears – usually in two to three days. Attention to blood loss and fluid overload, serum electrolytes, and potential medical complications are necessary to keep morbidity and mortality at a minimum.

X. MORTALITY AND MORBIDITY OF PROSTATECTOMY

A. Mortality

The mortality rates for all forms of prostatectomy have gradually decreased. The mortality rates for open prostatectomy are comparable, fluctuating around one percent (Grayhack et al. 1975). The risk of death with transurethral resection is even less. An increased risk seems to be associated with azotemia (Melchor et al. 1974), older age (Melchior et al. 1974), and larger prostates.

Ten years of experience at the University of Kansas with over 4,000 transurethral resection of the prostate procedures sums up the causes quite nicely (Table 2. Holtgrewe and Valk 1962; Melchior et al. 1974).

B. Morbidity

1. Incontinence

Prevention of incontinence starts with the preoperative assessment of the patient. If the patient has had a bulbomembranous stricture treated by an inlay procedure, the urologist should be cautious about performing prostatectomy because often the patient's external sphincter mechanism is impaired by the inlay urethroplasty. If there is a history of urgency incontinence, especially with Parkinson's disease, a preoperative cystometrogram should be done to exclude uninhibited neurogenic bladder disease. Intraoperatively the position of the external sphincter must be ascertained and the verumontanum is a good guide to this. The surgeon should remain on the bladder side of the verumontanum to insure complete control. Incontinence following retropubic prostatectomy has improved from 4.5 percent in an older series (Millin et al. 1949) to one percent by 1972 (Salvatierra et al. 1972) and is probably related to the increased familiarity of the operation over the years. Supra-pubic prostatectomy seems to have had a better record throughout with a report of 0.7 percent in 1954 (Caine 1954) and in 1966 (Cooper et al. 1966).

For perineal prostatectomy, a study reported 1.9 percent in 1964 (Turner and Belt 1957). A complication incidence of 5.5 percent was reported in 840 transurethral resections in 1964 (Hollgrewe and Valk 1964), of which 1.4 percent were severe enough to warrant having an incontinence device.

2. Impotence

The incidence of impotence varies with multiple reports in the literature. This incidence is difficult

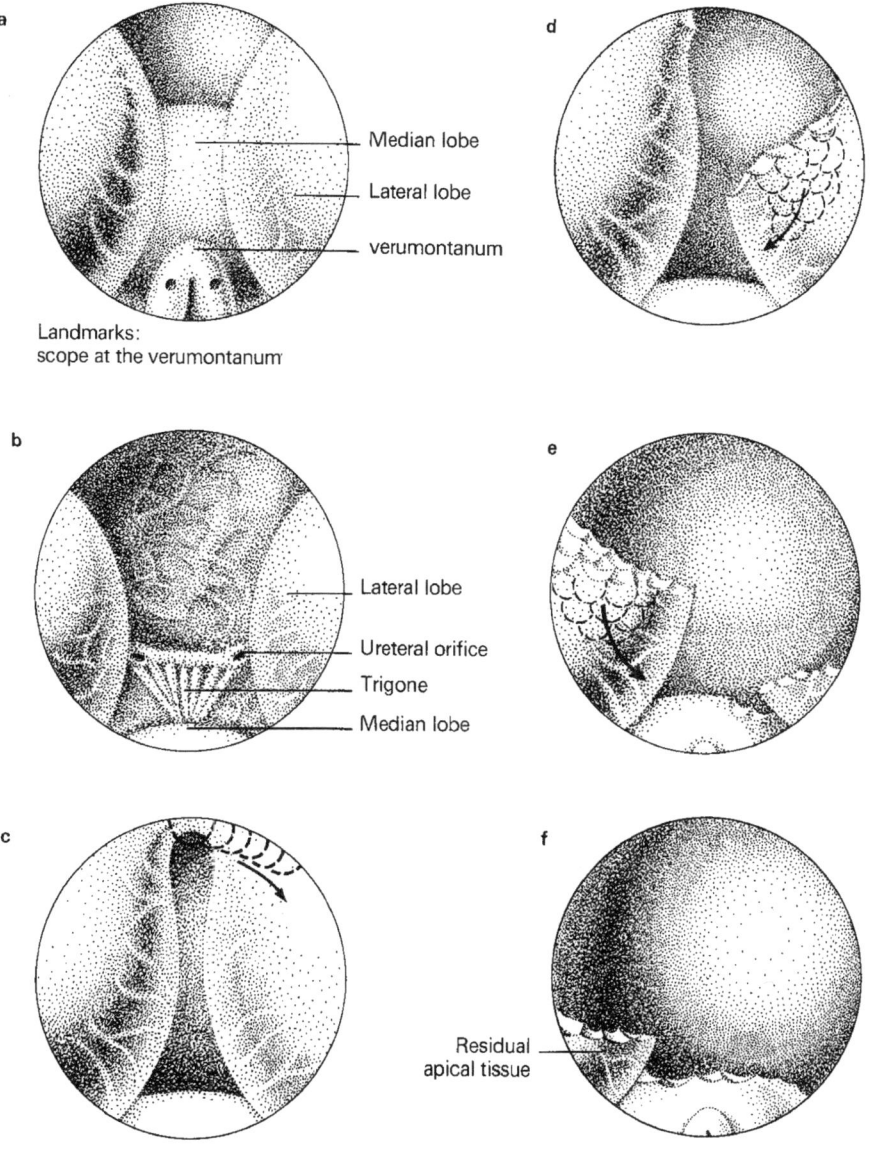

Figure 4. Landmarks: scope at the verumontanum.

Table 2. Causes of mortality in prostatectomy (percentage).

	1955-60 (2015 cases)	1965-71 (2223 cases)
Myocardial infarct	0.9	9.5
Pulmonary embolus	0.5	0.1
Cerebrovascular accident	0.2	
Pyelonephritis and sepsis	0.2	0.1
Pneumonia	0.2	
Hemorrhage	0.1	
Acute renal failure	0.1	0.1
G.I. bleeding	—	0.2
Congestive heart failure	—	0.2
Respiration failure	—	0.1
Ruptured aneurysm	0.1	0.1
Mesenteric artery thrombosis	0.05	01.
Total	2.5	1.3

to determine due to multiple variables and the patient's willingness to blame the surgical procedure. The open procedures may have a higher incidence than transurethral resection with perineal being the highest. An exact incidence figure is impossible to quote because of the variance of reports and unreliability of the data. Postoperative impotence following prostatic surgery is rather more dependent upon the patient's preoperative interest in intercourse rather than in the type of operation performed (Finkel and Priam 1966). They reported potency in 79 percent for perineal, 87 percent for suprapubic, and 95 percent for transurethral prostatectomy: others (Lilien et al. 1968) gave rather depressing figures of 26 percent for perineal and 61 percent for suprapubic, but the perineal cases were in highly debilitated cases and preoperative potency was not noted. With the use of an electroencephalogram and penile phletysmography in a sleep laboratory, there was no change in pre- and postoperative patterns in 14 cases studied (Madorsky et al. 1976).

3. Stricture

The highest incidence is undoubtedly with transurethral resection. Some strictures seem to be transient and respond to one or two soundings shortly after surgery. Other strictures remain and their seriousness depends on their location and response to treatment. Bladder neck contractures can be very difficult to relieve and may need further surgery to neutralize. Strictures of the membranous urethra and deep bulbous urethra hopefully

will respond to treatment because surgical correction can be quite difficult. Fossa navicularis or meatal strictures are the most common and usually can be fairly easily handled.

4. Hemorrhage

Immediate hemorrhage from the prostatic fossa can usually be controlled in the immediate postoperative period by traction on the catheter.

Amicar is used by some as a routine, but we have never found any need for this (Herr 1973). If the patient has much bleeding from the wound, then the patient should be checked for intravascular coagulopathy (Kernoff 1972). If the bleeding does not stop by conservative means, then it may be necessary to either insert the resectoscope to deal with the bleeding vessels or if an open prostatectomy is performed, to reopen the main wound and pack the fossa. More recently, selective bilateral hypogastric embolization has been performed for the rare case where morbid bleeding occurs in a very sick postoperative case unresponsive to conservative measures (Mitchell et al. 1976). Other acute morbidity has been well summarized by the Kansas articles (Table 3: Holtgrewe and Valk 1962; Melchior et al. 1974).

Table 3. Transurethral morbidity associated with prostatectomy for BPH (percentage).

	1955-60 (2015 cases)	1965-71 (2223 cases)
Hemorrhage	0.5	2.3
Myocardial infarct	0.2	0.8
Congestive failure	0.4	0.2
Pulmonary embolism	0.3	0.2
Renal failure	0.7	0.3
Epididymitis	6.0	2.6
Pyelonephritis	1.1	0.4
Pneumonia	1.3	0.7
Thrombophlebitis	0.7	0.4
Endotoxin shock	0.5	X
G.I. bleeding	0.2	0.3
Extravasation	1.1	0.6
Suprapubic fistula	—	—
Secondary resection	3.4	0.9
Total	18	17.3

REFERENCES

Ahluwalia MS and Tandon HD: Nodular hyperplasia of the prostate in North India: An autopsy study. J Urol 93: 94, 1965.

Anikwe RM: Urodynamics in benign prostatic hypertrophy. Br J Urol 50: 20, 1978.

Ashley DJB: Observations on the epidemiology of prostatic hyperplasia in Wales. Br J Urol 38: 567, 1966.

Birkhoff JD, et al: Natural history of benign prostatic hypertrophy and acute urinary retention. Urol VII(1): 48, 1976.

Blandy JP: Benign enlargement of the prostate gland. In: Urology, vol 2 John Blandy (ed), Oxford, Blackwell Scientific Publications, 1976.

Brooks MB, Lytton B, et al: Vasectomy in the control of epididymitis after prostatectomy following urethral catheter drainage. J Urol 105: 694, 1971.

Burns E: Prostatic obstruction in negroes. J Urol 44: 177, 1940.

Caine MO: The late results and sequelae of prostatectomy. Br J Urol 26: 205, 1954.

Chang HL and Char GY: Benign hypertrophy of the prostate. Chinese Med J 50: 1707, 1936.

Cooper JF, Ashamanna G and Cobbs R: A survey of 302 transvesical prostatectomies with primary closure technique. Surg Gyn Obst 123: 277, 1966.

Culp DA: Benign prostatic hyperplasia. The Urology Clinics of North America, 2(1): 29, 1975.

D'Aunoy R, Schenken JR and Burns EL: Relative incidence of hyperplasia of prostate in white and colored races in Louisiana: An analysis of 325 glands removed at operation. South Med J 32: 47, 1939.

Day GH: Urological and venereal idiosyncrasies presented by the negro. J Urol 5: 19, 1921.

Dodge OG: Carcinoma of the prostate in Uganda Africans. Cancer 16: 1264, 1963.

Drake WH Jr: The uroflowmeter. J Urol 59: 650, 1948.

Emmett JL, Rouse SN, et al: Primary internal urethrotomy in 1,036 cases to prevent urethral stricture following transurethral resection: caliber of normal adult male urethra. J Urol 89: 829, 1963.

Finkel AL and Prian DV: Sexual potency in elderly men before and after prostatectomy. JAMA 196: 139, 1966.

Franks LM: Benign nodular hyperplasia of the prostate: A review. Ann Royal Coll Surg (Eng) 14: 92, 1954.

Giesecki AH Jr, Cale JO and Jenkins MT: The prostate: ventilation and anesthesia. JAMA 203: 389, 1968.

Goldstein AE: Bilateral ligation of the vas deferens in prostatectomy. J Urol 17: 25, 1927.

Grayhack JT, Wilson JD, et al: Benign prostatic hyperplasia, NIAMDD Workshop Proceedings, NIH. Bethesda, Feb. 20-21, 101-103, 1975.

Harvard BM and White RR: A technique for transvesical prostatectomy. Conn Med 24: 286, 1960.

Herr HW: Use of prophylactic antibiotics in the high risk patient undergoing prostatectomy: Effect on morbidity. J Urol 110: 686, 1973.

Hirsch EW: Prostatic enlargement in the black and white races. Urol & Cutan Rev 36: 821, 1932.

Hodges CV and Barry JM: Suprapubic and retropubic prostatectomy. The Urology Clinics of North America. 2(1): 49, 1975.

Holtgrewe HL and Valk WL: Factors influencing the morbidity and mortality of TUR prostatectomy. A study of 2015 cases. J Urol 87: 450, 1962.

Hudson PB: Perineal prostatectomy. In Urology, vol 3, Campbell MF and Harrison JH (eds), Philadelphia, WB Saunders Company, 1970.

Hunt VC: Benign prostatic hypertrophy: a review of 1000 cases. Surg Gyn & Obstet 46: 769, 1928.

Kernoff PA: Prostatectomy in haemophilia and Christmas Disease. Br J Urol 44: 51, 1972.

Lapides J: Principles of treatment of persistent post-prostatectomy hemorrhage. J Urol 106: 913, 1971.

Lilien OM, Schaefer JA, et al: The case for perineal prostatectomy. J Urol 99: 79, 1968.

Lisoos I: Simple prostatic hyperplasia in the Bantu. S Afr Med J 47: 389, 1973.

Lowsley OS: The development of the human prostate gland with reference to the development of the structures of the urinary bladder. Amer J Anat 13: 299, 1912.

Lytton B, Emery JM, et al: The incidence of benign prostatic obstruction. J Urol 99: 639, 1968.

Madorsky ML, et al: Post-prostatectomy impotence. J Urol 115: 401, 1976.

Marshall A: Retropubic prostatectomy: A review of 761 patients with special reference to urinary infection. Br J Urol 39: 307, 1967.

Meares EM, Jr and Stamey TA: Bacteriologic localization patterns in bacterial prostatitis and urethritis. Invest Urol 5: 492, 1968.

Melchior J, Valk WL, et al: TUR prostatectomy: computerized analysis of 2223 consecutive cases. J Urol 112: 634, 1974.

Millin T: Retropubic prostatectomy – a new extravesical technique – a report on 20 cases. Lancet 2: 693, 1945.

Millin T, McAlister CLO, et al: Retropubic prostatectomy. Experience based on 751 cases. Lancet 1: 381, 1949.

Mitchell ME, et al: Control of massive prostatic bleeding with angiographic techniques. J Urol 115: 692, 1976.

Moore RA: Benign hypertrophy and carcinoma of the prostate. Occurrence and experimental production in animals. Surgery 16: 152, 1944.

Mostofi FK and Price EB: Tumors of the male genital system. The Armed Forces Institute of Pathology, Wash DC, 1973.

Nesbit RM: Transurethral prostatic resection. In: Urology, vol III, Campbell MF and Harrison JH (eds), Philadelphia, WB Saunders Company, 1970.

Oomura J, Ookita K, et al: Clinical observation on prostatic hypertrophy and cancer: Okayama University Medical School in the recent eight years. Jap J Urol 56: 583, 1966.

Randall A: Surgical pathology of prostatitis obstructions. Baltimore, Williams and Wilkins Co, 1931.

Robinson MC: The incidence of benign prostatic hyperplasia and prostatic carcinoma in cirrhosis of the liver. J Urol 92: 307, 1964.

Rodman WL: In: Keen's Surgery. Philadelphia, WB Saunders Company vol 4: 1150, 1919.

Salvaris M: Retropubic prostatectomy: An evaluation of 1200 operations. Med J Aust 47: 370, 1960.

Salvatierra O Jr, Rigdon WO, et al: Modified retropubic prostatectomy: A new technique. J Urol 108: 126, 1972.

Semple JE: Surgical capsule of the enlargement of the prostate. Br Med J 2: 1640, 1963.

Singh M, Blandy JP, et al: The evaluation of transurethral resection for benign enlargement of the prostate. Br J Urol 45: 93, 1973.

Smart CJ and Jenkins JD: The role of transurethral prostatectomy in chronic prostatitis. Br. J Urol 45: 654, 1973.

Smith KJ and Jaffe RH: The comparative frequency of prostatic hypertrophy in the white and colored races. Urol & Cutan Rev 36: 661, 1932.

Susset JG, Picker P, et al: Critical evaluation of uroflowmeters and analysis of normal curves. J Urol 109: 874, 1973.

Tan RE: Prostatic disease in Indonesia. J Urol 86: 428, 1961.

Turner RD and Belt E: The results of 1694 consecutive simple perineal prostatectomies. J Urol 77: 853, 1957.

Valk WL: Present status of transurethral resection of the prostate for benign prostatic hypertrophy, The Urological Clinics of North America, 2(1): 85, 1975.

Walker KM: Nature and cause of old age enlargement of the prostate. Br Med J 1: 297, 1922.

Ward RO: Vesicocapsular prostatectomy – a new extravesical technique – a report on 20 cases. Lancet 2: 693, 1948.

Wear JB and Haley T: Transurethral prostatectomy without antibiotics. J Urol 110: 436, 1973.

Weyrauch HM: Surgery of the Prostate. Philadelphia, WB Saunders Company, 1959.

Whitfield HJ: Prostatism in the negro with clinical and pathological studies. J Urol 64: 106, 1950.

17. EPIDIDYMECTOMY, SEMINAL VESICULECTOMY AND HYDROCELECTOMY FOR EPIDIDYMITIS, SEMINAL VESICULITIS AND HYDROCELE

M.A. SILVERT and T.H. STANISIC

I. EPIDIDYMECTOMY

Epididymectomy was first described by Bardenheuer in 1887 for the treatment of tubercular epididymitis. Since that time, epididymectomy has been performed for a number of other indications although tuberculosis has been the most common reason. The era of antitubercular chemotherapy has now made epididymectomy a relatively uncommon operative procedure.

A. Diagnosis and Indications

Epididymitis includes the acute and chronic manifestations of inflammatory lesions of the epididymis. As summarized in Table 1, these lesions may be infective or idiopathic. Since the appropriate treatment, whether medical or surgical, is, to a large extent, a function of the etiology, a closer evaluation of these causes is warranted.

Table 1. Etiologies of epididymitis.

Infective
    Pyogenic infections
    Chlamydia
    Gonorrhea
    Syphilis
    Tuberculosis
    Fungal
    Brucellosis
    Friedländer's Bacillus
    Amoeba
    Schistosomiasis
    Filaria
Idiopathic
    Traumatic
    ? Chemical irritation
    ? Immunologic
    Unidentified infective agents
        Chlamydia
        Virus

Pyogenic epididymal infections are caused by common bacteria including aerobic enteric organisms, staphylococcus, and streptococcus. Anaerobic organisms are not commonly believed to contribute to acute epididymitis although the role of corynebacterium and chlamydia are still being elucidated. Typically, the symptoms of acute epididymitis include epididymal enlargement, tenderness, and fever. Predisposing factors include urethral strictures and manipulation of an infected genitourinary system. Most differential diagnostic problems involve torsion of the testis or one of the appendages, although testicular tumors are occasionally misdiagnosed as epididymitis. A careful scrotal examination with or without local spermatic cord anesthetic usually suffices to make the diagnosis, although Prehn's sign, scrotal thermography, nuclear scans, and Doppler stethoscopes can be useful adjuvants.

Classic treatment of acute epididymitis includes rest, scrotal elevation and support, an ice pack and antibiotics. If the urine culture is positive, the selection of the appropriate antibiotic should be based on the antibiotic sensitivity pattern of the urinary organism. Epididymectomy is generally reserved for epididymal abscesses or for chronic painful epididymitis or a painful epididymis. However, a strong argument for early surgical intervention has been made (Wilson et al. 1974). Prompt intervention allows almost immediate relief of pain, a benign postoperative course, decreased length of hospitalization, and a decreased convalescent period (patient returned to work in an average of 15 days instead of 30 days). In addition, further attacks of epididymitis are totally eliminated – at least on the removed side. Despite the theoretical advantages cited, we rely almost entirely upon medical treatment in the usual case of acute epididymitis. Surgical therapy, of course, should be routinely considered only for men not interested in their future fertility.

Prior to the antibiotic era, up to 25 percent of patients with gonorrheal urethritis had concurrent epididymitis. Fortunately, epididymal involvement is now rare due to early antibiotic therapy. The signs and symptoms are virtually identical to other pyogenic infections with the critical addition of the urethral symptoms associated with the gonorrheal urethritis. Although the testis was rarely involved, infertility occurred in 50-80 percent of the patients with extensive epididymal involvement.

Syphilitic epididymitis involvement is usually asymptomatic and may occur either in early secondary syphilis or as late as eight or nine years post onset. However, congenital syphilitic epididymitis has been reported in a two year old. Tertiary or gummatous epididymitis is extremely rare although extension from a testicular gumma is not uncommon. The diagnosis is usually made presumptively. Treatment is based on the stage of disease rather than the epididymal site of involvement.

When the lower genitourinary tract is involved with tuberculosis, the kidney is almost always involved also. Although the prostate and seminal vesicle are more commonly secondarily involved than the epididymis in male genitourinary tuberculosis, approximately 63-75 percent of involved patients have subclinical microscopic epididymal involvement (Boyce and Politano 1970). When clinical tuberculous epididymitis occurs, the epididymis usually is a slowly enlarging, painless mass. Classically, the testis is not involved in the granulomatous process although exceptions to this rule have been reported (Stanisic et al. 1978). This 'sparing of the testis' made epididymectomy the treatment of choice for tubercular epididymitis prior to the development of effective chemotherapeutic agents. As with the fungal infections, formation of a chronically draining fistula is common. With the advent of antitubercular chemotherapy, epididymal involvement is now rarely seen and can often be treated medically. However, surgical treatment is occasionally warranted, although exteriorization of the proximal vas deferens is no longer necessary.

The idiopathic causes of epididymitis are not well understood. Various etiologies have been proposed to explain those cases in which an infective agent is not found. Some of these are due to agents which are difficult to culture routinely, such as chlamydia, or due to infections restricted to the epididymis. However, the importance of chemical inflammation from urinary reflux of the vas deferens or nonspecific inflammation from immunologic mechanisms cannot be discounted. Treatment of idiopathic epididymitis is almost identical to that of pyogenic infections, although anti-inflammatory agents are a common therapeutic addition.

In addition to epididymitis, epididymectomy is occasionally indicated for a number of other pathologic conditions. Recurrent spermatoceles certainly justify surgical intervention. Epididymal tumors are fortunately a rare indication for surgery. In 1968, 75 percent of 278 reported epididymal tumors were benign (usually adenomatoid tumors). Of the malignant tumors, 28 percent were carcinomas, 48 percent were sarcomas and 24 percent were metastatic lesions (Broth et al. 1968). Treatment of the malignant lesions usually involved orchiectomy as well as epididymectomy. Due to the rarity of these tumors, very little is known about the role of chemotherapy and radiotherapy in postoperative care of these patients.

B. Surgery and Surgical Anatomy

The normal epididymis receives spermatozoa from the testes via the ductuli efferentes or rete testes. As shown in Figure 1a, the ductuli efferentes coalesce into a single conduit in the globus major. The duct then follows a serpentine course through the corpus of the epididymis to the globus minor where the duct forms the vas deferens. Note that the blood supply is primarily from the vas deferens and from a branch of the testicular artery.

The original epididymectomy in 1887 was performed through an oblique inguinal incision. The testicle was then delivered from the scrotum prior to performing the epididymectomy. Due to a significant complication rate of atrophic testicles, tubercular fistulas and severe wound infections, a transcrotal approach was popularized in the 1930s. Currently, the preferred technique is the scrotal approach through a vertical incision. This allows extension of the incision without contaminating the contralateral hemiscrotum. Anesthesia is usually general or regional in nature, but a local anesthetic can also be effective.

After delivering the testicle through the scrotum, much the same as in a simple orchiectomy, the dissection is generally initiated at the lower pole. Lightly incising the epididymo-testicular junction significantly aids the dissection (Figure 1b). Careful attention must be paid to the spermatic vessels which enter between the testes and epididymis at their lateral junction. As the upper pole is reached, the bifurcating spermatic artery can be seen. After ligating *only* the branch to the epididymis, the upper pole can easily be freed (Figure 1c). After obtaining adequate hemostasis, the tunica vaginalis

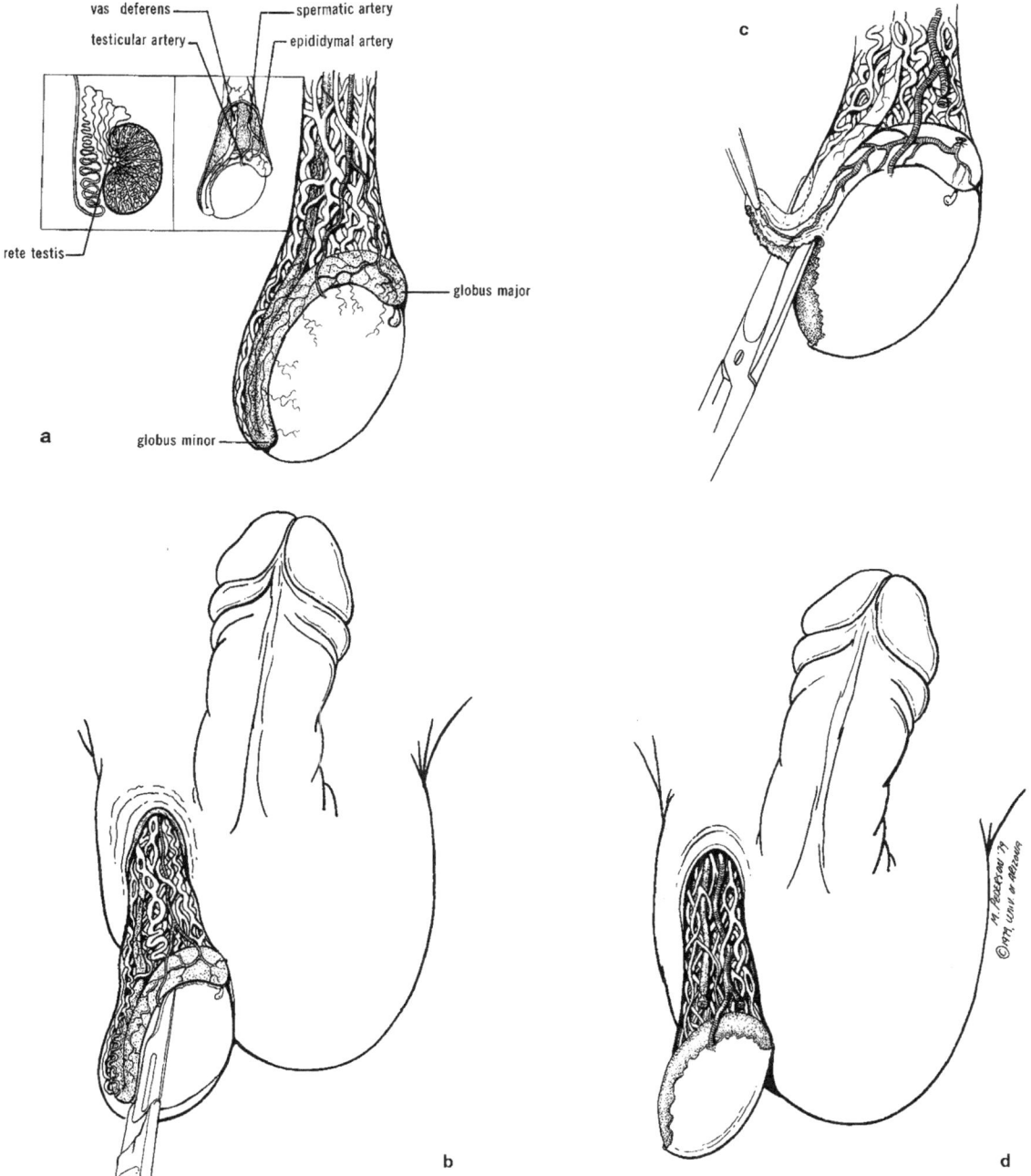

Figure 1. Epididymectomy: a. Normal epididymal anatomy. b. Beginning the dissection with a superficial incision of the epididymo-testicular junction. c. The epididymal artery is ligated as the epididymis is sharply dissected from the testicle. Note the preservation of the testicular artery lateral to the epididymis. d. Completed epididymectomy including ligation of the vas deferens.

can be closed over the epididymal defect (Figure 1d) and the vas deferens and its vessels can be divided. The testes should be replaced in the scrotum, following which a dependent penrose drain is inserted. The scrotum is then closed with interrupted chromic sutures.

If a draining sinus is present, an elliptical incision excising the sinus tract should be performed when the initial skin incision is made. If an abscess has caused extensive scrotal damage, debridement of additional necrotic tissue may be necessary. The elliptical wound is then allowed to heal secondarily.

C. Complications

In general, removal of a normal epididymis is not difficult. However, when tumor, infection or abscess is present, the anatomy becomes very distorted, thereby increasing the chances of a surgical misadventure. In addition to the expected risks of infection and bleeding, testicular atrophy due to damage to the spermatic artery may occur. After sacrificing the artery of the vas deferens, the testes cannot tolerate loss of the remaining blood supply. Only careful dissection and attention to detail can prevent testicular infarction.

II. SEMINAL VESICULECTOMY

A. Introduction

The seminal vesicles were originally described by Herophilus and first illustrated by Leonardo da Vinci (Murphy 1972). However the first seminal vesiculectomy was not described until 1889 by Ullmann (Murphy 1972; Politano et al. 1974). Ullman utilized a perineal approach in his treatment of a man with tubercular seminal vesiculitis. In subsequent years over a dozen techniques of performing seminal vesiculotomies and vesiculectomies were described (Table 2).

Although the first seminal vesiculectomy was performed for tuberculosis, the indications in later years included impotence, infections, nervous conditions and rheumatic arthritis – all reportedly with great success (Fuller 1912). From 1910 to 1930 the operation was very popular among surgeons but that popularity was without a firm

Table 2. History of the seminal vesiculectomy.

1889	Lloyd	First seminal vesiculotomy
1889	Ullmann	First seminal vesiculectomy via perineal approach for tuberculosis
1893	Schede	Transischial approach with coccygeal resection
1894	Schede	Transsacral approach
1895	Klotz	Catheterized ejaculatomy duct and injected silver nitrate
1900	Young	Suprapubic approach
1901	Futter	Utilized perineal seminal vesiculotomy for treatment of impotence, neurologic disorders, infection, tuberculosis and arthritis
1905	Cholyoff	Transischial approach with temporary resection of coccyx
1908	Voelcker	Ischiorectal approach
1909	Marion	Inguinoperineal approach
1911	Fiolle	Coccygeoperineal approach
1913	Belfield	Seminal vesiculography by vasotomy
1920	Young & Waters	Seminal vesiculography by catheterization of the ejaculatory ducts
1922	Soposhkoff	Transrectal approach
1922	Young	Perineal approach
1924	Thomson-Walker	Transvesical approach
1926	Young & Davis	Advocated radical seminal vesiculectomy for tuberculosis
1928	Hunt	Anococcygeal approach
1932	Seymour	Transperitoneal approach
1952	De Assis	Suprapubic, retrovesical, transperitoneal approach
1974	Politano et al.	Transvesical approach with complete division of bladder neck

scientific basis. With the advent of antibiotics, antitubercular agents, and, perhaps, better evaluation of results of therapy, seminal vesiculectomy is now an uncommon operation. Acceptable modern indications (Table 3) for a seminal vesiculectomy include calculi, chronic seminal vesiculitis, tumors and cysts. Seminal vesiculotomies are usually reserved for acute abscesses or occasionally for the treatment of chronic seminal vesiculitis.

B. Diagnosis and Indications

Pathological conditions of the seminal vesicles rarely have presenting signs. Approximately 2 percent of all reported seminal vesicle tumors have indicated hematospermia as a presenting sign. Hematospermia is much more common in benign diseases such as seminal vesiculitis but often cannot be linked with any definable pathologic process. Urinary obstruction, hematuria and perineal or low back pain can be presenting symptoms, although they are also relatively uncommon. The mainstay of diagnosis remains palpation of a tubular mass superior to the prostate. Once a suspicion of seminal vesicle pathology has been raised, an intravenous pyelogram, seminal vesiculography (either retrograde catheterization of the ejaculatory ducts, antegrade vasography, or transperineal injection of a cystic structure) and needle biopsy can be utilized to define the abnormality. If a tumor is suspected, an evaluation to rule out primary tumors is mandatory.

Benign masses are easily evaluated. Abscesses usually present as a tender, inflamed mass associated with fever and chills. If a trial period of antibiotic administration is unsuccessful, seminal vesiculotomy and, occasionally, seminal vesiculectomy can be definitive treatment. The cystic lesions are usually diagnosed in patients in the third decade of life and must be separated from Mullerian cysts. Mullerian cysts are usually found in the midline and cyst fluids characteristically are devoid of sperm when aspirated. Seminal vesicular retention cysts, on the other hand, are always lateral in origin although a large cyst can cross the midline, thus making the origin difficult to ascertain. However, fluid removed from a retention cyst usually contains spermatozoa and vesiculography demonstrates a connection to the vas deferens. Benign cysts have been reported in 25 cases as of 1975 (Bagley et al. 1975). Treatment must be tailored to the individual patient since appropriate therapy may take various forms, from simple observation to periodical cyst aspiration or even seminal vesiculotomy or seminal vesiculectomy.

The prostate and seminal vesicle are both androgen-dependent organs with similar embryologic origins. However, while prostatic malignancy is extremely common, primary seminal vesicle cancer is exceedingly rare. The peculiar resistance of the organ to malignant degeneration is unexplained. Seminal vesicle malignancies are usually seen in the elderly age group. Unfortunately, few tumors have been discovered early enough for curative surgery. Of the 44 carcinomas reported up to 1976 or the 5 sarcomas reported up to 1972, prognosis has been poor due to the advanced stage of the lesions. The effectiveness of chemotherapy, lymph node dissection and radiation therapy is also essentially an unknown quantity due to the rarity of the tumors. Estrogen hormonal therapy has been shown to be effective in one patient (Kees 1964), but absolutely ruling out that this represents a hormonally sensitive prostate tumor cannot be done with assurance. If the tumor is found early, radical seminal vesiculectomy, usually with a concurrent prostatectomy, is the operation of choice. For example, transcoccygeal seminal vesiculectomy has been curative in a 39 year-old with adenocarcinoma of the seminal vesicle (Lathem 1975). Treatment of metastatic lesions to the seminal vesicle should be based on the natural history and therapeutic peculiarities of the primary tumor.

Calculi, if symptomatic, can be treated by seminal vesiculotomy or vesiculectomy. Seminal vesiculitis is a benign condition that is usually self-limited. Only in rare cases is operative intervention indicated. Tubercular seminal vesiculitis, once the primary indication for a seminal vesiculectomy, rarely fails to respond to antitubercular therapy. An ectopic ureter inserting in the seminal vesicle is a rare congenital abnormality that is usually treated by reimplantation of the ureter or a nephroureterectomy, depending on the remaining function of the involved renal unit. Occasionally, a seminal vesiculectomy will also be required in conjunction with the primary ureteral operation.

Table 3. Indications for seminal vesiculectomy.

Masses

    Benign
       Abscess
       Congenital cysts
       Retention cysts

    Malignant
       Primary
          Carcinoma
          Sarcoma
       Metastatic
          Prostate
          Bladder
          Rectum
          Stomach

Infection

    Chronic Seminal Vesiculitis
    Tuberculosis

Calculi

Ectopic Ureters

C. Surgery and Surgical Anatomy

A multitude of approaches to the seminal vesicles have been described; not surprisingly, most of these techniques have fallen by the wayside, leaving only a few proven techniques. The perineal approach is the standard by which all other techniques must be judged. However, due to a fear of inducing impotence and the relative unfamiliarity most recently trained urologists have with the perineal approach, other procedures have become popular. The transcoccygeal or transsacral methods give excellent exposure, although this technique is not familiar to most urologists. In addition, the surgery is performed through very vascular tissues and can cause considerable postoperative coccygeal pain.

The extravesical, transperitoneal approaches tend to be relatively difficult forms of surgery that have a significant chance of interrupting the vascular pedicle to the bladder and prostate. The transvesical approach (Politano et al 1974) utilizes knowledge that is familiar to most urologists from their experience with radical retropubic prostatectomies. The seminal vesicles can easily be exposed, the rectum is always under direct vision, and there is minimal prostatic disturbance.

The key to using any of these approaches well lies in a clear understanding of the anatomic relationships of the bladder, prostate, seminal vesicles, rectum, as well as their blood and nerve supplies (Figure 2). The seminal vesicles arise embryologically from the lower end of the mesonephric ducts. The ampulla of the vas deferens joins the distal seminal vesicle to form the ejaculatory duct which lies almost completely within the prostate. The ureters usually cross the seminal vesicles medially. Posteriorly, the obliterated peritoneal reflection of Denonvilliers' fascia is encountered. The rectum is the next posterior structure. Anteriorly, the seminal vesicles are attached to the posterior bladder wall. The medial and inferior vesical arteries supply the seminal vesicles. Lymphatic drainage is the same as the prostate, initially to the obturator nodes and thence to the internal iliac chain. The nerve supply is derived from the inferior hypogastric plexus.

1. Perineal Approach. Young's classic descriptions of radical prostatectomy and seminal vesiculectomy require little modification (Young 1922; Hodgins

and Hancock 1972). It is almost mandatory to have available a set of Young perineal instruments and a Lowsley retractor. The patient is given a modified bowel preparation before surgery in case of inadvertent rectal injury.

In the operating room, careful attention is paid to operative position. The patient should be in an exaggerated lithotomy position with a sandbag under the sacrum. The use of shoulder braces aids the final positioning which results in the perineum being parallel to the floor. An inverted U incision is made between the medial aspects of the ischial tuberosities and approximately 2-3 cm anterior to the anus. Avoidance of continuing the incision over the ischial tuberosities will help decrease postoperative pain (Figure 3a).

At this point, the surgeon may, depending on his preference and training, continue the dissection either in a presphincter manner as described originally by Young or in a subsphincter manner as later described by Belt (1942). In Young's classical approach, the central perineal tendon can easily be divided. After displacing the levator ani from the anterior rectal wall, the rectourethralis muscle is divided (Figure 3b). The posterior layer of Denonvilliers' fascia can then be divided exposing the 'pearly' gates (Figure 3c). Retraction with the Lowsley retractor should enable the seminal vesicle to be visualized easily. After freeing the anterior prostate, a combination of sharp and blunt dissection can be utilized to mobilize the seminal vesicles completely. If only a seminal vesiculectomy is being performed, prostatic tissue surrounding the ejaculatory ducts can be excised with the specimen. The defect is closed with interrupted 00 chromic sutures (Figure 3d). The wound is then closed in layers with or without a drain depending on the original indications for the seminal vesiculectomy.

2. Transcoccygeal Approach. After placing the patient in a prone, slight jackknife position with the pelvis elevated, an incision is made in the midline from the sacrococcygeal junction to approximately 2-3 cm from the anus (Figure 4a). Sharp dissection is utilized to expose the levators ani which are then divided in the anococcygeal raphe. The rectum is then easily exposed by lateral retraction of the levator ani following which the tip of the coccyx is excised (Figure 4b). In order to provide access, the

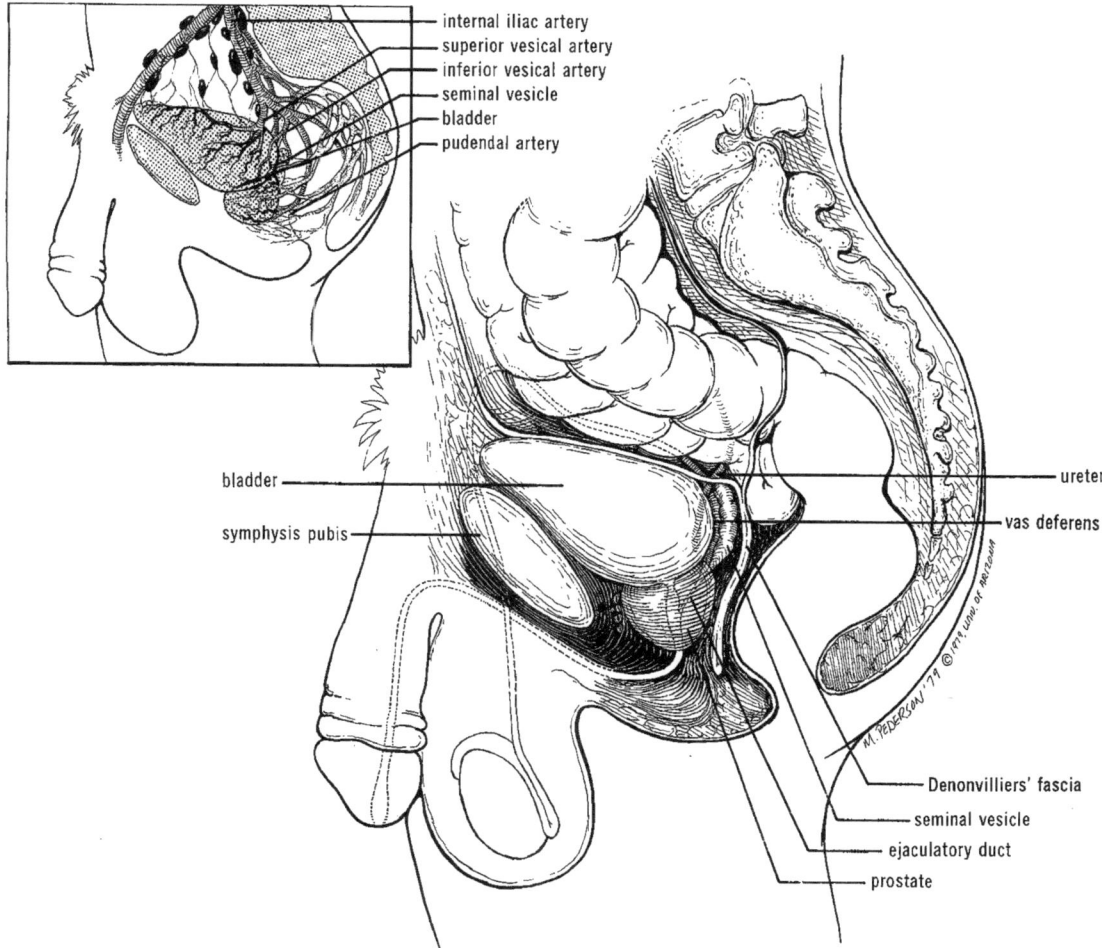

internal iliac artery
superior vesical artery
inferior vesical artery
seminal vesicle
bladder
pudendal artery

bladder

symphysis pubis

ureter

vas deferens

Denonvilliers' fascia
seminal vesicle
ejaculatory duct
prostate

Figure 2. Normal surgical anatomy of the seminal vesicles.

seminal vesicles, the rectum and lower sigmoid are dissected and retracted laterally (Figure 4c). Division of the rectovesical fascia allows reflection of the fascia superiorly, completing the exposure of the seminal vesicles. The seminal vesicle may then be dissected sharply under direct vision. Ligation of the vas deferens is optimal. Drainage is utilized as required due to vascular oozing or to the primary indication for surgery. Closure is easily accomplished in layers.

3. Extravesicular, Transperitoneal Approach. After placing the patient in a supine position, a Pfannenstiel's or vertical midline incision is made. If a unilateral seminal vesicle excision is to be performed, an extraperitoneal approach can be utilized. The bladder is dissected medially by a combination of blunt and sharp dissection until the lower ureter and seminal vesicle are visualized.

Further dissection will allow removal of the seminal vesicle (Figure 5a).

However, if a bilateral seminal vesiculectomy is indicated, a transperitoneal approach to reduce the amount of perivesical dissection should be utilized. After opening the peritoneum (Figure 5b), the posterior peritoneum between the rectum and bladder is incised. As in a radical cystectomy, this plane can easily be developed to expose the seminal vesicles. Further sharp dissection is required to mobilize the seminal vesicles completely prior to their removal (Figure 5c). After completing seminal vesiculectomy, a standard abdominal closure is performed.

4. Transvesical Approach. Because radical retropubic prostatectomies are familiar to most urologists, and excellent exposure is afforded by this procedure, the transvesical approach is often the opera-

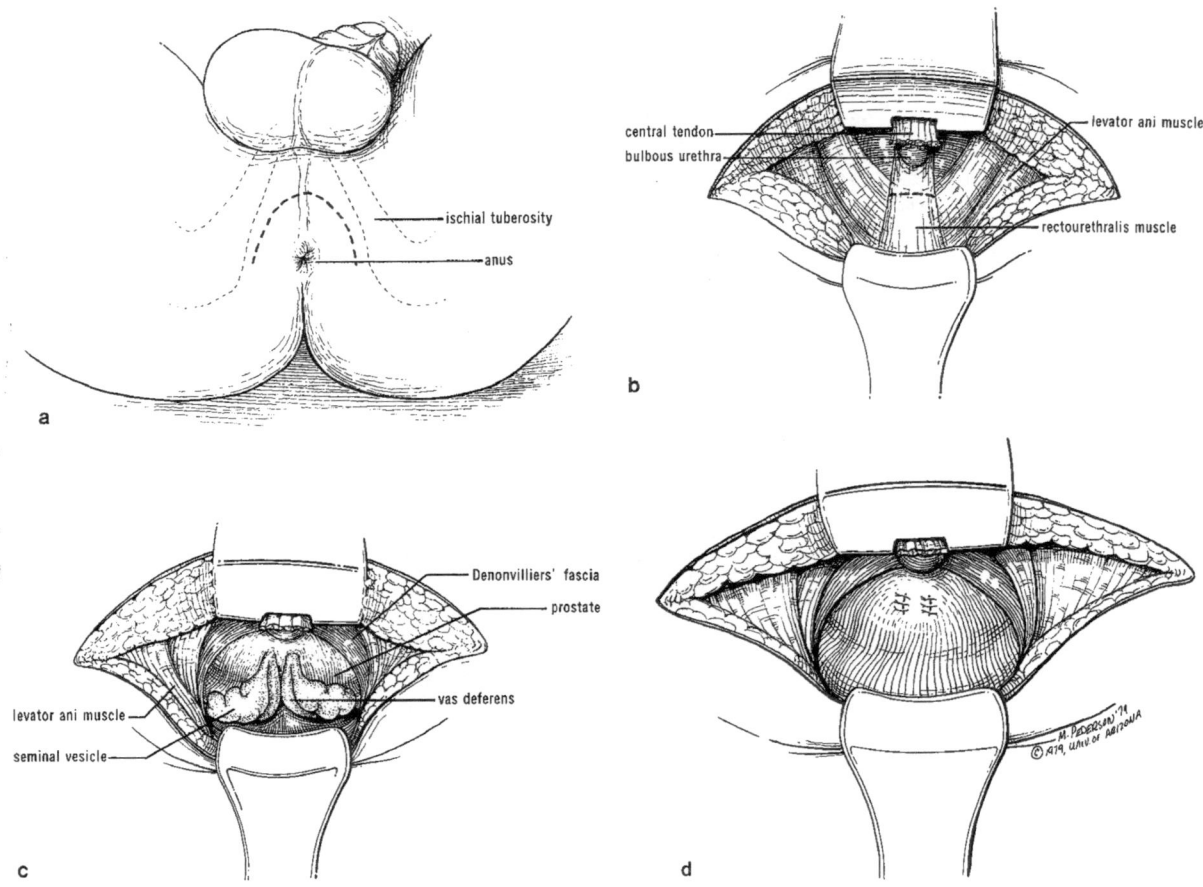

Figure 3. Perineal approach to seminal vesiculectomy: a. Classical inverted-U incision. b. Presphincteric approach after division of central tendon illustrating incision of rectourethralis muscle. c. Exposure of seminal vesicles and prostate after division of overlying muscles and appropriate retraction with the Lowsley retractor. d. Closure of the prostatic capsular defect after removal of seminal vesicles.

tive procedure of choice. After a suprapubic incision is utilized to expose the bladder, a transverse incision is made approximately 1-2 cm superior to the bladder neck (Figure 6a). Ureteral catheters are inserted following which the incision is carried posteriorly completely dividing the posterior bladder distal to the ureteral orifices as in a radical retropubic prostatectomy (Figure 6b).

The floor of the bladder can be dissected superiorly allowing visualization of the anterior seminal vesicles. After ligating both vas deferens, the seminal vesicles are mobilized under direct vision. As in the other procedure, the ejaculatory ducts are transected deep in the prostate following which the prostatic defects are closed with interrupted chromic sutures (Figure 6c). The bladder is then closed in two layers. A urethral catheter and drain should be left seven to ten days postoperatively.

D. Complications

All of the foregoing procedures are occasionally accompanied by complications due to bleeding, infection and/or injuries to adjacent organs. Obviously, careful surgical techniques and knowledge of surgical anatomy can minimize these problems. The single morbidity which is a function of the surgical approach is the incidence of postoperative impotency. Although numerous studies (Cunningham 1919; Dillon and Blaisdell 1923) show no loss of potency with the perineal approach, most urologists avoid extensive perineal surgery whenever preservation of potency is a factor. The transvesical seminal vesiculectomy seems to be the procedure least likely to disturb potency.

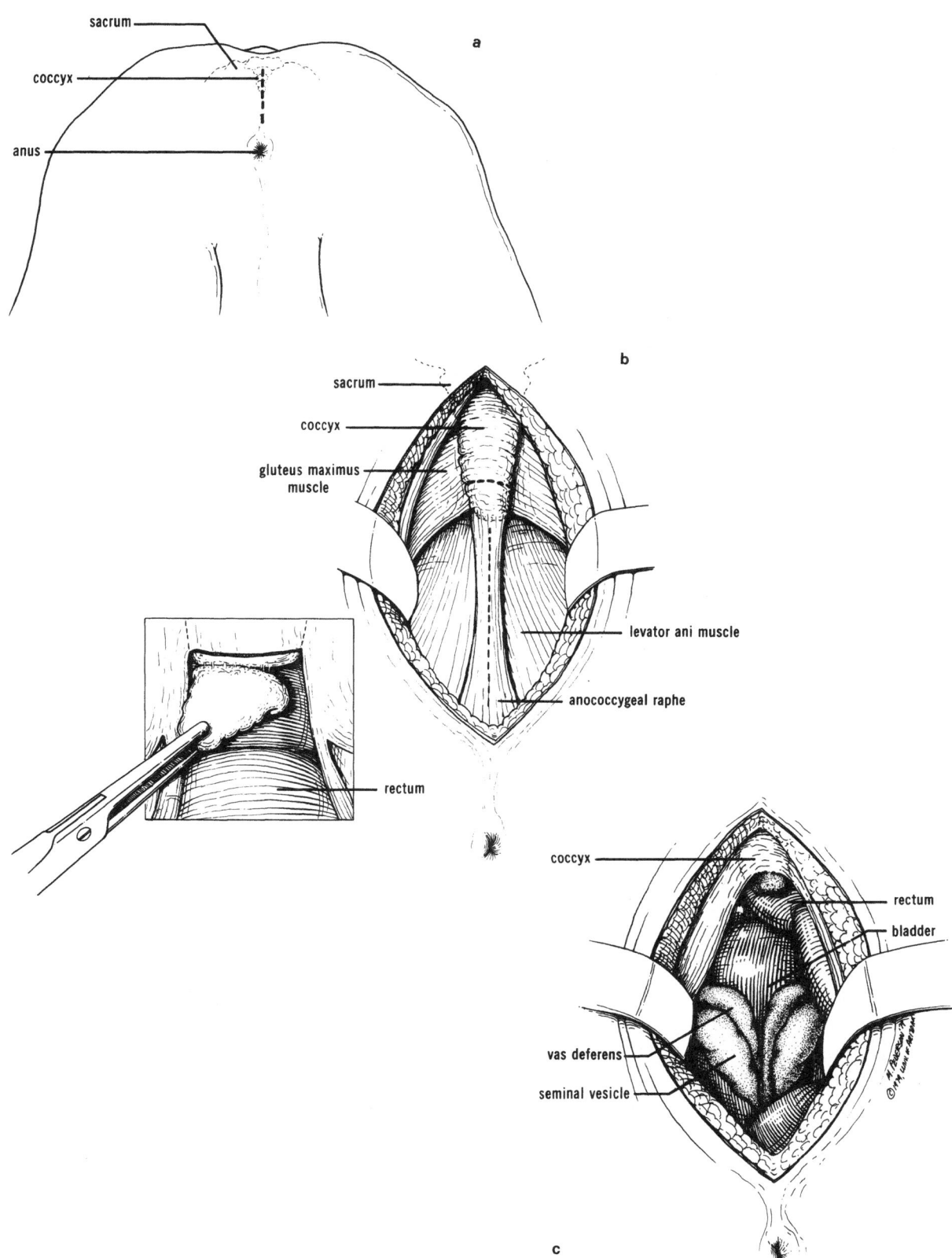

Figure 4. Transcoccygeal approach to seminal vesiculectomy: a. Midline skin incision.
b. Division of levator ani in midline. Inset illustrates removal of the tip of the coccyx.
c. The rectum is retracted to expose the seminal vesicles.

III. HYDROCELECTOMY

A 'hydrocele' is an appreciable increase in the amount of fluid within the scrotal tunica vaginalis testis. In infants, a scrotal hydrocele is usually associated with a patent processus vaginalis, while the 'idiopathic' hydrocele of the adult rarely communicates with the peritoneal cavity. Our discussion deals primarily with this latter noncommunicating hydrocele.

Hydrocele is a common affliction that has commanded the attention of physicians since ancient times. John Hunter perhaps best summarized the particulars of the history of hydrocele therapy when he wrote: 'No disease affecting the human body and requiring an operation for its cure has called forth the opinions and pens of surgeons so much as this disease. Each finds that every mode of operating but his own has failed.' Physicians of antiquity treated the lesion by simple drainage. Galen, and later Paré and Pott, advocated the percutaneous introduction of silk threads into the hydrocele via a seton (needle) and left the silk temporarily in place to act as a wick for slow drainage of sequestered fluid. Avicenna was more direct, simply creating a cutaneous fistula with red hot cautery. Later, workers combined drainage with either packing or injection of materials designed to provoke suppuration or sclerosis, thereby destroying the secretory membrane and obliterating the space within the hydrocele sac. At various times, arsenic, sea sponges, wine (full and half strength), linseed meal, brandy, sublimate of mercury, quinine and urethane have each been injected or packed into the

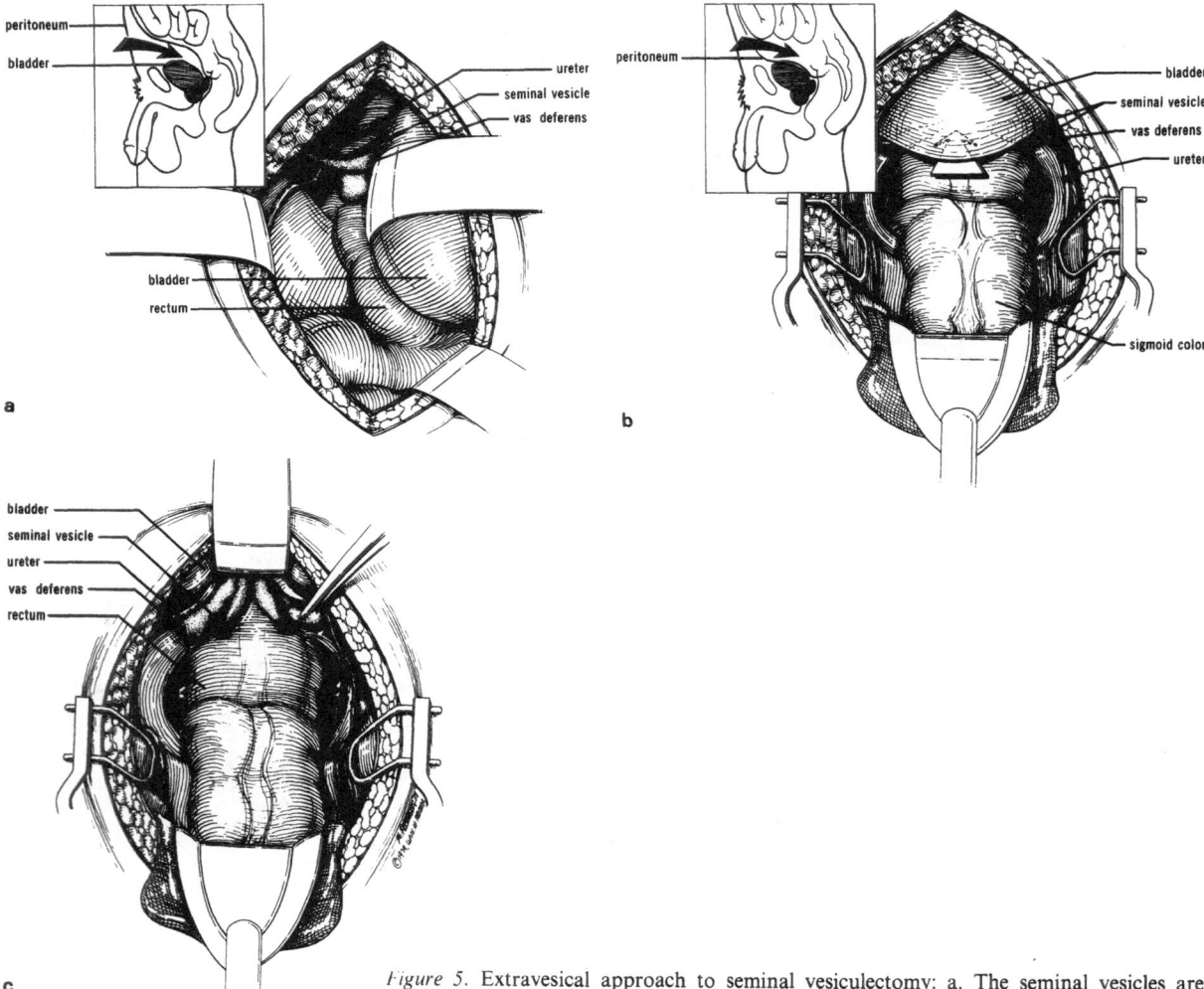

Figure 5. Extravesical approach to seminal vesiculectomy: a. The seminal vesicles are exposed with difficulty by medial retraction of the bladder. b. Proposed plane of dissection between bladder and rectum for transperitoneal bilateral seminal vesiculectomies. c. Exposure of seminal vesicles and ligation of vasa after bladder and rectum are separated.

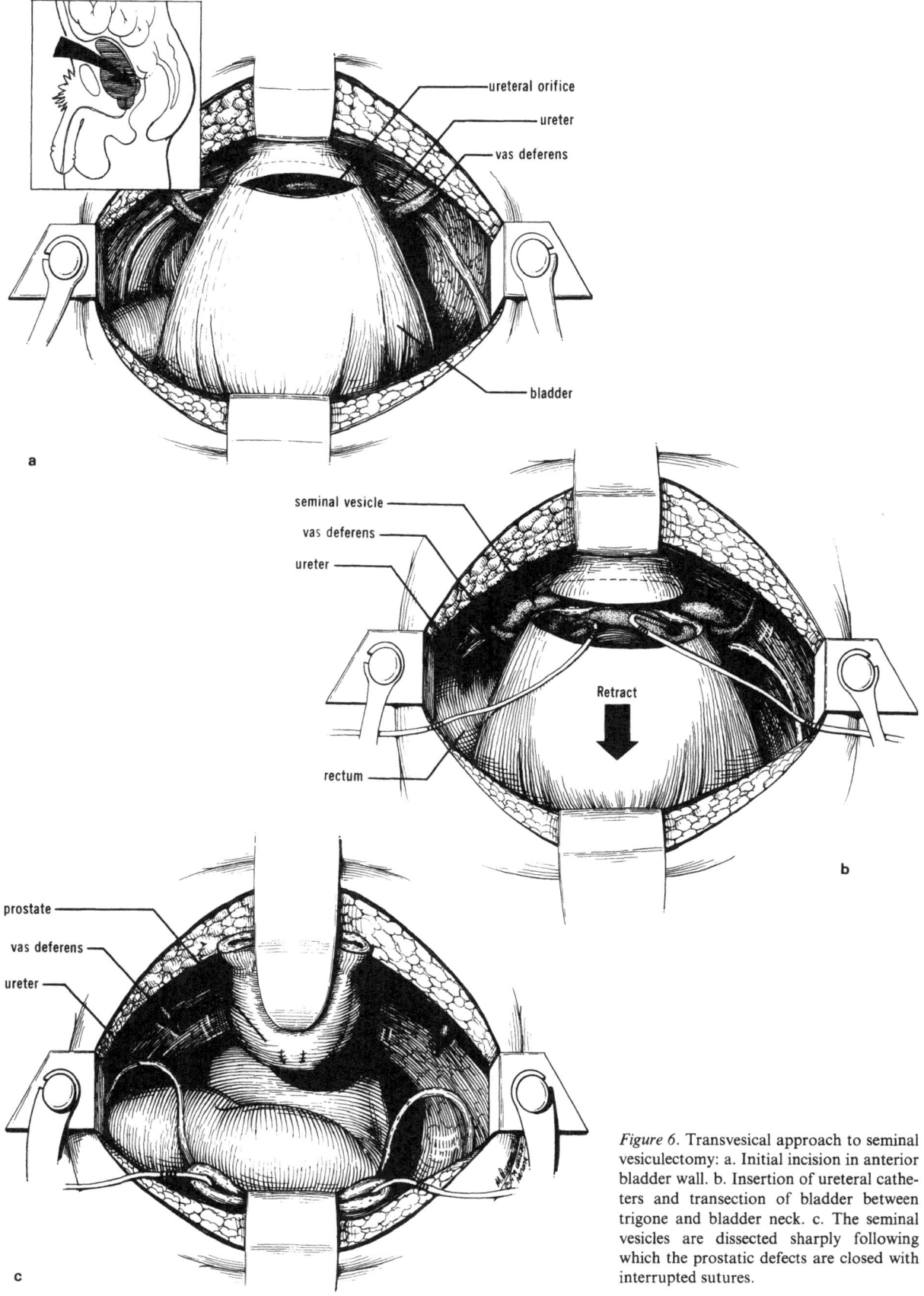

ureteral orifice

ureter

vas deferens

bladder

a

seminal vesicle

vas deferens

ureter

Retract

rectum

b

prostate

vas deferens

ureter

c

Figure 6. Transvesical approach to seminal vesiculectomy: a. Initial incision in anterior bladder wall. b. Insertion of ureteral catheters and transection of bladder between trigone and bladder neck. c. The seminal vesicles are dissected sharply following which the prostatic defects are closed with interrupted sutures.

hydrocele sac, presumably in an effort to prevent recurrence. Detailed information concerning the success of most such efforts is, not surprisingly, unavailable. Today, except under unusual circumstances, such methods have given way to more direct surgical treatment. However, we refer the interested reader to Landes and Leonhardt's fascinating review of the history of hydrocele for a more detailed accounting of the varied modes of treatment employed over the past eighteen centuries in an attempt to deal with this common lesion.

A. Physiology

The excessive accumulation of fluid present in a hydrocele has long been rather vaguely attributed to an 'imbalance' between the secretory and reabsorptive functions of the serous lining of the cavity. Early experiments were performed in the 1930s which clearly indicated that reabsorption of secreted fluid is inadequate in hydrocele. This was demonstrated by studies in which phenolsulfonphthalein was injected into the tunica vaginalis of normal males and patients with hydrocele. A marked delay in appearance and recovery time of the dye in the urine of the men with hydrocele was evidenced (Huggins and Entz 1931). It is now accepted that the responsible defect is one of lymphatic reabsorption. Absorption of materials injected into the hydrocele sac is much slower than would be expected if blood capillaries were responsible for reabsorption of the fluid (Huggins and Entz 1931). Histologic studies of hydrocele specimens injected with India ink in vivo have demonstrated a deficiency in subserous lymphatics beneath the parietal tunica vaginalis (Rinker and Allen 1951). Similarly, lymphographic studies in a limited number of hydrocele patients have demonstrated deficient drainage via the iliac lymphatic chain (McBrien et al. 1972). Practical clinical experience with hydrocele in renal transplant patients would also support the theory that a lymphatic defect is a primary cause of hydrocele formation. In such surgery, the cord structures were, at one time, routinely divided, and, of course, the iliac lymphatics were also compromised during the vascular dissection. Not surprisingly, 67 percent of individuals so treated developed hydroceles postoperatively (Penn et al. 1972). Similarly, hydroceles

commonly occur when retroperitoneal lymphatics are disrupted during irradiation therapy and retroperitoneal node dissection for testis tumor (Streit et al. 1978). In the typical hydrocele encountered in daily practice, however, the precise cause of the lymphatic abnormality is usually unknown. One theory is that a low-grade inflammatory lesion of the epididymis, or perhaps the minor trauma of daily activity, damages the lymphatic vessels as they pass over and near the epididymis on their way to the cord. The result is an idiopathic hydrocele (Wallace 1960).

B. Diagnosis and Indications

Hydroceles come in all shapes and sizes, but certain clinical features remain constant. Pain is not a prominent feature except in acute hydroceles secondary to testicular or epididymal pathology (e.g., epididymitis, orchitis, trauma, testis tumor, or after postoperative surgical procedures which disrupt the lymphatic drainage). Most hydroceles transilluminate, although long-standing lesions with thickened fibrotic sacs may fail to exhibit this classical clinical sign. We have found the fiberoptic light source used for routine cystoscopy most useful in the examination of scrotal masses. The light source must be held flush against the scrotal skin and the examining room must be quite dark for an adequate examination. The typical flashlight with semi-exhausted batteries found in the hospital ward is generally inadequate. Similarly, the typical patient's room with sunlight streaming in the window is not the place for attempted transillumination. The hydrocele is generally smooth in contour and the mass feels distinctly cystic. However, in long-standing lesions, the sac may become multiloculated and its contours correspondingly irregular. In most instances, if the examiner supports the mass in his left hand and gently palpates the posterior, inferior aspect of the sac with the right hand, a normal testis can be identified.

Typically, the diagnosis of idiopathic hydrocele is not difficult and surgical correction is purely elective. Large hydroceles extending into the superior aspect of the scrotum may sometimes be difficult to distinguish from hernias on initial inspection. However, in noncommunicating hydroceles, no impulse is felt at the external ring with coughing or straining. No bowel sounds are present within the scrotum on auscultation and the sac does not empty when the patient is supine. When hydroceles arise acutely and/or are associated with a great deal of pain, especially in men under the age of 35, the clinician must be certain to rule out associated testicular torsion or testis tumor – conditions requiring urgent diagnosis and treatment. When the history suggests torsion and the hemiscrotum is tender and the testicular outline cannot be appreciated adequately through the tense hydrocele sac, prompt exploration is indicated. Similarly, when the testis is felt to be irregular or large through the hydrocele sac, we advise exploration via the inguinal route clamping the cord before delivering the testis into the wound. We do not practice or advocate diagnostic aspiration because of the definite, though small, danger of piercing a possible neoplasm and seeding the scrotum with tumor cells.

C. Surgery and Surgical Anatomy

With few exceptions, open operation is the treatment of choice for the symptomatic, idiopathic adult hydrocele. In debilitated elderly males or individuals who are symptomatic, yet reluctant to undergo a formal surgical procedure, an attempt at aspiration under aseptic conditions is warranted, although rapid recurrence is common. Under such circumstances, we use the Bard Angiocath for aspiration to minimize trauma. The scrotum is prepped with povidone-iodine, a small area of skin is infiltrated with 1 percent xylocaine and the scrotum is gently compressed with the left hand until the skin over the anterior scrotum is tense. The Angiocath is introduced into the hydrocele cavity, the inner trocar removed, and the hollow plastic sheath is used to aspirate the contained fluid with a syringe (Veenema and Ehrlich 1971). In the past, aspiration has been combined with the injection of sclerosing solutions (quinine or urethane). We have little experience with this technique and agree with critics who oppose its use because of the danger of inducing a reactive epididymitis or orchitis, or of misplacing the injection. Since a variety of procedures have been devised to deal with hydrocele under direct vision with minimal morbidity, we feel the injection procedures are obsolete.

A detailed discussion of the anatomy of the scrotum and its contents has been presented in Section I. However, a brief re-emphasis of certain obvious and important anatomic features is warranted before considering specific surgical techniques of hydrocele repair. Figure 7 illustrates the multilayered nature of the scrotal wall. Obviously, any scrotal incision designed to expose the innermost tissue layer, the tunica vaginalis and the testis,

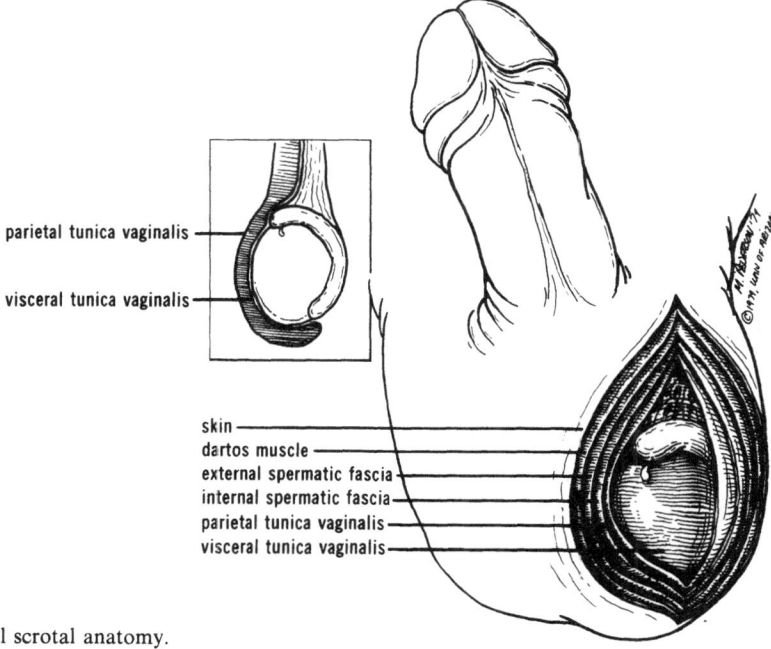

parietal tunica vaginalis

visceral tunica vaginalis

skin
dartos muscle
external spermatic fascia
internal spermatic fascia
parietal tunica vaginalis
visceral tunica vaginalis

Figure 7. Normal scrotal anatomy.

must necessarily transect all of the outer layers and expose the multiple potential tissue planes between layers. Should these planes be opened during extensive intraoperative dissection, one must expect rather extensive postoperative swelling and discomfort as blood and reactive exudate dissect within these spaces. This process is, of course, aided by the relative laxity and elasticity of the scrotal tissues. Keeping these anatomic features in mind, the surgeon can minimize his patient's postoperative discomfort by (1) minimizing extensive intrascrotal dissection, and (2) exercising extreme care in obtaining adequate hemostasis.

All effective procedures designed to cure hydrocele do so by essentially the same basic means: (1) permanently disrupting the continuity of the hydrocele sac by excision or eversion and (2) exposing the testis and its overlying serous membranes to the scrotal lymphatics external to the parietal tunica vaginalis testis, thus allowing for adequate reabsorption of subsequent serous secretions.

No single procedure is applicable to all clinical situations, but we find that most lesions can be dealt with by either an excision operation similar to that described by Young, Winkleman or Jauboulay or by the eversion procedure popularized by Lord. Both procedures are performed through a vertical scrotal incision.

1. The Excision Operation. When the hydrocele sac is thick walled and bulky, excision of all or part of it is indicated to avoid leaving a large amount of tissue within the scrotum. The operation is made much easier if all the scrotal layers are divided superficially to the thin tunica vaginalis testes and the sac is dissected intact out of the surrounding tissues. We favor a vertical incision on the anterior surface of the scrotum, its length varying with the size of the sac. The upper extent of the incision should be at least 1 cm lateral to the base of the penis to avoid involving this organ in scar formation postoperatively.

The surgeon or first assistant compresses the scrotum posteriorly to place the tissues to be incised under tension. The incision is carried down through the skin, dartos and multiple fascial layers of the scrotal wall until the parietal tunica vaginalis comes into view. It is important to use the belly, rather than the point of the knife for the incision to avoid

puncturing the sac. Also, continuous pressure on the posterior aspect of the scrotum while the incision is made will 'spring' each layer apart as it is incised, thus exposing the next innermost layer. The endpoint of the incision's depth, the tunica vaginalis, can often be identified by its slightly blue color and by the absence of blood vessels in this layer (Figure 8a).

After bleeders are meticulously clamped and tied with 0000 chromic ligatures or electrocoagulated, the intact sac can be bluntly shelled out of the scrotum by using a finger or by wiping the surrounding tissues from the sac with a dry sponge. Usually, a few tenacious adhesions must be sharply divided, especially in long-standing hydroceles (Figure 8b).

The testis is identified by palpation and the sac is opened anteriorly, the fluid aspirated and the excess tunica vaginalis is excised a distance of 1-1.5 cm from the testis (Figure 8c). Spot bleeders are electrocoagulated, or tied if large, and the edge of the sac is oversewn with running locking suture of 0000 chromic (Figure 8d). Any testicular or epididymal appendages are ligated at their base and removed. A stab wound is made over a clamp in the most dependent portion of the scrotum and a $^1/_4$-inch penrose drain is pulled into the scrotal cavity and loosely sutured to the skin (Figure 8e). The testis and remaining tunica vaginalis are again inspected for hemostasis and returned to the scrotal cavity. The scrotum is closed in two layers using 0000 chromic sutures with the knots inverted.

Unfortunately, on many occasions, dense inflammatory adhesions make the operation more difficult than that described above. Often it is impossible to separate the parietal tunica vaginalis from its surrounding fascial investments. In such cases the sac is opened (often inadvertently) and as much of it as possible is excised. Again, the edge is oversewn to secure hemostasis and the edges of the remaining tunica, with as little surrounding tissue as possible, are folded behind the testis and sutured together, thus maintaining eversion of the serous membrane and preventing reformation of a closed cystic space (Figure 8f). Closure is as described above. We usually cover the skin incision with collodion and dress the wound with a scrotal support packed tightly with fluffs.

2. The Lord Extrusion Procedure. The standard

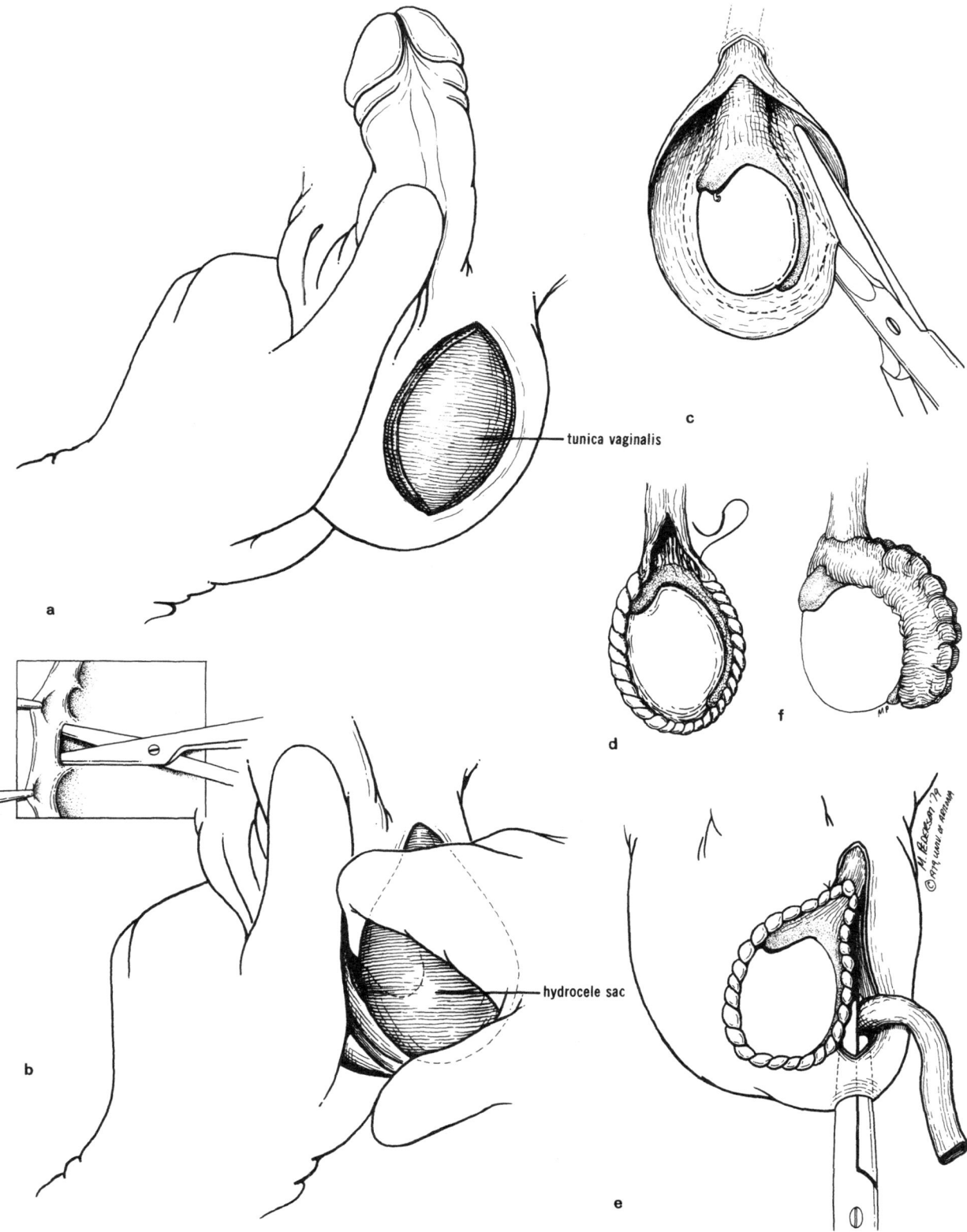

Figure 8. The excision operation for hydrocelectomy: a. The scrotum is steadily compressed posteriorly while the multiple layers of the scrotum are incised anteriorly until the bulging avascular parietal tunica vaginalis is exposed. b. Blunt digital dissection of hydrocele sac. Inset illustrates sharp division of adhesions between hydrocele sac and scrotum. c. Excision of hydrocele sac. d. The edge of the hydrocele sac is oversewn. e. The scrotum is drained by a small penrose drain inserted through a stab wound in the dependent scrotum. f. Eversion of remnants of the hydrocele sac behind the epididymis.

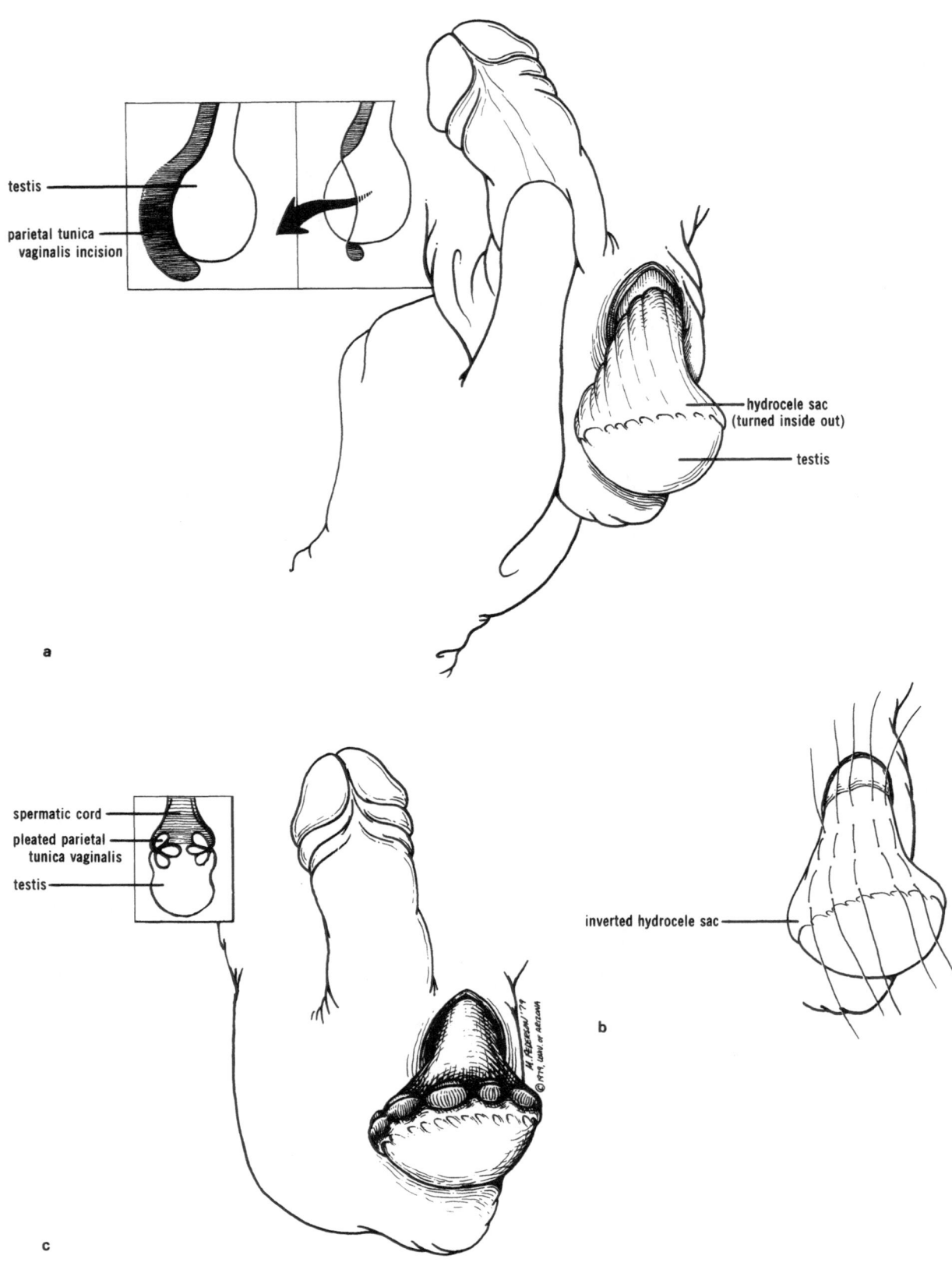

Figure 9. The Lord extrusion operation for hydrocelectomy: a. The testis is extruded through an incision in the hydrocele sac, thus turning the sac inside out. b. Plication of hydrocele sac. c. The plicating sutures have been tied thereby obliterating the sac.

excision operation requires complete mobilization of the tunica vaginalis, an exercise which often opens multiple tissue planes and is sometimes associated with considerable oozing from small vessels when inflammatory reaction makes the dissection difficult. Considerable scrotal swelling and hematoma formation may result.

In 1964, Lord described a simple operation which eliminated extensive dissection of the tunica vaginalis, yet still obliterated the hydrocele sac and exposed the testis and its coverings to new lymphatic drainage via the more superficial scrotal tissues. Variations of the technique have been described by other authors (Solomon 1955; McGowan and Howley 1969). We perform the procedure largely as originally described by Lord.

The incision is the same as for the excision operation, except that the tunica vaginalis is incised initially along with the other layers of the scrotum. The fluid within is then aspirated. The testis is grasped and pulled out of the scrotum, thus turning the parietal tunica vaginalis inside out (Figure 9a). Next, eight to ten sutures of 000 chromic gut are utilized to gather or plicate the tunica vaginalis (Figure 9b). Each stitch is begun at the junction of the testis and epididymis and the suture is radially extended to the cut edge of the tunica by taking small shallow bites of the tunica 1 cm apart. The process is repeated around the circumference of the junction of the visceral and parietal tunica vaginalis and after all sutures are placed, each is tied, thereby gathering or pleating the parietal tunica and obliterating the sac (Figure 9c). The surgeon stretches the subcutaneous tissues with his fingers to make a pouch for the testis. Replacing the testis in the scrotum is often difficult and may require a moderate amount of slow, steady, inward pressure on the testis while the edges of the incision are held apart by Allis clamps applied to the dartos. No drain is needed. The dartos is closed with 000 chromic and the skin with a subcuticular chromic suture. A scrotal support packed with fluffs is used as a dressing.

Numerous authors have reported a favorable experience with the Lord procedure or slight variations of the technique (Solomon 1955; Lord 1964; Efron and Sharkey 1967; Dahl et al. 1972; McGowan and Howley 1969; Wechsler 1975). Of 193 cases reported and followed for varying periods, only two recurrences were noted. Hospitalization time, when compared to that required for the standard operation in the same institution, was halved, averaging three to five days. Since dissection is minimal and localized, the procedure is readily performed under local anesthesia in elderly patients. The procedure is not recommended for thick-walled hydroceles, however, because of the bulky tissue left in place in such cases.

REFERENCES

Bagley DH, Javadpour N, Witebsky FG and Thomas LB: Seminal vesicle cyst. Urology 5: 147, 1975.

Belt E: Radical perineal prostatectomy in early carcinoma of the prostate. J Urol 48: 287, 1942.

Boyce WH and Politano VA: Infections & diseases of the scrotum and its contents: epididymitis. In: Urology, 3rd edition, Campbell MF and Harrison JHH (eds), Volume 1, chapter 16, p 609, Phila, Pa, WB Saunders Co, 1970.

Broth G, Bullock WK and Morrow J: Epididymal tumors, J Urol 100: 530, 1968.

Buck AC and Shaw RE: Primary tumors of the retro-vesical region with special reference to mesenchymal tumors of the seminal vesicles. Br J Urol 44: 47, 1972.

Campbell MF: Hydrocele of the tunica vaginalis: A study of 502 cases. Surg Gynecol Obstet 45: 192, 1927.

Cunningham JH: Operative treatment of seminal vesiculitis. J Urol 3: 175, 1919.

Dahl DS, Singh M, O'Connor VJ Jr, Sokol JK and Bulkley GJ: Lord's operation for hydrocele compared with conventional techniques. Arch Surg 104: 40, 1972.

De Assis JS: Seminal vesiculectomy, J Urol 68: 747, 1952.

Dillon JR and Blaisdell FE: Surgical pathology of the seminal vesicles. J Urol 10: 353, 1923.

Efron G and Sharkey GG: The Lord operation for hydrocele. Surg Gynecol Obstet 125: 603, 1967.

Fuller E: Seminal vesiculectomy. Its purpose and accomplishments. JAMA 59: 1959, 1912.

Hodgins TE and Hancock RA: Technic of radical perineal prostatectomy. South Med J 65: 1437, 1972.

Huggins CB and Entz FH: Absorption from normal tunica vaginalis testis, hydrocele and spermatocele. J Urol 25: 447, 1931.

Hunt VC: Posterior excision of the seminal vesicles. Ann Surg 87: 257, 1928.

Kees OS: Clinical improvement following estrogenic therapy in a case of primary adenocarcinoma of the seminal vesicle. J Urol 91: 665, 1964.

Kreager JA Jr and Jordan WP Jr: Transcoccygeal approach to the seminal vesicles. Am Surg 31: 126, 1965.

Landes RR and Leonhardt KO: The history of hydrocele. Urol Surv 17: 135, 1967.

Lathem JE: Carcinoma of the seminal vesicle. South Med J 68: 473, 1975.

Lord PH: A bloodless operation for the radical cure of idiopathic hydrocele. Br J Surg 51: 914, 1964.

McBrien MP, Edwards JM, Kinmonth JB: Lymphography of the testis and its adnexa in the normal and in idiopathic hydrocele. Arch Surg 104: 820, 1972.

McGowan AJ and Howley TF: Experiences with the extrusion operation for hydrocele. J Urol 101: 366, 1969.

Murphy LJG: The History of Urology, p 439, Springfield, Ill, Charles C Thomas, 1972.

Penn I, Mackie G, Halgrimson CG and Starzl T: Testicular complications following renal transplantation. Ann Surg 176: 697, 1972.

Politano VA, Lankford RW and Susaeta R: A transvesical approach to total seminal vesiculectomy: A case report. Trans Am Assoc Genitourin Surg 66: 116, 1974.

Rinker JR and Allen L: A lymphatic defect in hydrocele. Am Surg 17: 681, 1951.

Solomon AA: The extrusion operation for hydrocele. NY State J Med 55: 1885, 1955.

Stanisic TH, Kolbusz W and Carter M: Unusual presentation of genital tuberculosis. Urology 12: 351, 1978.

Streit CC, Richie JP, Clyde HR and Sargent CR: Hydrocele formation after sandwich irradiation therapy for testicular tumor. Urology 12: 222, 1978.

Veenema RJ and Ehrlich RM: A new method for aspiration of hydroceles. J Urol 105: 112, 1971.

Walker WC and Bowles WT: Transvesical seminal vesiculectomy in treatment of congenital obstruction of seminal vesicles: A case report. J Urol 99: 324, 1968.

Wallace F: Aetiology of the idiopathic hydrocele. Br J Urol 32: 79, 1960.

Wechsler M: Hydrocelectomy: Evaluation of Lord's operation. NY State J Med 75: 2165, 1975.

Wilson SK, Hagan KW and Rhamy RK: Epididymectomy for acute and chronic disease. J Urol 112: 357, 1974.

Witherington R and Rinker JR: Retropubic seminal vesiculectomy for chronic seminal vesiculitis with preservation of potency. J Urol 104: 463, 1970.

Woodruff MW, Marden HE Jr and Schoenfeld LV: Benign and malignant tumors of the penis, urethra, epididymis and seminal vesicles. In: Urology, Karafin and Kendall (eds) vol 2, chapter 9, p 16, Hagerstown, Maryland, Harper & Row 1975.

Young HH: Radical cure of hydrocele by excision of serous layer of sac. Surg Gynecol Obstet 70: 807, 1940.

Young HH: The radical cure of tuberculosis of the seminal tract: I. A brief survey of the literature. Arch Surg 4: 334, 1922.

VI. ONCOLOGICAL SURGERY

18. PENECTOMY AND GROIN DISSECTION FOR CARCINOMA OF THE PENIS

T.R. MALLOY and A.J. WEIN

I. PENECTOMY

Carcinoma of the penis is a highly significant health problem in many areas of the world. Surgery remains the primary treatment modality for this disease. Certainly controversies exist over the optimal extent and timing of primary surgical intervention (Hoppman and Fraley 1978; De Kernion and Persky 1978), but in any case, a thorough understanding of the surgical anatomy of the penis is mandatory for deciding on a proper therapeutic approach.

A. Surgical Anatomy of the Penis

The penis is primarily a sexual organ with erectile capacity and secondarily, a urinary conduit. Cylindrically shaped, it contains the paired corpora cavernosa and the urethra surrounded by the corpus spongiosum. The penis is attached to the pubic rami and ischii by the crura of the corpora cavernosa to the urogenital diaphragm by Buck's fascia, and to the linea alba by the suspensory ligament. The corpus spongiosum rests in the ventral groove formed by the corpora cavernosa. The distal corpus spongiosum expands into the glans penis in which are embedded the distal extensions of the corpora cavernosa. Buck's fascia invests the corpora in a dense fibrous sheath which terminates posteriorly at the urogenital diaphragm and anteriorly in the suspensory ligament of the penis.

The arterial blood supply originates from the internal iliac artery which terminates in an anterior trunk, the internal pudendal artery. The internal pudendal artery distal to its perineal branch becomes the penile artery, which divides into the deep and dorsal arteries of the penis. A deep penile artery enters the crus of each corpus and traverses the corpus cavernosum in a central position to axially supply blood to the erectile tissue. The dorsal arteries of the penis ascend between the corpora cavernosa to course forward on the dorsal surface of the penis deep to the fascia and lateral to the deep dorsal vein. Terminal branches of these arteries supply the glans and the prepuce. The dorsal arteries further supply the penile skin and the fibrous sheath of the corpus cavernosum, sending anastomotic branches through the sheath to the deep penile artery.

Veins drain the cavernous tissue by a series of vessels. Some of these emerge from the base of the glans penis to converge on the dorsum of the penis and form the deep dorsal vein. Other veins pass through the upper surface of the corpora cavernosa and join the deep dorsal vein. Additional vessels from the inferior surface, receiving blood from the corpus spongiosum, travel around the side of the penis to end in the deep dorsal vein. Other veins pass out the root of the penis to join the prostatic plexus. The superficial dorsal vein drains the prepuce and skin of the penis. It joins the external pudendal vein, a tributary of the great saphenous vein. The deep dorsal vein passes through the suspensory ligament to divide into branches to the prostatic plexus and the internal pudendal vein.

Nerves to the penis descend from the second, third, and fourth sacral spinal nerves through the pudendal nerve and the pelvic plexuses.

Of maximum importance in dealing with carcinoma of the penis is a thorough understanding of the lymphatic drainage system of the penis, which is the primary path for metastasis. The prepuce and the skin of penis are drained largely by lymphatics that drain into the superficial inguinal nodes. The glans penis and the corpora drain to the deep inguinal nodes and to the external iliac nodes

(Young 1931; Daseler et al. 1943; Hovnanian 1967; Warwick and Williams 1973). The lymphatics decussate along the penis and at the base of the penis. Nodes from both sides may be involved by metastases from a tumor at any location on the penis.

B. Preoperative Evaluation

Careful physical examination of any penile lesion is mandatory. Any fungating or diffuse lesion should be considered penile carcinoma until proven otherwise. Certain premalignant lesions (Table 1) are often difficult to diagnose, and biopsy is required to differentiate early carcinoma. Thorough palpation of the inguinal region is necessary to ascertain the extent of adenopathy.

The staging system for carcinoma of the penis most commonly used by urologists is that of Jackson. An alternative system has been proposed by Johnson et al. (Table 2).

All clinical staging systems are somewhat inaccurate in that the clinical stage and the pathological stage of the disease are often not the same. Hardner found 16 percent of his clinical Stage I or II patients were actually pathologically Stage III. Similarly Hoppman and Fraley found 18 percent of their clinical Stage I and II patients to be pathologically Stage III. On the other hand, of the 37 patients judged to be clinically Stage III, Hardner found 40 percent to have nodes free of tumor on

Table 1. Possible premalignant lesions of the penis.

Lesion	Characteristics	Therapy
Erythroplasia of Queyrat	Flat, ill-defined erythema	1. Circumcision 2. Radiation 3. 5-Fluorouracil
Leukoplakia	Glans irritated, scondary to lack of hygiene	Excision
Bowen's Disease (Intraepithelial carcinoma)	Flat, not painful	1. Excision 2. 5-Fluorouracil
Buschke-Löwenstein Tumor	Giant penile condyloma; may have areas of carcinoma within it	1. Partial penectomy 2. Excision
Balanitis Xerotica Obliterans	Burning and pruritus of glans; obstruction of meatus	1. Local excision 2. Circumcision 3. Meatotomy 4. Steroid Injection

Table 2. Staging for cancer of the penis.

Stage	(Jackson 1966)	(Johnson 1973)
I	Lesions confined to glans and/or prepuce	Malignant disease confined to penis
II	Lesions extending onto shaft of penis or into corpora	Clinical suspicion of tumor extension beyond penis but not beyond regional (ilio-inguinal) nodes
III	Lesions with malignant but operable groin nodes	Disseminated disease as seen in generalized abdominal (visceral) or pulmonary metastasis
IV	Primary tumor extending off shaft of penis and/or those with inoperable groin nodes or distant metastases	

pathologic examination. In 24 patients with clinical Stage III, DeKernion and Persky found 33 percent to be pathologically Stage I or II. Obviously, a high incidence of clinical understaging and overstaging is present in most series. Hardner, in his group of 82 patients, found 27 percent were initially clinically mis-staged.

All suspected lesions should be cultured, as most are infected. A biopsy is also required, and in a large lesion, multiple biopsies may be required. A thin needle aspiration biopsy may be performed on any significant lymph nodes that are palpable. Cabanas, in 1977, identified a 'sentinel node' that he feels represents the primary node involved in metastases from carcinoma of the penis. In his experience, noninvolvement of this node by carcinoma indicates that the inguinal and iliac nodes are free of tumor.

Radiologic studies should include a chest Roentgenogram and a bone scan. Lymphangiography may reveal involvement of the internal iliac or paraaortic nodes. However, most authors feel that this technique is of little value in assessing the inguinal lymph nodes (DeKernion and Persky 1978; Hoppman and Fraley 1978). Corpus cavernosography may delineate invasion of the corpora. If invasion has occurred, there exists the possibility of hematogenous metastasis to lung and bone. Computerized axial tomography (CAT) scans of the pelvis may reveal massive involvement of lymph nodes in the pelvis or retroperitoneum that would contraindicate radical surgery.

Antibiotic therapy should be instituted as soon as

the culture of the lesions is reported so that the operative site will not become infected. Therapy also decreases the inguinal adenopathy which is usually present due to lymphadenitis and which may be confused with metastatic involvement.

C. Partial Penectomy

Primary tumors are usually on the prepuce or glans of the penis. However, 10 to 20 percent can occur on the shaft. Although preservation of length and function is desirable from a psychological and functional aspect, oncological surgical principles should not be compromised. Conservative surgery, i.e., excisions or circumcision, has been associated with local recurrences (Johnson et al. 1973; Hardner et al. 1972). Hanash et al. found that 40 percent of locally excised glandular lesions recurred. Although circumcision for lesions of the prepuce in the younger patient is sometimes advocated, careful postoperative assessment is mandatory for many years. The patient population that develops carcinoma of the penis is frequently unreliable in seeking early or continued medical care. Definitive surgical therapy is the treatment of choice in most cases.

Proper surgical technique in performing partial penectomy is extremely important. The patient should be adequately prepped prior to surgery. The lesions should be covered with a condom or rubber finger cot so that possible metastases will not be implanted into the wound and secondary infection of the incision will not occur. A penrose drain is wrapped around the base of the penis and clamped to occlude the blood supply (Figure 1a). The skin incision should be made a minimum of 2.5 cm from the edge of the lesion. This circumferential incision is extended to Buck's fascia and the skin is retracted proximally. The deep dorsal arteries and veins are ligated. The corpus spongiosum urethra is divided in the plane of the original incision and separated from the corpus cavernosa. The urethra is spatu-

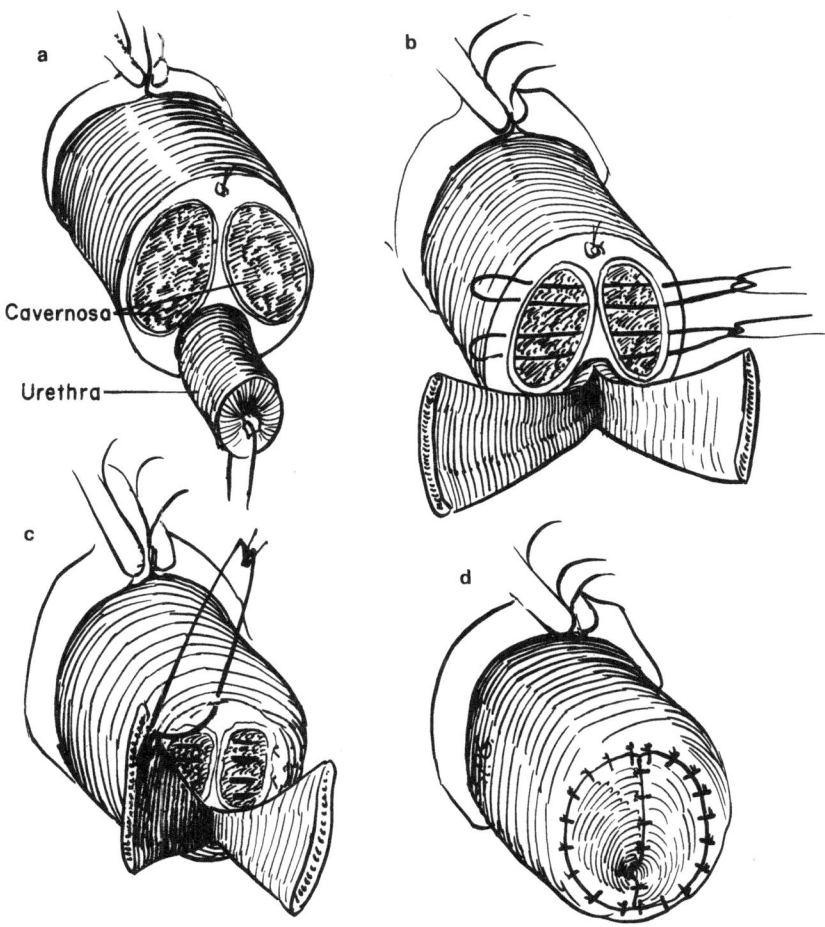

Cavernosa

Urethra

Figure 1.

lated so that the neo-meatus will not be stenotic (Figure 1b). The corpora are divided in a plane 6-8 mm proximal to that used to sever the urethra. Each corporal body is individually ligated with mattress sutures for hemostasis. The spatulated urethra is anastomosed to the tunica albuginea and the skin of the penis (Figure 1c, d).

Postoperatively, a Foley catheter is left in place for two to three days. This allows an occlusive hemostatic dressing to be applied to the incision for 48 hours. Appropriate antibiotics administered on the basis of the results from cultures of the primary lesion are continued for several weeks. This therapy prevents wound infection and allows resolution of adenopathy secondary to infection.

The principal complication to be avoided in partial penectomy is recurrence of the primary tumor. A frozen section should be performed to verify that the line of incision is free of tumor. With careful placement of the initial incision, at least 2.5 cm from any visible tumor, recurrence should not occur. Meatal stenosis may occur, but with adequate spatulation of the urethra, this complication should be avoidable. Proper antibiotic administration aids in preventing infection and promotes healing.

D. Total (Radical) Penectomy

The majority of carcinomas of the penis are amenable to partial penectomy. The major postoperative benefits of partial amputation are that the patient can urinate in the standing position, direct his stream, and potentially retain his ability to have sexual intercourse.

When lesions extensively invade the shaft of the penis, the surgeon should not hesitate to perform a total (radical) penectomy. Sound oncologic surgical principles should be observed in making a decision as to the extent of the penectomy required. A penile stump which is too short will cause spraying of the urinary stream with resulting personal hygiene problems. Extensive penile lesions have usually already precluded sexual activity for years, so the patient is generally not overly concerned with erectile function at the time of operation.

Young described a technique of radical penectomy combined with a lymph node dissection in 1931. The majority of surgeons today prefer to limit

the initial procedure to penectomy, delaying any lymphadenectomy procedures in order to lessen the possibility of wound infection from the primary lesion and to allow resolution of inguinal adenopathy secondary to infection and not tumor.

Preoperatively, the patient's lesion is cultured so that appropriate antibiotics may be instituted. The patient is placed in the lithotomy position. The penile lesion is covered with a condom or gauze packing to lessen the opportunity for tumor implantation into the surgical wound. A midline perineal incision is made and extended to expose both corpora cavernosa and the corpus spongiosum urethra (Figure 2a). The urethra is freed from the corpora and severed. The distal end is sent for frozen section to assure no evidence of tumor involvement. A circular incision is extended around the base of the penis and extended to the suspensory ligament of the penis (Figure 2b). The deep dorsal arteries and vein of the penis are severed (Figure 2c). The suspensory ligament of the penis is incised. The corpora are divided at the crus using mattress sutures to ligate the deep penile artery (Figure 2d, e). Hemostatic mattress sutures are placed through Buck's fascia to prevent delayed bleeding (Figure 2f). The penis is removed. The urethra is spatulated and brought into the perineum as a perineal urethrostomy (Figure 2g). The wound is closed with a perineal drain in place (Figure 2h). If the lesion extends into the scrotum, the scrotum should be excised. Removal of both testicles and cord structures may be required in well advanced cases.

Postoperative care requires catheter drainage for five to seven days. An occlusive perineal dressing will decrease hematoma formation under the skin flap. Antibiotic coverage is continued for several weeks to prevent wound infection and to decrease the lymphadenopathy produced by the chronic infection of the penile lesion.

Hematoma, wound infection and delayed healing are the most common postoperative complications encountered. Local recurrence may occur if the surgery was conservative. Tumor free margins should be substantiated by frozen sections on all the specimens removed. In case of doubt, the dissection should be extended.

II. LYMPHADENECTOMY

Lymphadenectomy for carcinoma of the penis is controversial. Its necessity, timing and extent have been debated by urologists since Sir William Mac-Cormic in 1886 reported five cases of radical penectomy followed by inguinal node dissections (Hovnanian 1967; Skinner et al. 1972).

Between 35 and 50 percent of patients with carcinoma of the penis have palpable inguinal adenopathy on the initial examination (Beggs and Spratt 1964; DeKernion et al. 1973); infection of the primary tumor accounts for much of this adenopathy. However, 50 percent of these patients with adenopathy have carcinoma in the nodes while the remainder have adenopathy due primarily to inflammatory changes (Kossow et al. 1973; De Kernion et al. 1973). After the primary lesion is removed, a period of at least three to six weeks should be allowed before considering lymphadenectomy and/or biopsy. During this period, the patient should be treated vigorously with appropriate antibiotics.

When regional adenopathy persists more than three to six weeks postoperatively, lymphadenectomy should be considered. Cabanas (1977) reported that the 'sentinel' lymph node was the primary site of metastases from penile carcinoma. He felt that this should be biopsied bilaterally and, if positive, extensive lymphadenectomy should be performed. If the nodes were negative for tumor, no further surgical procedure was immediately required. Patients with negative sentinel lymph node biopsies had a five-year survival of 90 percent.

When involvement of regional lymph nodes is present, a lymphadenectomy should be performed. Overall, approximately 30 to 40 percent of patients with nodal involvement can be cured by lymphadenectomy (Hardner et al. 1972; Skinner et al. 1972; DeKernion et al. 1973). Untreated patients usually die of their disease within two to three years.

Further controversy concerns prophylactic node dissection in patients without clinical evidence of nodal involvement versus a program of observation and subsequent surgery only if nodes become clinically positive. The stage of the primary tumor is important in this decision. In patients with clinical Stage I carcinoma of the penis, positive lymph nodes have been reported in 25 percent by Hardner

et al. Kurvilla et al. found 20 percent of clinical State I and II tumors had positive lymph node metastases. Others, however, have found a low incidence of occult metastases in Stage I desease (Beggs and Spratt 1964; Skinner et al. 1972; De Kernion et al. 1973). They suggest considering superficial inguinal node dissection and frozen section examination (Figure 3a, b, c). If the nodes are positive for tumor, a deep ilio-inguinal dissection is performed. If Cabanas' sentinel node biopsy results are confirmed by other surgeons' experience, this procedure may supersede a formal groin dissection.

Stage II disease has a higher mortality rate than Stage I. Those who favor a palliative lymphadenectomy note that 16 to 20 percent of patients may develop tumor in regional nodes (Hardner et al. 1972; Kossow et al. 1973). Other authors have found that even when nodes develop while under observation, subsequent lymphadenectomy can be successful. Frew et al. found no deaths due to observation of initially clinically negative nodes. Ekstrom and Edsmyr reported a 50 percent cure rate in patients who had node dissection only when nodes became clinically apparent.

In Stage III disease, obvious clinical involvement of the nodes necessitates definitive treatment of the superficial and deep inguinal nodes. Radiation therapy has been advocated by Staubitz, who reported a 40 percent five year survival. Murrel and Williams also reported a 41 percent success rate, but others found little success with this treatment (Hanash et al. 1970; Johnson et al. 1973). Most urologists favor a lymphadenectomy which includes the superficial and deep inguinal nodes plus the iliac nodes. It should be noted, however, that a five-year survival in patients with positive iliac lymph nodes is a rarity.

The object of a radical ileo-inguinal lymphadenectomy is to do an en bloc dissection of all lymphatic tissue from the aortic bifurcation to the area where the femoral artery enters Hunter's canal. Precise knowledge of the anatomy is mandatory for successful surgery. The skin of the inguinal area is supplied by the superficial pudendal, iliocircumflex and superficial epigastric arteries. These vessels run in Camper's fascia parallel to the inguinal ligament. The transverse orientation of the blood supply mitigates against vertical incisions in this area.

The femoral triangle contains the majority of the

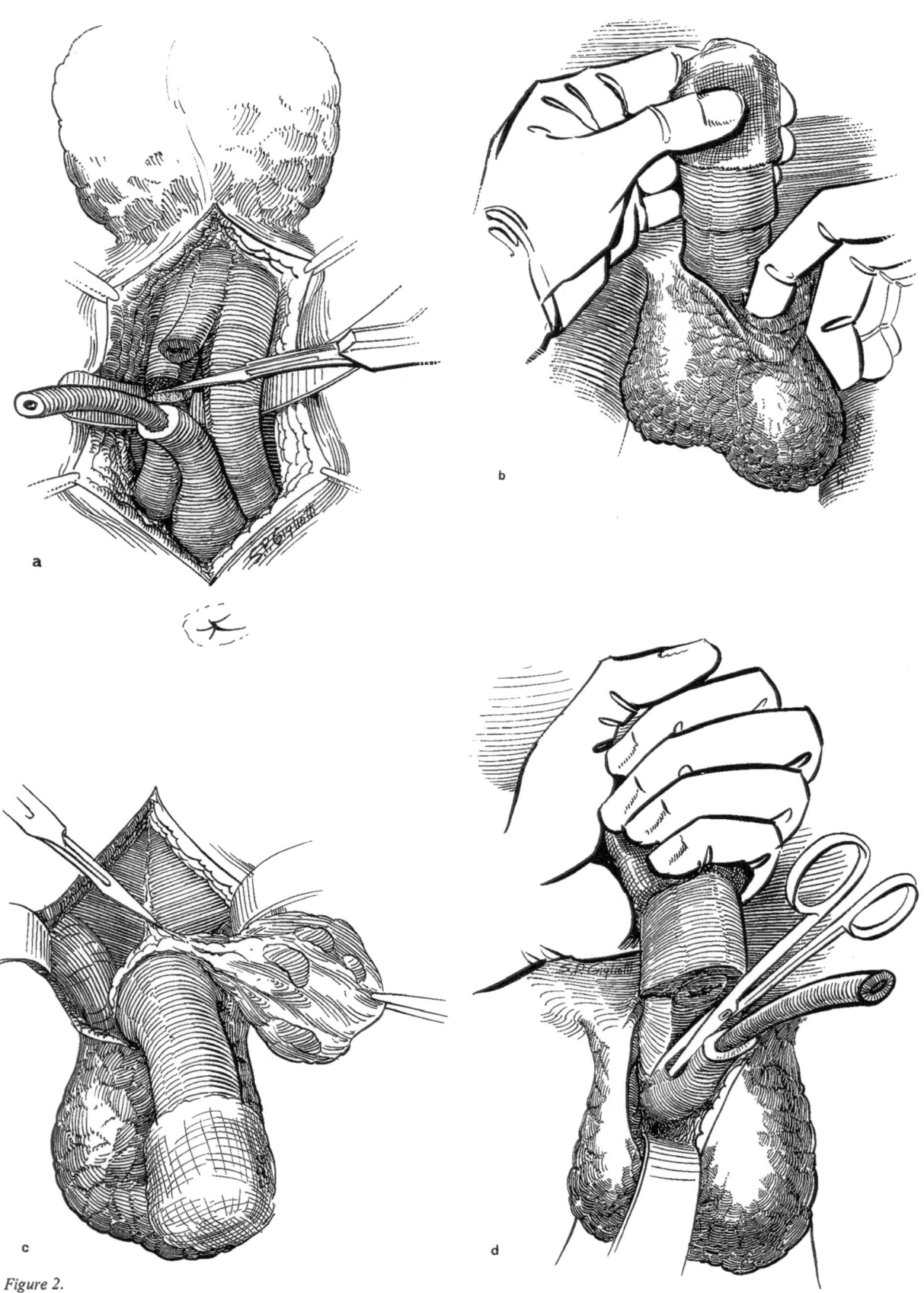

Figure 2.

lymph nodes in the groin. It is bounded superiorly by the inguinal ligament, medially by the adductor longus muscle, and laterally by the sartorius (Figure 4a). The floor of the femoral triangle is formed by iliopsoas and pectineus muscles. The lymph nodes in the inguinal area are divided by the fascia lata into superficial and deep nodes. They are found either overlying the femoral triangle or attached to the femoral vessels. The superficial nodes (4-25) lie in Camper's fascia and drain into both deep in-

guinal and iliac nodes. The deep inguinal nodes are fewer in number and form a continuous chain with the iliac nodes (Figure 4b).

Various surgical techniques have been applied in performing ilioinguinal lymphadenectomies (Young 1931; Daseler et al. 1943; Hovnanian 1967; Skinner et al. 1972). In 1972, Fraley and Hutchens described the skin bridge technique. This allowed exposure to the superficial and deep inguinal nodes plus the iliac nodes without compromising the

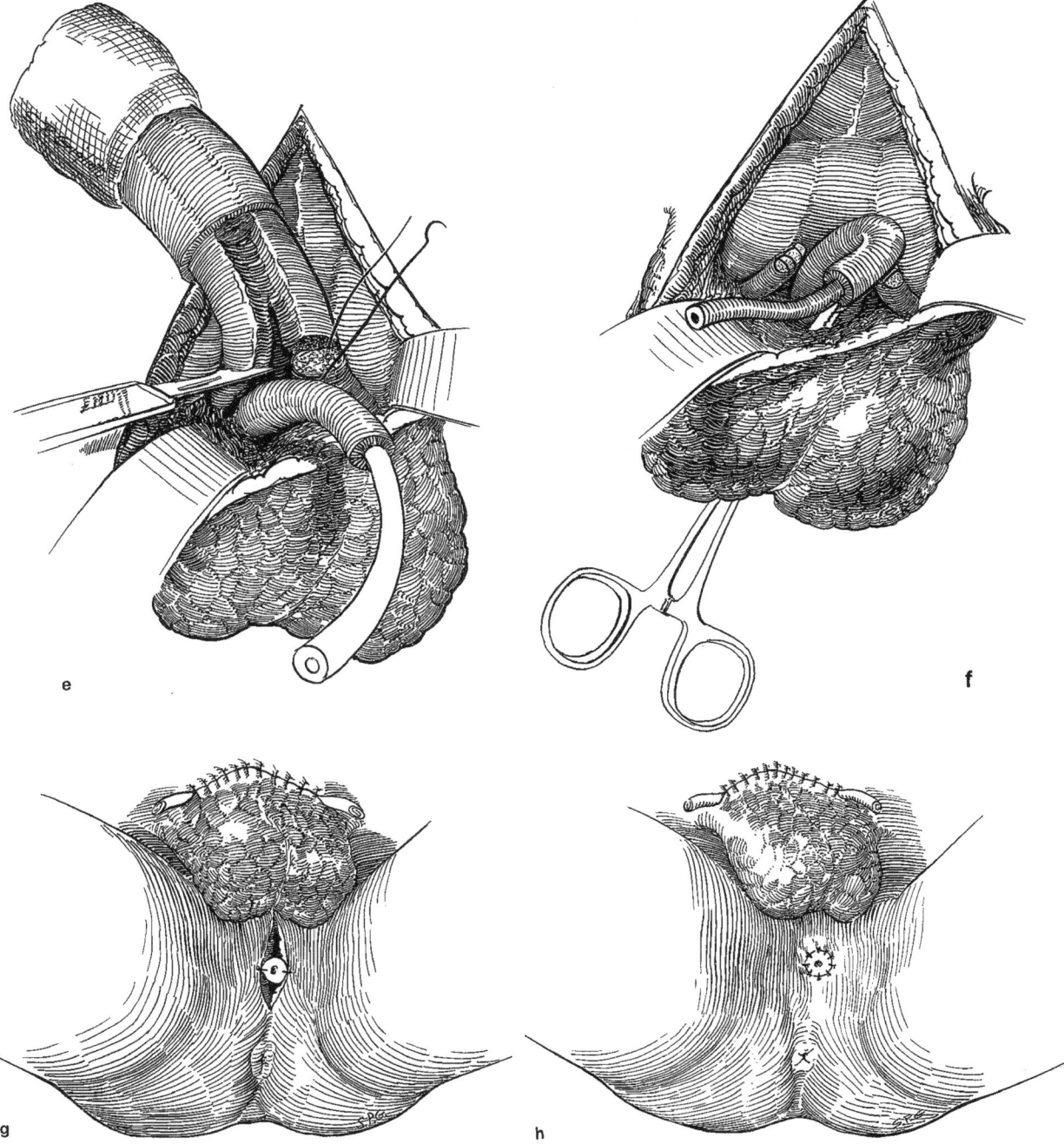

e

f

g

h

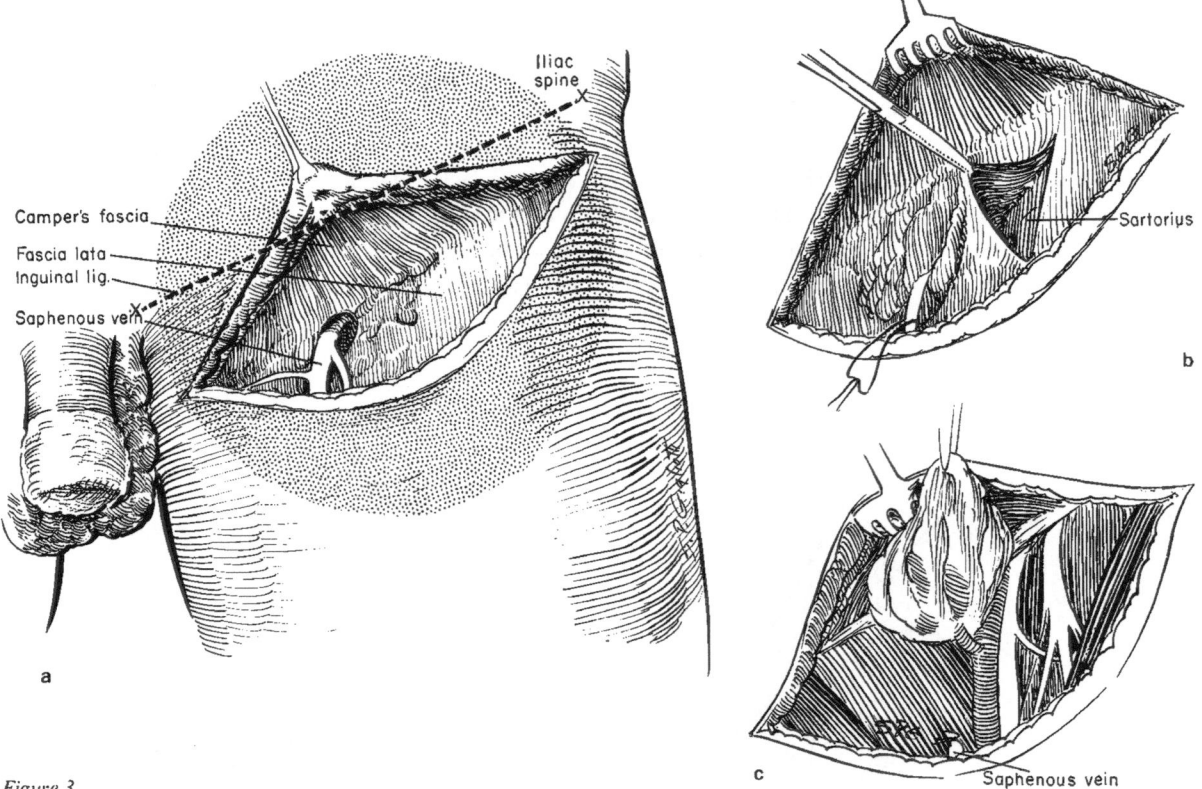

Figure 3.

blood supply to the skin flaps. Earlier techniques had resulted in sepsis, skin necrosis and slough in a high percentage of patients. In 1978, Hoppman & Fraley modified their skin bridge procedure to use three incisions instead of four. A midline incision exposes the iliac vessels and can be used both times if the two groin dissections are done at separate operations.

The surgical procedure is usually performed three to six weeks after the primary excision of the penile carcinoma. The patient is placed in a supine position with the leg held in moderate external rotation (Figure 5a). The entire groin, proximal thigh and distal two-thirds of the abdominal wall are prepped and exposed. A midline abdominal incision is made from the symphysis to umbilicus, and two parallel incisions above and below the inguinal ligament are made (Figure 5b). The proximal dissection is initiated so that the extent of tumor can be assessed. If extensive metastases are present, the lower incision is not made. The proximal lymphatics are ligated early so that embolization does not take place in the dissection of the lymph nodes in the femoral triangle. Skin and subcutaneous tissue are sepa-

rated carefully. The proximal incision provides exposure for the iliac vessels when the peritoneum is retracted medially. The proximal dissection begins with incising the endopelvic fascia medial to the genitalfemoral nerve from the inguinal ligament to the aortic bifurcation. All fat and adventitial tissue with lymph nodes that surround the major vessels are excised. The dissection commences at the level of the aortic bifurcation and should include the superficial and deep iliac and obturator lymph nodes. The proximal en bloc dissection terminates when the iliac vessels are completely free. The lymphatic and connective tissue are passed under the inguinal ligament in the femoral canal (Figure 5b).

The second skin incision is made 10 cm below the inguinal ligament. The ends of the incision are curved away from the inguinal ligament to preserve blood supply of the skin. A skin flap 2-4 mm in width is developed from the incision to a point just below the inguinal ligament. This portion of dissection should include the prepubic nodes. All efforts should be made not to devascularize the skin bridge. The fatty subcutaneous tissue beneath the skin flap is then dissected off the underlying abdominal wall and the inguinal ligament. The distal skin flap over the femoral triangle is developed. At the limits of the dissection the subcutaneous tissue is incised through the fascia lata and down to the muscle. The saphenous vein is ligated at the distal margin of the dissection. The lymphatic tissue is dissected cephalad to the inguinal ligament. The femoral vessels are cleaned of all tissues. The saphenous vein is ligated again in the region of the inguinal ligament. The floor of the femoral triangle is dissected to free all lymphatic tissue. The specimen is dissected from the femoral vessels and inguinal ligament so it becomes continuous with the dissection that has been done from above the inguinal ligament. The specimen is labelled as to the anatomical location and sent to pathology. The sartorius muscle is sectioned at its origin near the anterior superior iliac spine and transposed to cover the femoral vessels (Figure 5c). The end of the muscle is sutured to the medial aspect of the inguinal ligament (Figure 5d). The medial borders are attached to the adductor longus muscle. This technique covers femoral vessels to prevent potential subsequent vessel erosion. It also eliminates dead space and provides a floor on which the skin bridge may heal. The shelving portion of the inguinal ligament is sutured to Cooper's ligament in an effort to prevent postoperative wound hernias. Fraley and Hutchens further advise resecting a small strip from the distal skin flap to prevent postoperative necrosis. Suction catheters are placed in the wound in the area of the femoral dissection. They exit in the mid-portion of the thigh away from the distal skin flap. Careful clipping of all lymphatics should be pursued throughout the procedure to eliminate postoperative lymphorrhea and seroma. The skin closure should be without tension.

Postoperatively, the leg should be wrapped with occlusive dressings and elevated. The patient should be immobilized for six to seven days. Skinner et al. (1972) recommend administration of anticoagulants commencing on the second postoperative day and continuing for six weeks. Antibiotic coverage is continued in the postoperative period to prevent wound infection and skin slough.

The contralateral dissection is usually performed four to six weeks after the initial lymphadenectomy.

Postoperative complications potentially include

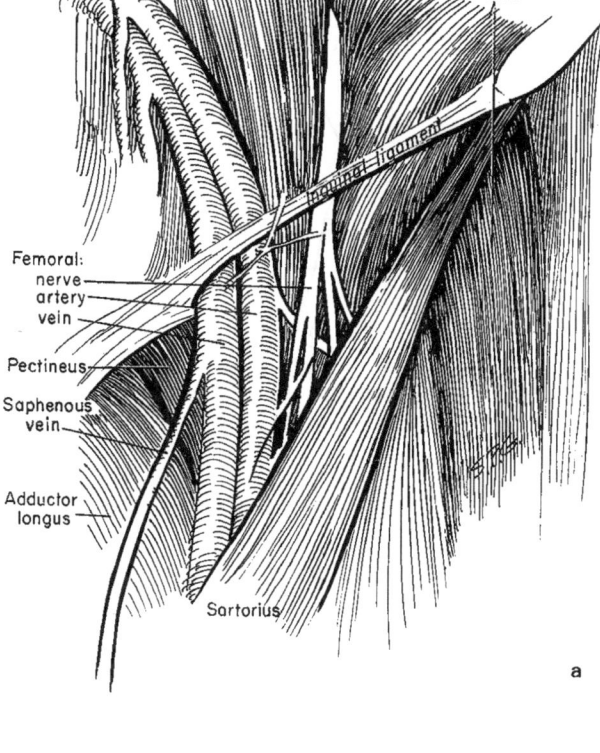

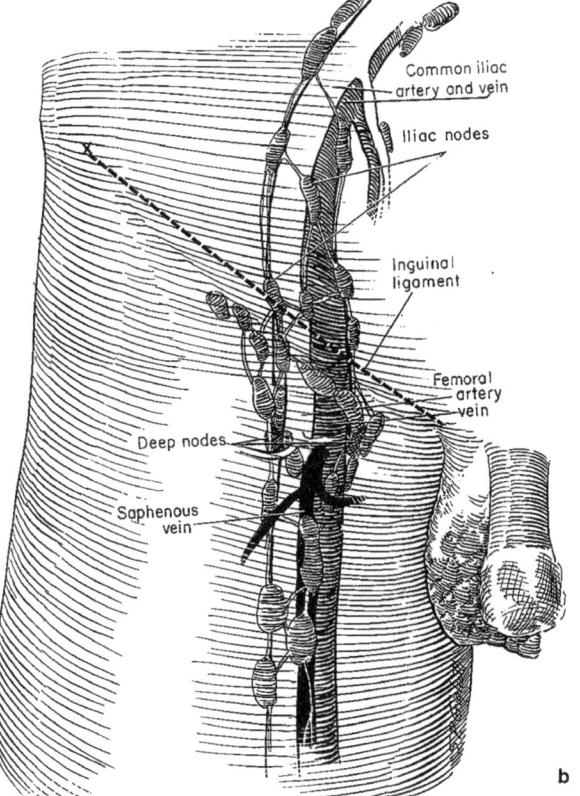

Figure 4.

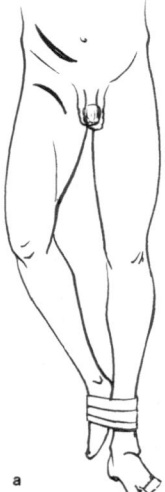

Figure 5.   a

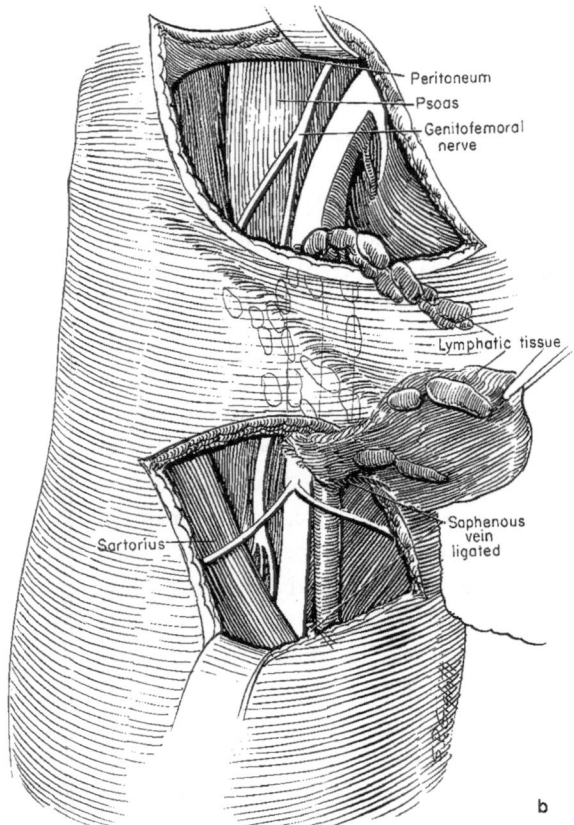

b

wound necrosis, lymphedema, hemorrhage, hematoma and herniation. With precise surgical technique, these complications should occur infrequently.

III. RESULTS OF SURGICAL TREATMENT

The five-year survival rates for carcinoma of the penis treated with penectomy (partial or total) plus lymphadenectomy are presented in Table 3. The rates vary from 48-69 percent.

Proponents of radiation therapy for carcinoma of the penis point to the results of Murrel and Williams and Englestad who reported, respectively, 40 and 67 percent five-year survival rates. However, in most series of patients treated only with radiation, clinical staging is not precise and never confirmed by histologic staging. Terms such as control are often substituted for cure.

The advantages of surgical therapy still appear

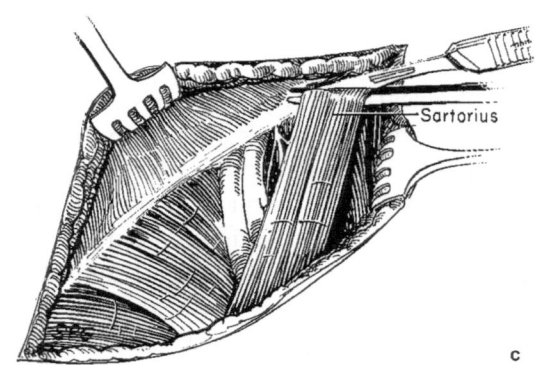

c

Table 3. Surgical 5-year survival for carcinoma of penis (all stages)

Year	Author	No. patients	5-year survival rate
1958	Ekstrom and Edsmyr	177	69%
1964	Beggs and Spratt	79	46%
1967	Frew et al.	36	53%
1970	Hanash, et al.	141	54%
1972	Hardner et al.	100	48%
1972	Skinner et al.	34	59%

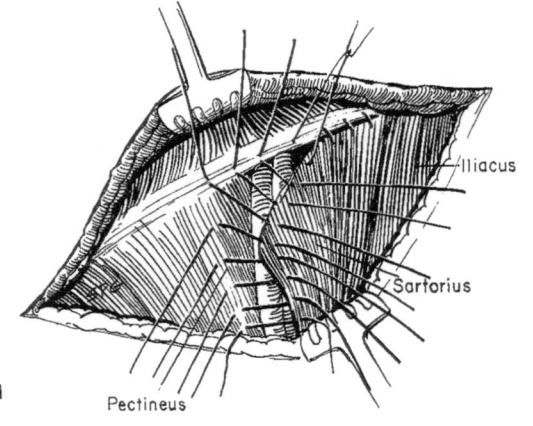

d

significant. Hoppman and Fraley listed five predominant reasons for favoring surgical therapy over radiation.

1. The morbidity and mortality rates of this operation have been reduced by improved surgical techniques.
2. The ilio-inguinal lymphadenectomy gives the best surgical margin, especially since metastasis may skip the inguinal lymph nodes and go directly to the iliac nodes.
3. If the patient has metastatic lymph nodes, extended operation appears to offer the most effective means of controlling the disease.
4. One of the most common causes of treatment failure in penile cancer is the development of inoperable lymph node metastases after penectomy while the patient is being followed.

5. There is no reliable method short of total extirpation of all ilio-inguinal lymph nodes of staging the tumors.

Block et al. reported in 1973 three survivals of seven patients treated with hemipelvectomy for recurrent penile carcinoma in the groin. Possibly this drastic surgery would not have been required if more aggressive surgical therapy was pursued initially. Several of the patients in their series were radiation treatment failures.

Chemotherapy for carcinoma of the penis in surgical failures has had minimal success (Ichikawa et al. 1969; Mills 1972). Bleomycin has been marginally successful in treating early carcinoma of the penis. However, pulmonary fibrosis is a serious potential complication of this therapy. Thus, surgery remains the treatment of choice.

REFERENCES

Beggs JH and Spratt JS: Epidermoid carcinoma of the penis. J Urol 91: 166, 1964.

Block NL, Rosen P, Whitmore WF: Hemipelvectomy for advance penile cancer. J Urol 110: 703, 1973.

Buddington WT, Kickham CJ, Smith WE: An assessment of malignant disease of the penis. J Urol 89: 442, 1963.

Cabanas RM: An approach for the treatment of penile carcinoma. Cancer 39: 456, 1977.

Daseler EH, Anson BJ, Reimann AF: Radical excision of the inguinal and iliac lymph glands: A study based upon 450 anatomical dissections and upon supportive clinical observations. Surg Gynec Obstet 87: 679, 1943.

DeKernion JB, Persky L: Neoplastic lesions of the penis. In: Genitourinary cancer, Skinner DG and DeKernion JB (eds), Philadelphia, WB Saunders Company, 1978, p 494-508.

DeKernion JB, Tynberg P, Persky L and Fegen JP: Carcinoma of the penis. Cancer 32: 1256, 1973.

Ekstrom T, Edsmyr F: Cancer of the penis – A clinical study of 229 cases. Acta Chir Scand 115: 25, 1958.

Engelstad RB: Treatment of cancer of the penis at the Norwegian Radium Hospital. Amer J Roentgenol 60: 801, 1948.

Fegen P, Persky L: Squamous cell carcinoma of the penis. Its treatment with special reference to radical node dissection. Arch Surg 99: 117, 1960.

Fraley EE, Hutchens HC: Radical ilio-inguinal node dissection: the skin bridge technique. A new procedure. J Urol 108: 279, 1972.

Frew IDO, Jefferies JD, Swinney J: Carcinoma of penis. Brit J Urol 39: 398, 1967.

Goette DK, Carson TE: Erythroplasia of Queyrat. Treatment with topical 5-fluorouracil. Cancer 38: 1498, 1976.

Hanash K, Furlow WL, Utz DC, Harrison EG: Carcinoma of the penis: A clinicopathologic study. J Urol 104: 291, 1970.

Hardner GJ, Bhanalaph T, Murphy GP, Albert DJ, Moore RH: Carcinoma of penis: analysis of therapy in 100 consecutive cases. J Urol 108: 428, 1972.

Hoppman HJ, Fraley EE: Squamous cell carcinoma of the penis. J Urol 120: 393, 1978.

Hovnanian AP: The evolution and present status of pelvi-inguinal lymphatic excision. Surg Gynec Obstet 124: 851, 1967.

Hueser JN, Pugh RP: Erythroplasia of Queyrat treated with topical 5-fluorouracil. J Urol 102: 595, 1969.

Ichikawa T, Nakano I, Hirokawa I: Bleomycin treatment of the tumors of penis and scrotum. J Urol 102: 699, 1969.

Jackson SM: The treatment of carcinoma of the penis. Brit J Surg 53: 33, 1966.

Johnson DE, Fuerst DE, Ayala AG: Carcinoma of the penis: experience with 153 cases. Urology 1: 404, 1973.

Kossow JH, Hotchkiss RS, Morales PA: Carcinoma of the penis treated surgically: analysis of 100 cases. Urology 2: 169, 1973.

McAninch JW, Moore CA: Precancerous penile lesions in young men. J Urol 104: 287, 1970.

McCarron DL, Carlton CE: Giant condyloma of the penis. J Urol 104: 730, 1970.

Murrel DS: Radiotherapy in the treatment of carcinoma of the penis. Brit J Urol 37: 211, 1965.

Mills EED: Intermittent intravenous methotrexate in the treatment of advanced epidermoid carcinoma. South African Med J 46: 398, 1972.

Skinner DG, Leadbetter F, Kelley SB: The surgical management of squamous cell carcinoma of the penis. J Urol 107: 273, 1972.

Staubitz WJ, Lent MH, Oberkircher OJ: Carcinoma of the penis. Cancer 8: 371, 1955.

Warwich R, Williams P: Gray's anatomy. Philadelphia, WB Saunders Company, 1973, p 741, 1346-48.

Young HH: A radical operation for the cure of cancer of the penis. J Urol 26: 285, 1931.

19. ORCHIECTOMY AND RETROPERITONEAL NODE DISSECTION FOR CARCINOMA OF THE TESTICLE

T.J. ROHNER, JR. and E.J. SANFORD

Although testicular carcinoma accounts for only one percent of all malignant tumors in men, it remains the leading cause of cancer death in males 25 to 35 years old. The survival rate of patients with testis cancer has greatly improved in recent years, due largely to more effective chemotherapeutic programs and radiation therapy techniques. Despite these advances in the treatment of patients with metastatic disease, early recognition and prompt surgical exploration of suspect testis mass lesions remains the foundation of testis cancer treatment.

The removal of tumor-bearing retroperitoneal lymph nodes has been shown (Walsh et al. 1971) to improve patient survival. The addition of lymphadenectomy to orchiectomy alone has improved the survival rate of pediatric patients with testis tumors from 47 to 84 percent (Sabio et al. 1974). Most importantly, retroperitoneal lymphadenectomy accurately establishes the stage or extent of the patient's disease and provides clear indications for subsequent chemotherapy or radiation therapy.

An increasingly useful indication for retroperitoneal lymph node dissection is the assessment of the nodal status of patients initially presenting with metastatic disease who have apparently responded well to chemotherapy. Evidence of residual retroperitoneal tumor in these patients clearly documents the need for further chemotherapy or radiation therapy. If the resected nodes are negative for cancer, continued observation alone may be indicated without subjecting the patient to further drug or radiation therapy.

the testicle mandates surgical exploration of the testicle through an inguinal incision. With this axiom in mind, the physician's careful physical examination of the scrotal contents should provide the proper information for suspicion of testicular carcinoma. There is perhaps no better clinical example in which the patient's history serves to confuse rather than aid the physician in diagnosis than testis tumors. For example, a patient history of mild trauma is common but it should not distract the physician from recommending exploration if the testicle is palpably abnormal.

The symptom that most often causes the patient to seek physician attention is a relatively painless hard scrotal lump or enlarged testicle. If there is a heavy, hard testicular mass, the diagnosis is usually made easily. The presence of pain, however, is not uncommon and in one report (Patton et al. 1959), 23 percent of the patients experienced painful scrotal symptoms. Both Stephen (1962) and Patton et al. (1959) demonstrated the coexistence of epididymitis and testis tumor in 5-16 percent of patients. In our experience, errors in diagnosis and delay of surgical exploration is most frequent in patients with associated epididymitis. A constantly high index of suspicion and awareness of this frequently occurring association should minimize delay. Although most common in the 18 to 35 year-old age group, testis tumors do occur in men of all ages. Our oldest patient was a 79 year-old gentleman with seminoma.

The variety of clinical presentations in patients with testicular tumor are listed in Table 1.

I. DIAGNOSIS

A hard scrotal mass that cannot be separated from

II. RADICAL INGUINAL ORCHIECTOMY

An inguinal approach should be used for the

Table 1. Clinical presentation of patients with testis tumor.

Painless scrotal mass
Hydrocele
Acute epididymitis
Trauma
Incidental finding on physical examination
Distant metastases

exploration of all testis mass lesions. There is no place in the diagnosis of these lesions for scrotal orchiectomy or transcrotal biopsy of testis tumors either by incision or needle aspiration. The hazards relating to these procedures have been described by Markland (1977) and include local tumor recurrence, which requires subsequent scrotectomy and inguinal lymphadenectomy. Rarely, a primary tumor may be so large as to preclude delivery of the testicle through the inguinal incision. An alternate approach to this problem will be described.

Radical inguinal orchiectomy is accomplished through an incision extending from the anterior-superior iliac spine to the pubic tubercle (Figure 1a). The aponeurosis of the external oblique is divided from the external to the internal inguinal ring and the inguinal canal is exposed. Using sharp and blunt dissection, the spermatic cord is mobilized and isolated to the level of the internal ring, and a noncrushing rubber shod clamp is immediately applied at this level (Figure 1b). The remainder of the spermatic cord and testis with their fascial investments intact is then freed up from the scrotum and delivered into the wound. At this point, if there is reasonable doubt of malignancy, the testis with its coverings can be placed outside the wound on a lap pad. The tunica vaginalis is opened, the lesion explored, and a biopsy is obtained for frozen section. If tumor is present the cord is then divided between Kocher clamps at the level of the internal

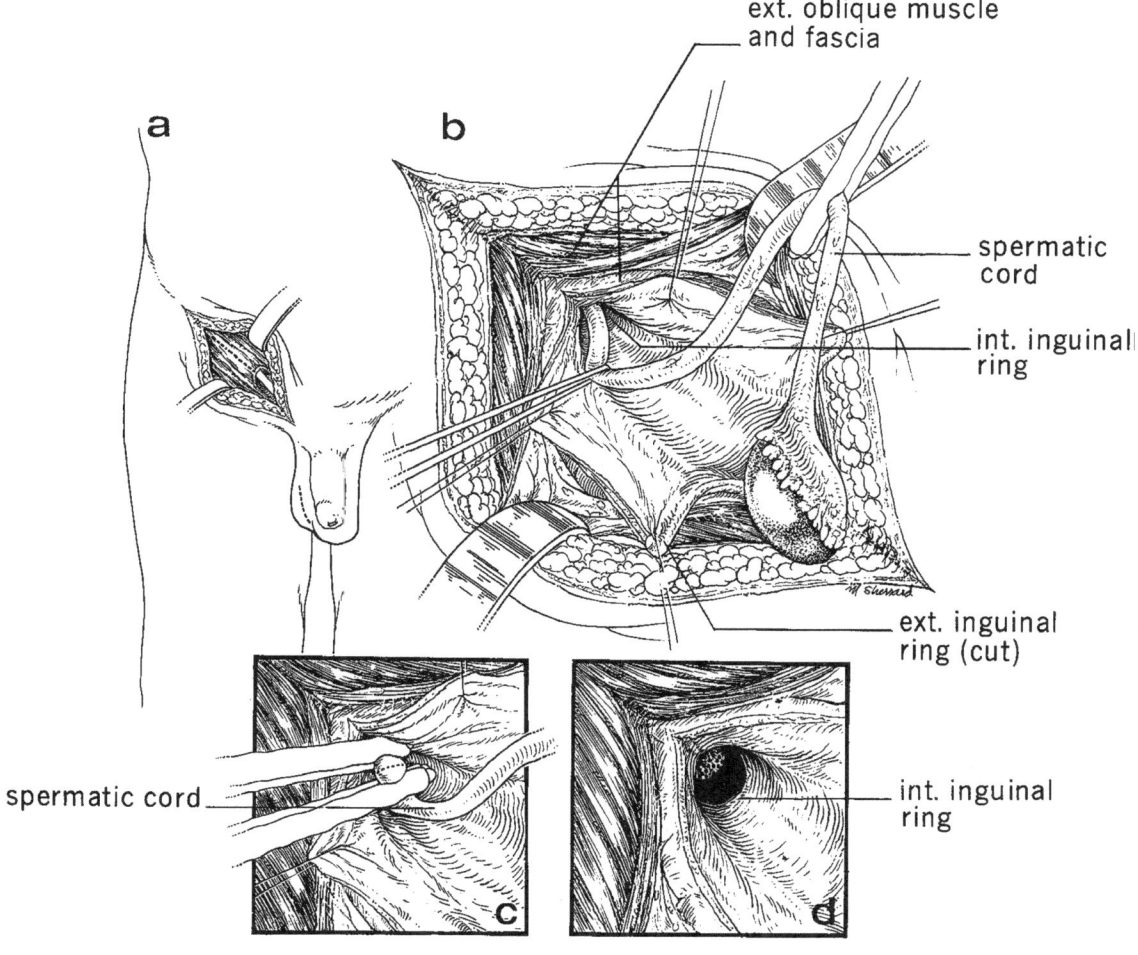

Figure 1. Radical inguinal orchiectomy.

ring, thus completing the radical inguinal orchi- ectomy (Figure 1c). Opening the tunica vaginalis and obtaining a biopsy specimen may be omitted in those patients in whom there is little doubt about the diagnosis. The stump of the cord is doubly ligated with a heavy 0-silk suture for easy identifi- cation if subsequent retroperitoneal lymph node dissection is required. After ligation, the spermatic cord generally retracts above the internal ring (Figure 1d). The external oblique aponeurosis is then reapproximated, using 2-0 silk sutures, and the remainder of the wound is closed in standard fashion. No drains are necessary.

If a testis mass is present but the pathologist cannot give a definite diagnosis, the surgeon should proceed with radical orchiectomy. The chances of a benign testis tumor are small and the risks of leaving a malignant tumor *in situ* are great. The safest course for the patient under these circum- stances is to remove the testis.

If the primary tumor is so large that it cannot be delivered easily through the inguinal incision or if a scrotal incision has been inadvertently used, the surgeon, upon recognizing a tumor, should im- mediately make an inguinal incision and clamp, divide, and ligate the spermatic cord at the level of the internal ring as described previously. The spermatic cord and testis can then be delivered through the scrotal incision.

III. PATHOLOGY AND STAGING OF TESTIS TUMORS

A. Pathology

Following radical orchiectomy, the management of the patient will depend on (1) tumor cell type(s) and (2) tumor stage or extent of disease. The germ cell tumors constitute about 96 percent of all testis tumors. The most commonly used classification of germ cell tumors of the testis is that of Dixon and Moore (1952). It is presented in Table 2 along with the percentage of relative frequency of occurrence. Careful multiple section histologic examination of the entire tumor is necessary to determine if more than one cell type is present. For example, the combination of embryonal and teratocarcinoma is relatively common. It is particularly important to

Table 2. Classification of testicular germ cell tumors (Dixon and Moore).

Seminoma	30-40%
Embryonal cell carcinoma	20%
Teratocarcinoma	20-30%
Adult teratoma	5-10%
Choriocarcinoma	0.3%

be certain that an apparent seminoma does not contain elements of teratocarcinoma or embryonal carcinoma, since there are major differences in the staging and treatment recommendations for semi- nomas and nonseminomatous tumors.

Yolk sac tumor of the testis, also known as orchioblastoma, an endodermal sinus tumor, is a malignancy occurring in infants and children which also arises from germ cell elements.

Non germ-cell tumors of the testis are uncom- mon (four percent), (Table 3).

Table 3. Non-germ cell tumors of the testis.

Sertoli cell tumor
Leydig cell tumor
Sarcomas of the testis and its tunica

B. Clinical Staging

When histologic classification of the tumor cell type(s) has been made, the physician must then determine the clinical stage or extent of tumor present to recommend appropriate treatment.

Testis tumors spread primarily by lymphatic extension although embryonal and choriocarci- noma in particular may demonstrate early hemato- genous dissemination. Unless altered by previous surgical procedures, such as orchiopexy, the tes- ticular lymphatics accompany the spermatic cord to the retroperitoneal area and then drain into the lymph nodes surrounding the vena cava and aorta from their bifurcation below to the level of the renal vessels above.

The most commonly used clinical staging system is outlined in Table 4. The procedures recom- mended for staging patients with seminoma are shown in Table 5.

An important advance in our capacity to deter- mine testis tumor staging is the serum tumor markers, beta human chorionic gonadotropin (B-

Table 4. Clinical staging of testis tumors.

Stage 1	Tumor confined to the testis
Stage 2	Tumor spread to the abdominal lymph nodes without supradiaphragmatic disease
Stage 3	Tumor spread to the supradiaphragmatic mediastinal and/or supraclavicular lymph nodes
Stage 4	Distant metastases

Table 5. Staging procedures for seminoma.

IVP
Pedal lymphangiogram
Serum alpha-fetoprotein (AFP) and beta-human chorionic gonadotropins (B-HCG)
Tomograms of the chest
Liver scan
Computerized axial tomography

Table 6. Staging procedures for nonseminomatous tumors.

IVP
Serum alpha-fetoprotein (AFP) and beta-human chorionic gonadotropins (B-HCG)
Tomograms of the chest
Retroperitoneal lymph node dissection

HCG) and alpha-fetoprotein (AFP). Current sensitive radioimmunoassay techniques permit accurate quantitative measurement of the serum levels of these two glycoproteins. It has been found that about 90 percent of patients with nonseminomatous tumor with lymph node metastases have elevated levels of one or both of these markers. Seminoma is always associated with normal serum levels of alpha-fetoprotein, although Javadpour (1978) found that four percent of patients with pure seminoma had elevated B-HCG levels. Serial determinations of both B-HCG and AFP are especially helpful in following tumor activity and response to surgery or chemotherapy, as described by Lange and Fraley (1977).

Seminoma is remarkably radiosensitive and thus retroperitoneal lymph node dissection is not performed in patients with this disease. As mentioned previously, only a small percentage of patients with seminoma will be found to have elevated serum levels of B-HCG. If the serum AFP is elevated in a patient with apparent seminoma, the patient should be considered to have nonseminomatous elements present in nodal metastases and the lesion should be staged as a nonseminomatous tumor. We have discontinued performing pedal lymphangiography in patients with nonseminomatous tumors since the results of the study would not alter clinical management, which always includes retroperitoneal lymph node dissection. The staging procedures for patients with nonseminomatous testis tumors are presented in Table 6.

C. Retroperitoneal Lymph Node Dissection

1. Indications. All patients with Stage 1 and Stage 2 nonseminomatous tumors should undergo retroperitoneal lymphadenectomy. Patients with clinical Stage 2 disease but who have large bulky retroperitoneal nodal metastases evidenced on an IVP or abdominal palpation are initially treated with chemotherapy prior to node dissection. Patients presenting with Stage 3 or Stage 4 disease are also treated initially with chemotherapy or radiotherapy. If response to chemotherapy is good, retroperitoneal lymph node dissection is usually done at a later time to remove residual nodal disease or conclusively demonstrate a complete response to therapy.

The management of germ cell testis tumors in children has been reviewed by Hopkins et al. (1978) and their evidence suggests that the indications for retroperitoneal lymphadenectomy in the adult are equally applicable in the pediatric patient.

2. Preoperative preparation. In addition to discussing the usual operative risks and complications the surgeon should inform the patient that although his erections will be preserved, he will probably experience infertility and loss of ejaculation as a result of lumbar sympathectomy.

A broad-spectrum antibiotic is started the night prior to surgery. Intravenous fluids are also begun that night, and the patient receives 20 ml/kg of 5 percent D&W in 0.25 percent saline during the 12 hours preceding surgery. Extensive retroperitoneal dissection involving mobilization and manipulation of the renal vessels and ureters and third space fluid losses require that the patient be well hydrated in order to avoid oliguria and possible renal failure.

3. Technique of Retroperitoneal Lymph Node Dissection. We have used the anterior transabdominal approach as described earlier by Patton et al. (1959), Staubitz et al. (1974) and Young (1975), including recent modifications by Donohue (1977).

There does appear to be a difference in the retroperitoneal lymph node drainage pattern between right and left testis tumors. Left testis tumors tend to drain primarily to lymph nodes in the region of the left renal vein just lateral to the aorta. Right testis tumors more commonly drain to the nodes lying between the vena cava and aorta just below the level of the left renal vein. Right tumors are more likely to cross the midline to involve contralateral para-aortic nodes. Because considerable variation in lymph node metastases occurs, we have continued to carry out extensive bilateral lymphadenectomy for both right and left testis tumors. The extent of dissection for right and left testis tumors is illustrated in Figure 2a. The dissection always includes both suprahilar areas from above the celiac axis to the origin of the external iliac artery on the ipsilateral side to just below the aortic bifurcation on the contralateral side. The ureters on both sides represent the lateral extent of dissection. Gerota's fascia and perirenal fat are resected on the ipsilateral side. On the contralateral side, Gerota's fascia and enclosed fat are removed anteriorly to the lateral border of the kidney.

Mobilization of the aorta and vena cava after division of the lumbar vessels is necessary for complete lymphadenectomy. Earlier techniques of lymphadenectomy did not advocate mobilization of the great vessels, and Tavel et al. (1963) documented that 25 percent of the retroperitoneal lymph nodes were not removed during dissection. More recently, Kaswick et al. (1976) has demonstrated it is possible to carry out a complete lymphadenectomy by removing the nodal tissue under and between these great vessels.

Figures 5 through 8 were drawn in the operating theater during a recent lymphadenectomy done for a patient with a right testis tumor. Numerous involved lymph nodes were encountered over the vena cava and right renal hilar and suprahilar areas. We do not routinely carry out ipsilateral adrenalectomy, but in this patient adrenalectomy was necessary to adequately resect the involved lymph nodes. The procedure is described below.

After induction of anesthesia, a nasogastric tube is passed and a No. 16 F. Foley catheter inserted and placed to urimeter drainage so that the anesthesiologist can monitor hourly urine outputs. The

patient is placed in the supine position and a midline incision extending from the xiphoid process to the pubis is made (Figure 2b). After opening the peritoneum, the abdominal cavity is carefully ex-

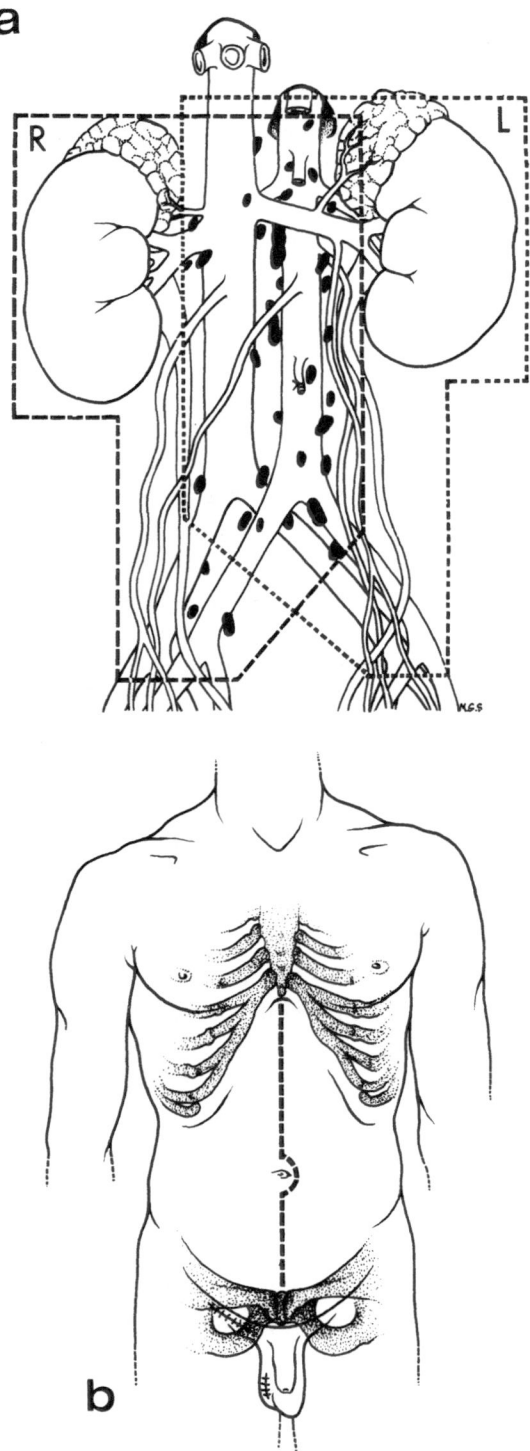

Figure 2. a. Extent of dissection for right and left testis tumors. b. Midline abdominal incision extending from xiphoid process to pubic symphysis.

plored. An incidental appendectomy is not performed. A deep Balfour retractor is placed in the wound and the right colon and hepatic flexure mobilized by incising the lateral peritoneal reflection and lesser omentum into the lesser sac (Figure 3).

Blunt and sharp dissection is used to separate Gerota's fascia anteriorly and the Kocher maneuver is used to free up the duodenum and head of the pancreas. Beginning at the cecum, the mesentery of the small bowel is divided from the cecum to the ligament of Treitz (Figure 4). At the upper extent of this incision it is important to identify, ligate and divide the inferior mesenteric vein. Division of the inferior mesenteric vein with extension of the incision into the colon mesentery is necessary to adequately expose the left suprahilar region. At this point the inferior mesenteric artery is

divided between 2-0 silk ties which further frees the colon. The large and small bowel are then packed in a plastic bowel bag and placed on the patient's chest (Figure 5). As Donohue (1977) has suggested, we find it easier to regard the right and left suprahilar dissections as separate procedures, removing the fat and nodal contents of each of these areas individually and without attempting to keep the entire retroperitoneal nodal specimen intact. The right suprahilar dissection is begun on the anteromedial surface of the vena cava just above the level of the celiac vessels (Figure 6). Additional superior and medial retraction of the duodenum and head of the pancreas with a sponge-protected Willauer retractor aids in exposing this area. Division of the areolar tissue over the vena cava is accomplished with scissors. The nodal and adventitial tissue can then be bluntly reflected laterally from the cava.

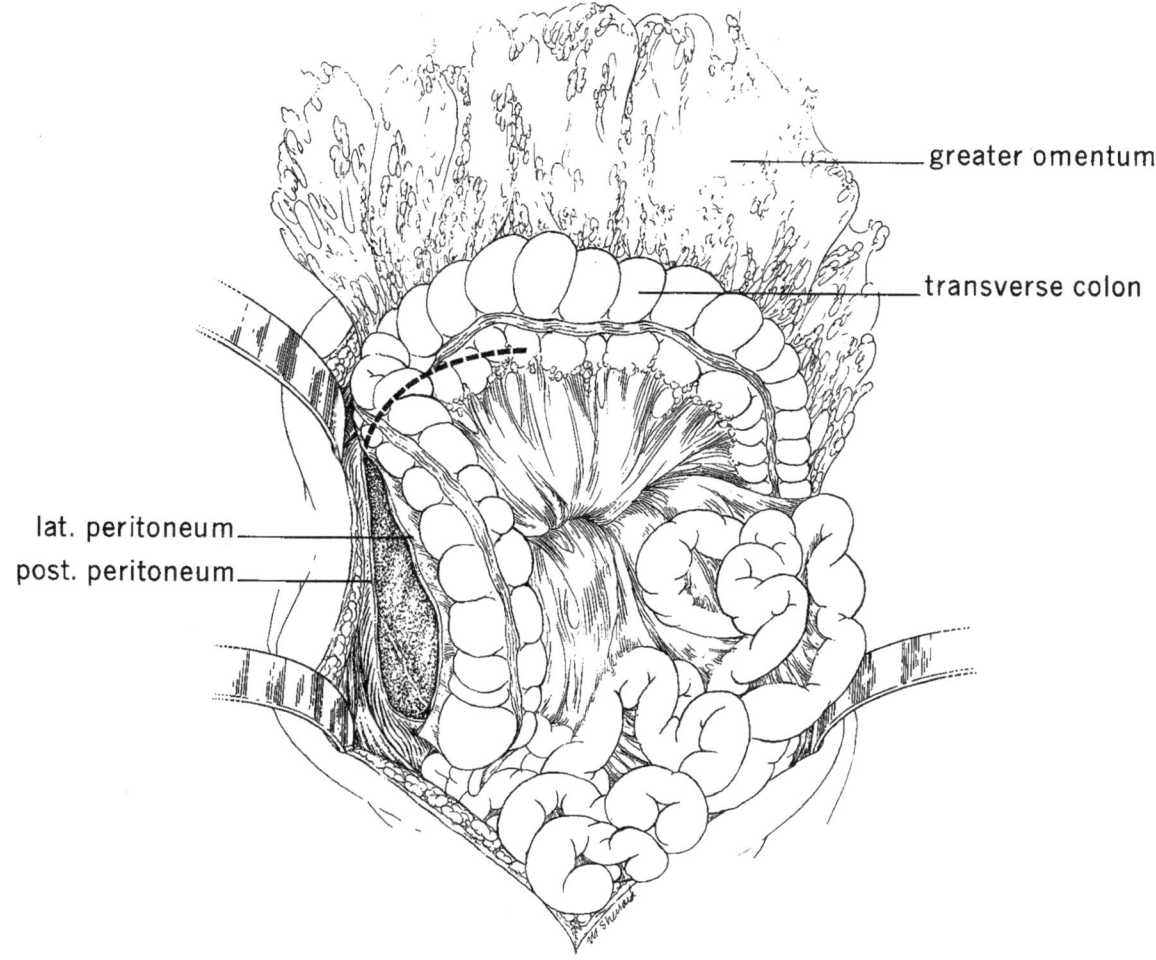

greater omentum

transverse colon

lat. peritoneum

post. peritoneum

Figure 3. An incision has been made along the lateral peritoneal reflection and the right colon mobilized. The incision will be extended along the dotted line to fully mobilize the hepatic flexure of colon.

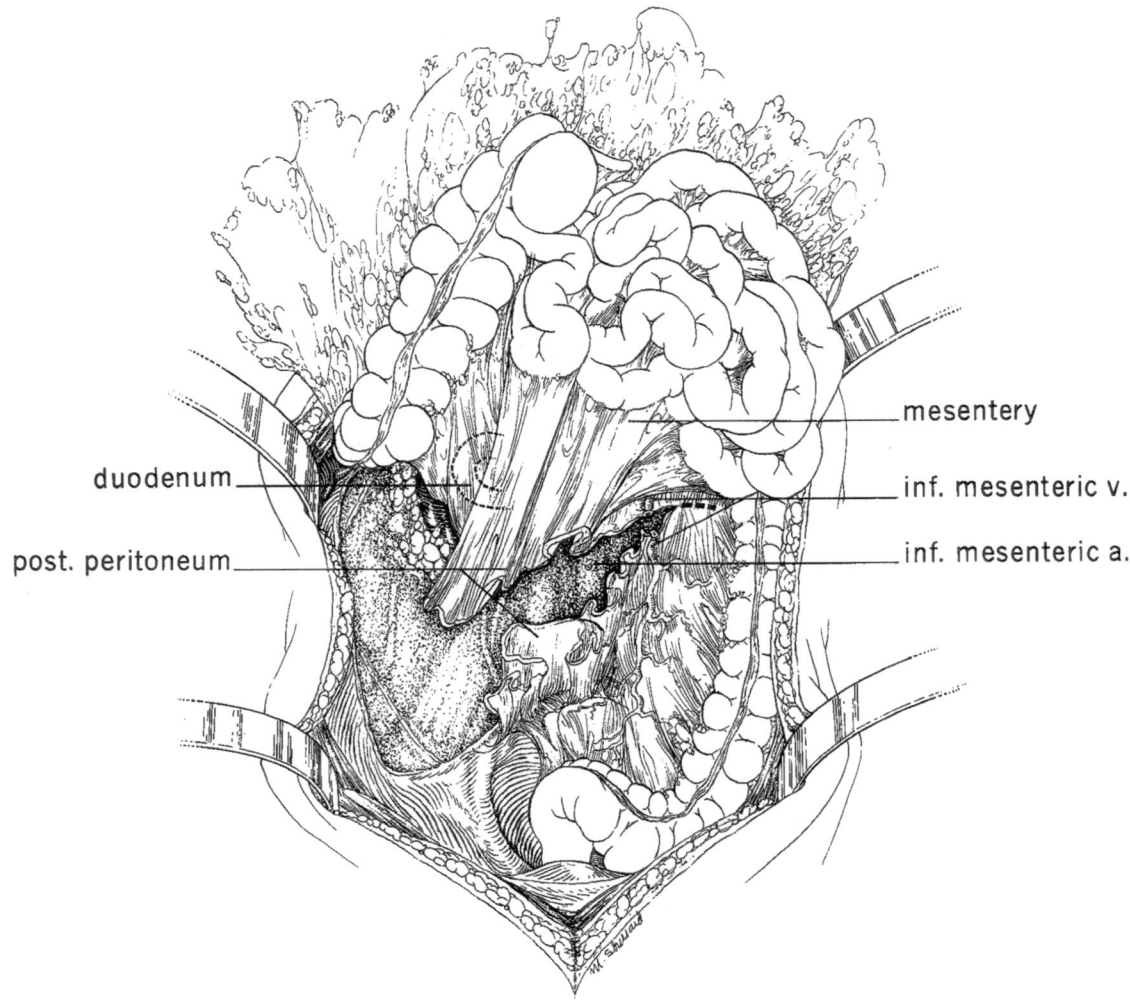

Figure 4. The posterior peritoneum has been incised from the cecum to above the ligament of Treitz. The inferior mesenteric vein and artery have been divided and the incision will be further extended into the left colon mesentery (dotted line). The duodenum (dotted line) on right will be mobilized.

Gentle forceps traction on this tissue allows one to identify lymphatic and splanchnic attachments which are clipped and divided. Small arterial branches to the adrenal vein coming from the renal artery are clipped and divided. The large right adrenal vein is usually preserved unless adrenalectomy is carried out. If extensive nodal tissue is present in this area, the adrenal vein is divided between the clips. A plane of dissection is developed under the adventitia surrounding the renal vein, and a vein retractor is helpful in visualizing the renal artery and deeper areas. This portion of the dissection is completed when all nodal and fatty tissue lateral to the midline and superior to the renal vessels has been removed.

The left suprahilar dissection is then carried out,

again with the aid of superomedial retraction of the tail of the pancreas and small bowel using a broad Willauer retractor. The plane of dissection is developed over the left renal vein and along the anteromedial surface of the aorta. The overlying anterior portion of Gerota's fascia and perirenal fat are resected. Again, the left inferior adrenal vein is clipped and divided at the renal vein and small arterial branches to the adrenal are sacrificed as the dissection is carried up along the medial aspect of the adrenal (Figure 7a).

After completion of the suprahilar dissection on both sides, the inferior dissection is carried out. This is begun by incising the adventitial tissue over both the vena cava and aorta using right-angle clamps and scissors. These incisions are extended

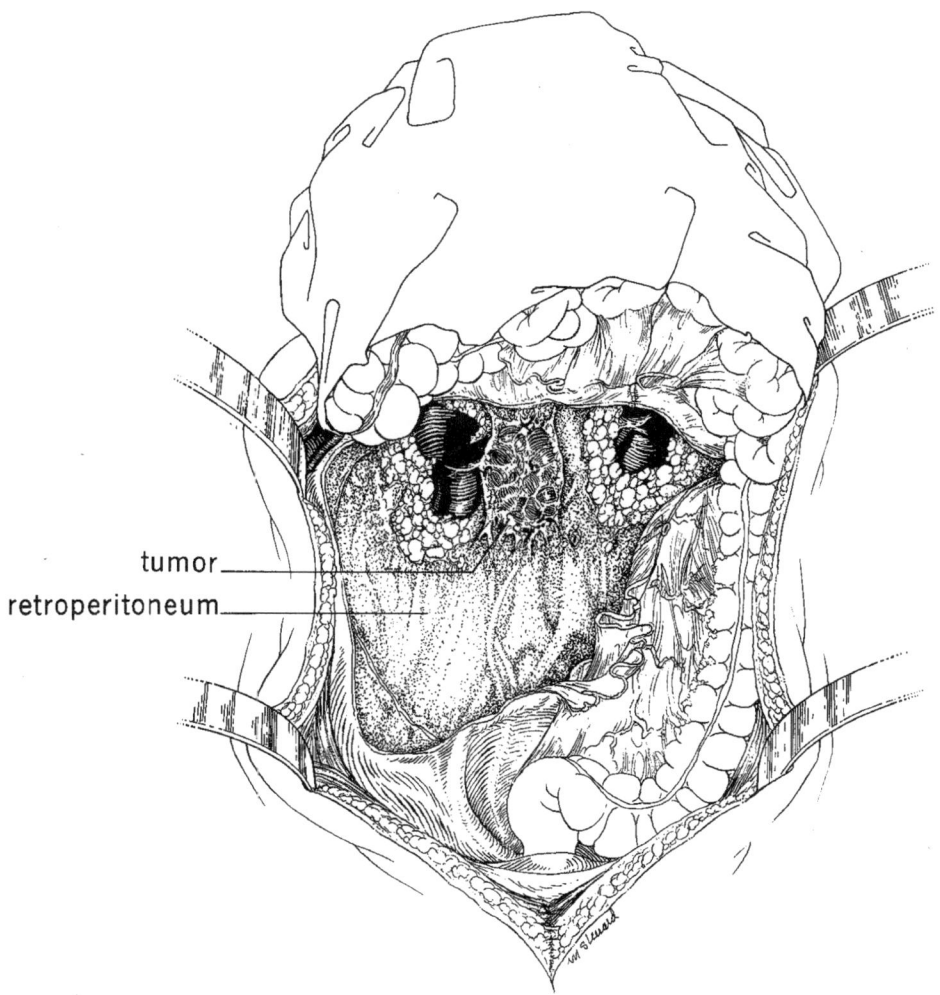

Figure 5. The colon and small bowel have been removed from the abdomen to expose the retroperitoneal region. A large group of involved lymph nodes is evident overlying the vena cava just medial to the right kidney.

superiorly to join the previously exposed and cleanly dissected renal vessels. All Gerota's fascia and fat are removed from around the ipsilateral kidney. Both testicular arteries are tied and divided at their origin from the aorta, along with the right testicular vein at its point of entrance into the vena cava (Figure 7b). The left testicular vein is divided at its junction with the left renal vein. These are preferably tied with 2-0 silk ties rather than clips. The tissue below and surrounding the renal vessels to the hilum of each kidney is dissected cleanly to the renal pelvis and ureter and reflected inferiorly. Posteriorly all tissue overlying the psoas fascia is removed. Later in the operation the ipsilateral testicular vein and artery will be traced to the internal inguinal ring and completely removed on

that side. The nodal and fatty tissue overlying the aorta and vena cava are bluntly reflected laterally. To accomplish complete removal of lymph nodes lying between and under the vena cava and aorta it is necessary to tie and divide the lumbar arteries and veins below the level of the renal arteries (Figure 8). After division of these lumbar vessels the underlying nodes can usually be swept below each great vessel to join the already laterally reflected anterior nodal tissue. There have been no reported instances of spinal cord ischemia resulting from division of the lumbar vessels below the renal arteries during the course of lymphadenectomy for testicular tumor. The dissection is terminated just below the bifurcation of the aorta on the contralateral side. The testicular vessels on the ipsilateral side are

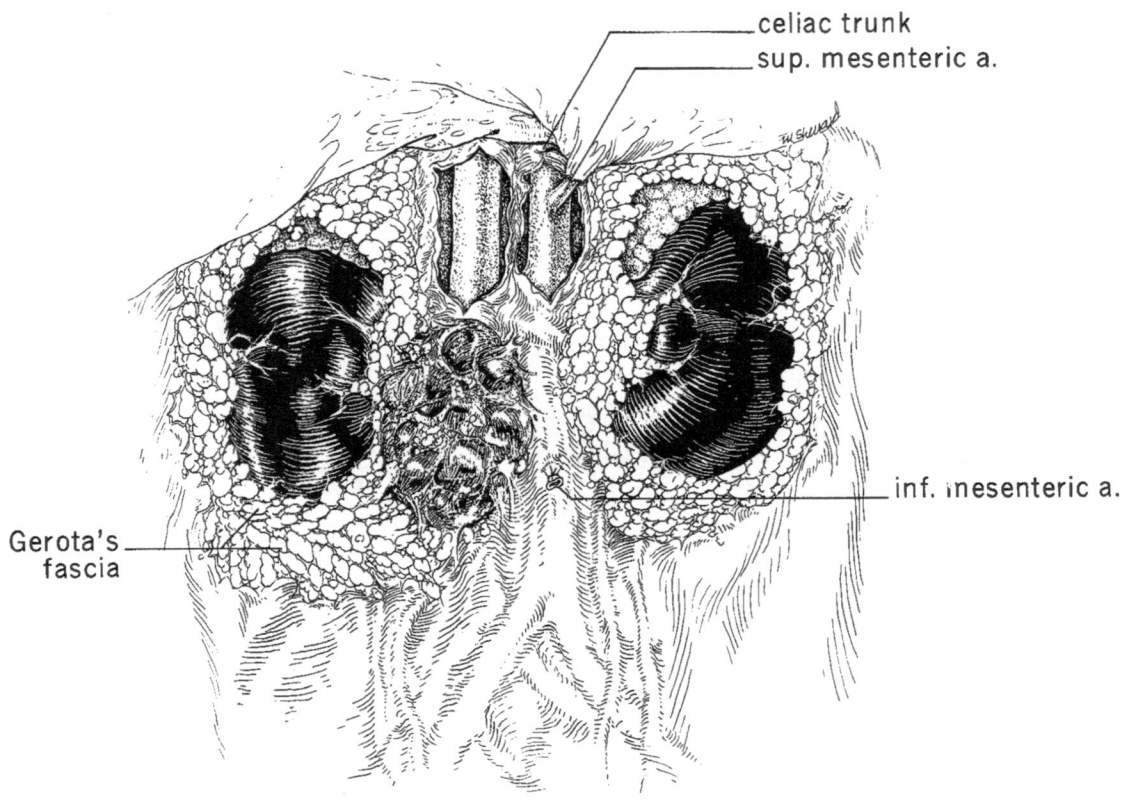

Figure 6. The suprahilar dissection extends from above the celiac vessels to the level of the renal vessels. The dissection is begun along the great vessels.

followed to the stump of the previously ligated spermatic cord which is identified by encountering the heavy silk ligature previously used. If the distal end of the spermatic cord cannot be mobilized easily, the surgeon should not hesitate to reopen the inguinal incision to free up the cord. On the left side, it is necessary to create a tunnel under the left colon mesentery to adequately remove the spermatic cord.

At the completion of lymphadenectomy (Figure 8) the psoas muscles and anterior longitudinal ligament are clearly evident.

The small bowel and colon are replaced in the abdomen and a running 0 chromic suture is used to reapproximate the posterior peritoneum. The abdominal incision is closed using through-and-through No. 26 wire or prolene single layer sutures including peritoneum, muscle, and fascia but excluding the skin.

The patient's urinary output during the procedure is monitored closely and if the level is less than 40 cc an hour, an intravenous injection of 40 mg Lasix is given.

Current treatment recommendations based on cell type and stage of testis tumors are presented in Tables 7-9.

Table 7. Summary of treatment of testicular tumors.

Seminoma

Stage 1	Radical inguinal orchiectomy, radiation therapy to the inguinal, iliac, and para-aortic lymph nodes to diaphragm.
Stage 2	Radical inguinal orchiectomy, radiation therapy to the abdominal, mediastinal, and supraclavicular lymph nodes.
Stage 3	Radical inguinal orchiectomy, radiation therapy to the abdominal, mediastinal, and supraclavicular lymph nodes, chemotherapy.
Stage 4	Radical inguinal orchiectomy, radiation therapy to the abdominal, mediastinal, and supraclavicular lymph nodes, chemotherapy.

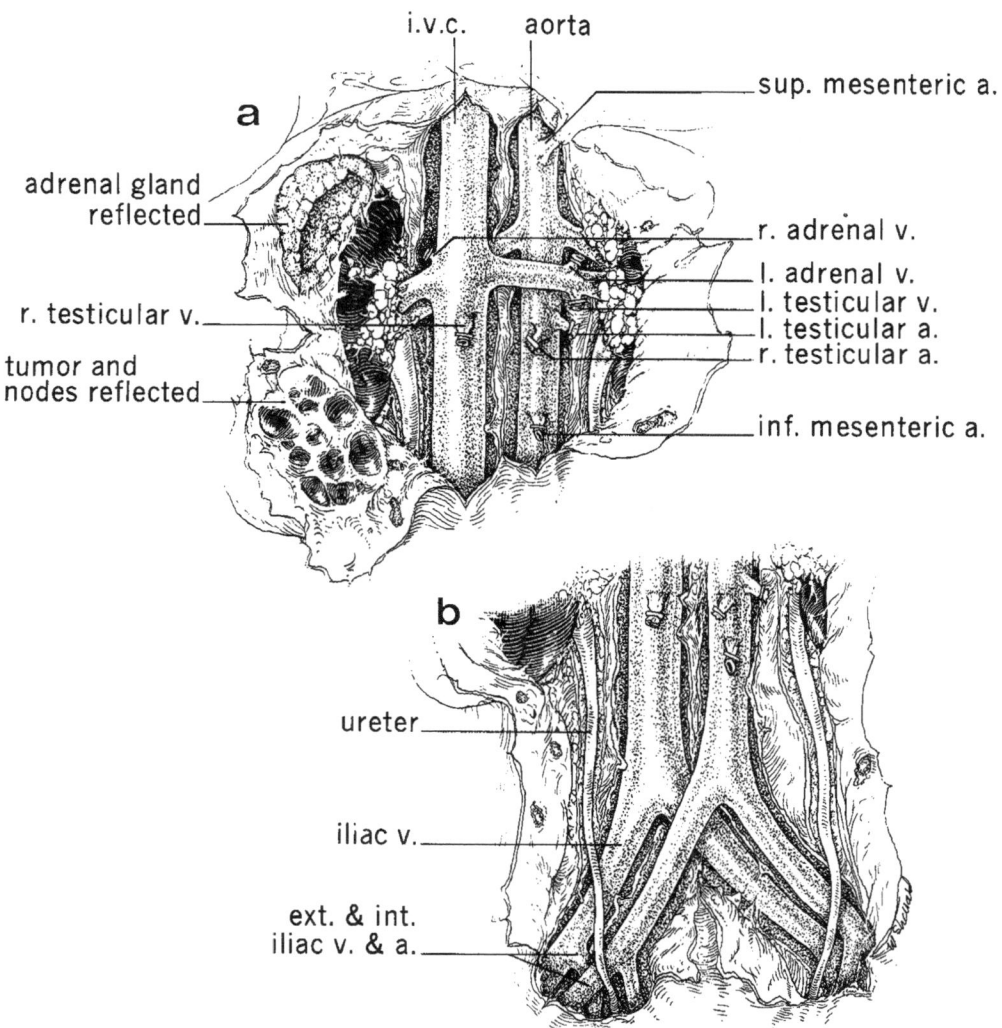

Figure 7. a. The suprahilar dissection on both sides has been completed and the lymph nodes overlying the vena cava and adrenal gland have been reflected laterally. b.The testicular arteries and veins have been divided. The anterior adventitia and nodal tissue overlying the aorta and vena cava have been incised and reflected laterally.

Table 8. Summary of treatment of testicular tumors.

Nonseminomatous germ cell tumors

Stage 1	Radical inguinal orchiectomy, retroperitoneal lymphadenectomy. Lymph nodes positive – further chemotherapy. Lymph nodes negative – close followup.
Stage 2	Radical inguinal orchiectomy, retroperitoneal lymphadenectomy, chemotherapy. In bulky Stage 2 tumors chemotherapy or radiotherapy is used preoperatively.
Stage 3	Radical inguinal orchiectomy, chemotherapy followed by retroperitoneal lymphadenectomy. Evidence of residual tumor – continued chemotherapy. No evidence of residual tumor – close followup.
Stage 4	Radical inguinal orchiectomy, chemotherapy followed by retroperitoneal lymphadenectomy. Evidence of residual tumor – continued chemotherapy. No evidence of residual tumor – close followup.

Table 9. Summary of treatment of testicular tumors.

Nongerm cell and other testis tumors

Leydig cell tumors – radical inguinal orchiectomy and retroperitoneal lymph node dissection.

Sertoli cell tumors – radical inguinal orchiectomy.

Yolk sac tumors – radical inguinal orchiectomy and retroperitoneal lymphadenectomy.

Sarcomas of the testis and adjacent structures – radical inguinal orchiectomy, retroperitoneal lymphadenectomy, adjuvant chemotherapy.

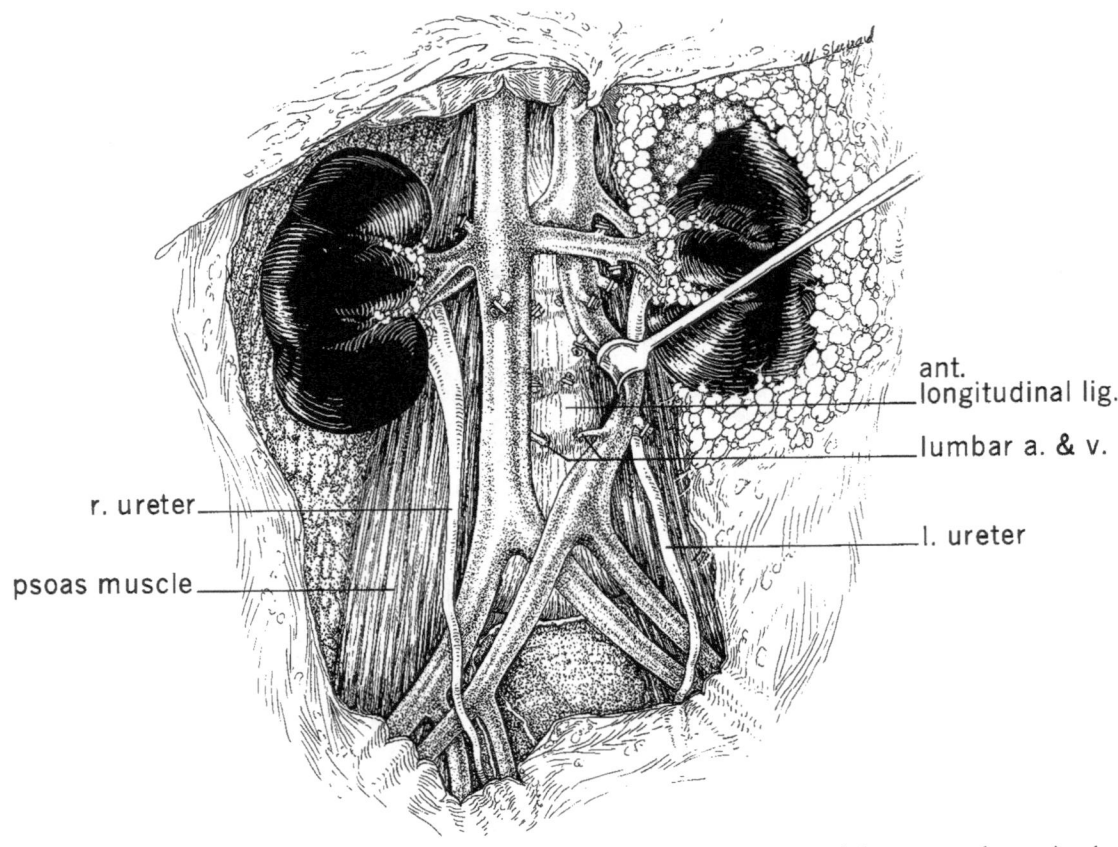

Figure 8. Completed lymph node dissection. All nodal tissue has been removed from behind the great vessels exposing the anterior longitudinal ligaments and psoas muscle.

Retroperitoneal lymph node dissection has played an important role in improving our understanding of testis cancer behavior and improving the patient survival rate during the past 20 years. As we gain more information about the diagnostic accuracy of serum tumor markers, the need for diagnostic lymphadenectomy may decrease. Similarly, improved chemotherapeutic drugs for testis cancer may diminish the therapeutic usefulness of this surgical procedure.

REFERENCES

Dixon FJ and Moore RA: Tumors of the male sex organs. Atlas of Tumor Pathology, Washington, DC. Armed Forces Institute of Pathology, 1952, vol 8, fasc 31b and 32.

Donohue JP: Retroperitoneal lymphadenectomy. Urol Clin N America 4: 509, 1977.

Hopkins TB, Jaffe N, Colodny A, Cassady JR and Filler RM: The management of testicular tumors in children. J Urol 120: 96, 1978.

Javadpour N: National Cancer Institute experience with testicular cancer, J Urol 120: 651, 1978.

Javadpour N and Bergman SM: Recent advances in testicular cancer. Curr Prob Surg 15: 1, 1978.

Kaswick JA, Bloomberg SD and Skinner DG: Radical retroperitoneal lymph node dissection: How effective in removal of all retroperitoneal nodes? J Urol 115: 70, 1976.

Lange PH and Fraley EE: Serum alpha-fetoprotein and human chorionic gonadotropin in the treatment of patients with testicular tumors. Urol Clin N America 4: 393, 1977.

Markland CA: Special problems in managing patients with testicular cancer. Urol Clin N America 4: 427, 1977.

Patton JF, Hewitt CB and Mallis N: Diagnosis and treatment of tumors of the testis. JAMA 117: 2194, 1959.

Sabio H, Burgert EO, Farrow GM and Kelalis PP: Embryonal carcinoma of the testis in childhood. Cancer 34: 2118, 1974.

Staubitz WJ, Early KS, Magoss IV and Murphy GP: Surgical management of testis tumor. J Urol 111: 205, 1974.

Stephen RA: The clinical presentation of testicular tumors. Brit J Urol 34: 448, 1962.

Tavel FR, Osius TG, Parker JW, Goodfriend RB, McGonigle DJ, Jassie MP, Simmons EL, Tobenkin MI, and Schulte JW: Retroperitoneal lymph node dissection. J Urol 89: 241, 1963.

Walsh PC, Kauffman JJ, Coulson WF and Goodwin WE: Retroperitoneal lymphadenectomy for testicular tumors. JAMA 217: 309, 1971.

Young JD: Retroperitoneal surgery. In: Urologic Surgery ed. 2, Glenn JF and Boyce WH (eds), New York, Harper and Row, 1975, p 848.

20. TOTAL PROSTATECTOMY FOR CARCINOMA OF THE PROSTATE

J.G. GREGORY

Carcinoma of the prostate is the second most common malignancy occurring in males and, in the United States, is responsible for over 23,000 cases per year (Silverberg and Holleb 1975). Despite this prevalence, therapy for all stages of carcinoma of the prostate is the subject of present controversy produced by factors inherent in the pathophysiology of the disease process. These factors include (1) the individual biologic variability of tumor course, (2) the difficulty of accurate clinical staging, (3) the inevitable variance between clinical and pathologic staging, (4) inaccurate disease survivor statistics in an age group prone to death by other causes and (5) the lack of easily compared therapeutic groups. In the face of these multiple variables, it is understandable that a definitive therapeutic plan should be the subject of debate.

Despite many areas of controversy and confusion, there is sufficient evidence available at present to strongly justify consideration of ablative surgery as definitive therapy in the early stages of carcinoma of the prostate. A comparison of two groups of patients, both thought by clinical staging techniques to have Stage B tumor (tumor confined to the prostate), shows (Figure 1) the group receiving total prostatectomy to have a far greater survival (Jewett 1975) than the group not treated for cure (Hanash et al. 1972). Likewise, Table 1 lists the survival rates of several large reported series and compares the results of surgery to those obtained by alternative therapeutic modalities. In reviewing these figures, it is important to remember the potential advantage that any surgical series has in being able to exclude with certainty cases that may have been clinically understaged, a figure which may be as high as 32 percent (Boxer et al. 1977). Such selection is avoided in Table 1 by comparing only patients grouped according to clinical stage. It

should also be noted that the number of patients receiving multiple therapies, either concurrently or sequentially, is not often clearly detailed in some of the studies listed. The 15-year survival figures in most groups are too small for a reasonable comparison and are nonexistent as regards ^{131}I instillation. In light of these considerations it is difficult to prove conclusively the superiority of the surgical approach. As is so often the case, the physician must call upon his skill in the art of medicine to determine the most advantageous therapy for a particular patient, bringing into consideration knowledge of the natural history of the disease, the patient's temperament and outlook on life, his longevity, the capabilities of the particular hospital and the extent of the surgeon's own skill in oncologic surgery.

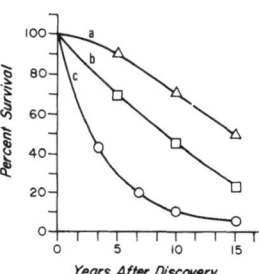

Figure 1. Survival of patients with clinical Stage B carcinoma of the prostate. a. Expected survival, general population. b. Survival of 182 patients with clinical Stage B carcinoma following ablative surgery (Jewett, 1975). c. Survival of 195 patients treated only with transurethral resection for relief of symptoms (Hanash et al. 1972).

I. PATIENT EVALUATION

A. Candidates for Surgery

We propose total prostatectomy done in conjunction with retropubic lymph node dissection in all patients with clinical Stage B disease who are under 75 years of age and who appear to have a life expectancy of six years, a figure roughly estimated by observation of the patient's general physical condition. In addition, recommendation for such surgery is also made to some patients with Stage A disease, which is defined as a clinically undetected tumor diagnosed histologically on tissue removed during either transurethral or open resection of the prostate. Such Stage A carcinomas are found in approximately 10 percent of prostates removed for benign disease (Bauer et al. 1960). Patients having a small focus of low grade tumor (one to two TUR chips) are carefully followed, but not subjected to total prostatectomy at this time. Patients having multiple chips filled with tumor, multiple foci of tumor, or high grade undifferentiated tumors are considered for total prostatic removal. In any attempt to assess the amount of tumor-involved prostate, it is essential that the hospital pathologist section and view the entire prostatic specimen. If such is not routinely done, on receiving a report indicating the presence of such an incidental carcinoma it is necessary to request such sections before a therapeutic decision can be made. In addition, it is felt by some that the palliative benefits of radical prostatectomy justify its use in patients with surgically incurable disease (Tomlinson et al. 1977).

B. Detection of Tumor

Because potentially curable carcinoma of the prostate is associated with no symptom complex, only on digital rectal examination can an early diagnosis of this disease be made. Males 45 years of age or older should be encouraged to have such examinations yearly, and preferably every six months. Recently developed methods for the measurement of prostatic acid phosphatase by radioimmunoassay (Foti et al. 1977) and counterimmunoelectrophoresis (Chu et al. 1978) offer the hope that early stages of prostatic carcinoma can be detected by such a screening test. Confirmation and extension of these early reports is now awaited. Following such a screening examination, all patients with prostatic nodules should be referred for urologic evaluation.

1. Patient Examination. The initial careful examination of such a patient must serve to rule out other urologic and nonurologic conditions which may influence any therapeutic approach. Time should be taken to gain patient rapport and confidence, especially if major ablative surgery is anticipated. Careful rectal examination is most important. It is not sufficient merely to feel the prostatic nodule. It is also important to assess the consistency of the lesion, the extent of glandular involvement, possible fixation of the gland, and possible involvement of the seminal vesicles. The smaller and more discrete the lesion, the better the prognosis (Jewett 1975), the less likely that spread has occurred and the greater the possibility that total prostatectomy will be recommended.

2. Prostatic Biopsy. Most prostatic nodules require biopsy. If on the basis of the office examination the rectal lesion is thought to represent an advanced lesion (Stage C or greater), the time of biopsy is not critical. If a B lesion is suspected, it is preferable to

Table 1. Survival rates of patients receiving various modes of therapy for carcinoma of the prostate.

Type of therapy	No. of patients	Clinical stage	Percent surviving 5 yr	10 yr	15 yr	Reference
Total prostatectomy with estrogen	329	A & B	79	52	—	Boxer et al. 1977
Total prostatectomy	182	B	70	50	33	Jewett 1975
Total prostatectomy	74	B	—	72	54	Culp & Meyer 1973
Total prostatectomy	148	B	—	50	—	Vickery & Kerr 1973
Total prostatectomy	132	B	76	61	39	Schroeder & Belt 1975
Estrogens			33	22	—	Emmett et al. 1960
External radiotherapy	193	B	75	47	—	Bagshaw 1978
^{128}I	100	B	79*	—	—	Whitmore 1976
^{148}Au and external radiotherapy	51	B	75	—	—	Carlton 1978

⁻ Actuarial prediction.

perform the biopsy and follow with total prostatectomy, usually within five days. Following prostatic biopsy, especially one done transrectally, a local reaction may occur which can cause the surgeon great difficulty in separating the prostate from the rectum, and can lead to rectal injury. In the same fashion, total prostatectomy is made more difficult by previous transurethral resection. In those cases of latent or unsuspected carcinoma requiring secondary ablative surgery, the second procedure should be done as soon as possible following the first prostatic resection, before the edema and fluid extravasation normally associated with transurethral resection results in an inflammatory reaction and possible fibrotic fixation. If radical surgery is not possible within a five-day period, it is thought preferable to delay surgery six weeks (Nichols et al. 1977).

C. Preoperative Evaluation and Preparation of the Candidate for Total Prostatectomy

The patient suspected of having an operatively curable carcinoma of the prostate is admitted to the hospital and there has performed, following routine admission studies, a cystoscopy and needle biopsy of his prostate. If the biopsy is negative for carcinoma, a repeat biopsy is obtained, and if still negative the patient is discharged and rebiopsied in three months. If the initial prostatic biopsy is positive, liver function studies, coagulogram, serum acid phosphatase, an IVP, a bone scan, and a urine culture with sensitivity are performed, followed by a lymphangiogram.

1. Lymphangiography. Lymphangiography is performed on most patients and definitely on patients with tumor thought to be present in more than one-half the gland, a figure based on an estimate made by rectal palpation. Because of the following facts we do not obtain lymphangiography on every patient suspected of having early disease: (1) Lymphangiographic accuracy is directly proportional to the familiarity of the radiologic staff with this procedure, and at best can be considered indicative. (2) Clinical Stage B disease is associated with nodal metastases in only 10 percent of cases (Glenn 1978). (3) Lymphangiograms can only detect metastatic lesions 5 mm or larger (Kohler

1976).

It is to be expected that in early carcinoma of the prostate lymphangiography will usually be negative. This study can be a helpful aid in detecting the possibility of metastatic spread in a more extensive clinical Stage B lesion. At the time of definitive surgery, early biopsy and frozen sections are obtained from any area appearing suspicious on lymphangiogram. In centers skilled in the technique of percutaneous lymph node aspiration (Perieras et al. 1978) such a followup to lymphangiography yields good predictive results.

2. Informed Consent. With the workup complete the physician must decide his course of action and present this to the patient. The physician should clearly tell the patient his preferred form of treatment, but should also outline alternative courses of therapy; endocrine manipulation, external radiation, or interstitial radiation. The particulars of this discussion should be detailed in the patient chart as documentation of informed consent to be used if total prostatectomy is the chosen course of therapy. In addition, it is important to discuss with the patient who has elected total prostatectomy, and to document in the chart that the following points were considered: (1) the possibility that the procedure will be abandoned if lymphatic involvement is found, (2) the 95 percent incidence of postoperative impotency, (3) the possibility of either partial or total urinary incontinence (10-30 percent), (4) the possibility of rectal injury necessitating temporary colostomy, (5) the possibility that the patient may develop osteitis pubis, and (6) the probable necessity of blood transfusion.

3. Immediate Preoperative Preparation. The patient is placed on clear liquids for 24 hours and undergoes a mechanical and antibacterial bowel preparation. He is typed and cross matched for five units of whole blood. Patients with positive urine cultures are treated with appropriate antibiotics prior to, during and following surgery. Patients with sterile urine are begun on a cephalosporin intraoperatively. The patient showers with a povidone-iodine soap preparation the night before and the morning of surgery. Adequate preoperative sedation is ordered and the patient prepared for general anesthesia.

II. SURGICAL PROCEDURE

A. Patient Positioning

The patient is placed supine on the operating table with his legs wrapped, separated and flexed at the knee over knee crutches (Figure 2). A sterile scrub is carried out from the costal margin to the mid-thigh, including the perineum. A sterile O'Connor sheath is placed in the rectum and the abdomen draped, allowing access to the midline and perineum. A No. 20 French 30 cc balloon catheter is placed in the bladder. The bladder is filled with 200 cc of a 20 percent povidone-iodine solution, drained, filled again and the catheter is clamped and kept sterile and available in the operative field.

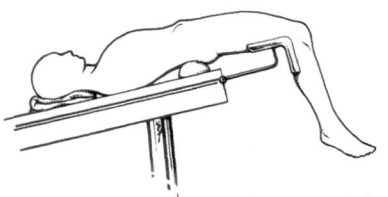

Figure 2. Patient position.

B. Surgical Approach

A midline incision (Figure 3) is made from the symphysis circumventing the umbilicus and ascending above the umbilicus for about 6 cm. The linea alba is incised, the rectus muscles divided in the midline, and the distal extension of the muscles detached from the symphysis bilaterally using an electrocautery. The retropubic, the suprapubic, the lateral and the retroperitoneal spaces are developed by careful blunt dissection. The inferior epigastric vessels are encountered and preserved if possible, or suture ligated and divided. Adequate retraction is essential and is best obtained by a large ring retractor with deep wide spatulated blades. Any areas that appeared suspicious on lymphangiography are now biopsied and sent for frozen section.

C. Bilateral Retroperitoneal Lymph Node Dissection

Beginning on the side ipsilateral to the positive prostatic biopsy, the bladder is retracted medially, and the peritoneal contents cranially. This retraction is facilitated by dividing and dissecting the vas

deferens near the internal ring, sharply separating the peritoneum from the spermatic vessels at this point, and then further bluntly removing the peritoneum from the iliac vessels and the psoas muscle as far cranially as possible. The ureter will be seen to be adherent to the posterior surface of the peritoneum and should be carefully retracted medially. Complete dissection of the fatty and lymphatic tissue from around the lateral pelvic vessels is then accomplished. An incision is made in the perivascular tissue over the common iliac artery, starting slightly proximal to the branching of the hypogastric artery (Figure 4a). This incision is continued to just beneath the inguinal ligament, where the circumflex iliac and inferior epigastric vessels are there dissected free. The external iliac vein lies directly inferior and slightly medial to the external iliac artery and a small amount of blunt dissection frees both artery and vein. Superior and medial retraction of these vessels allows blunt sweeping of the perivascular tissue beneath the vessels (Figure 4b). Small vascular branches encountered are divided between hemoclips. Progress is soon limited by a condensation of this fibrofatty tissue in the femoral canal. This tissue is divided between ligatures at the femoral ring and further dissection, mostly blunt, is then possible beneath

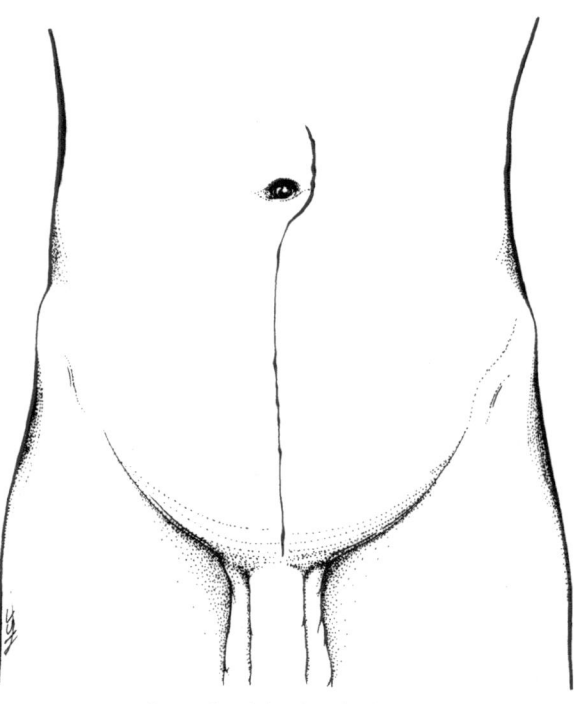

Figure 3. Abdominal incision.

the iliac vessels. The hypogastric vessels are cleared of perivascular tissue for 1 cm. The limits of dissection are now marked (Figure 4c): laterally, the genitofemoral nerve, lying on the psoas muscle; cranially the common iliac artery; and medially the hypogastric artery and the obturator nerve.

The tissue lying beyond these limits is divided and ligated. Blunt dissection continues toward the obturator fossa, where final separation of the specimen is made by digitally teasing the fatty tissue from around the obturator nerve. All tissue is carefully removed from the obturator fossa, if necessary sacrificing the obturator artery and vein. The obturator area deserves special attention, insofar as this is thought to be the first and most frequent site to which carcinoma of the prostate metastasizes, followed sequentially by the external iliac, hypogastric and common iliac lymph drainage systems (Whitmore 1976). Representative lymph nodes from these areas are sent for frozen section and the remaining tissue is anatomically arranged, labeled and sent for pathologic evaluation and paraffin sectioning. The wound is irrigated and packed, and a similar dissection performed on the opposite side. If the frozen sections reveal tumor, the prostatectomy is not carried out and wound closure with Hemovac drainage is immediately accomplished. The decision to abandon prostatectomy if lymph node invasion is found is an area of debate. It is felt by some that a lymph node dissection as described is therapeutic and in fact there are cases of patients with Stage D disease doing well following removal of a small volume of lymph node metastases (Barzell et al. 1977). Despite these instances, our course of action is based on the belief that lymph node dissection is purely diagnostic. We feel that metastatic disease found on frozen section most likely does not represent minimal metastatic disease. We also feel that the consequences and potential complications of total prostatectomy are not warranted if a good chance of cure cannot be afforded the patient.

D. Total Retropubic Prostatectomy

If frozen sections are negative total prostatectomy is carried out. Total retropubic prostatectomy can be approached either by dissecting distally from the bladder neck or cranially from that area of urethra just proximal to the membranous urethra. We prefer the latter method because that sequence allows careful severance of the distal urethra early in the procedure under direct vision in a relatively bloodfree field.

1. Initial Dissection. The ring retractor is adjusted to allow access to the retropubic area. If distended, the bladder is allowed to empty through the catheter and is retracted cranially with a well padded spatula retractor or bladder blade. The retropubic space is further enlarged by blunt dissection. Bleeding from superficial veins on the surface of the bladder and prostate is controlled by fulguration. The endopelvic fascia is excised at the point of reflection onto the prostate and the space lateral to the prostate bluntly developed. The puboprostatic ligaments, condensations of the endopelvic fascia lying between the symphysis and the anterior surface of the prostate, are suture ligated and severed (Figure 5). On occasion space does not permit accurate suturing of these structures and they must be blindly cut. Usually the dorsal penile vein can be identified lying between these ligaments on the surface of the distal prostate. It should be suture ligated.

Good exposure beneath the symphysis is essential for accurate vesico-urethral anastomosis following removal of the prostate. If it appears that the exposure is not adequate, the symphysis can be removed at this point (Figure 6).

2. Symphysectomy. Symphysectomy is accomplished by extending the skin incision to the base of the penis. Two large angulated clamps are passed around the symphysis on either side of it. Flexible Gigli blades are drawn into position and a wedge of pubic bone about 5 cm wide is removed. Following this maneuver, the apex of the prostate and the membranous urethra are well visualized. The removed bone is discarded and no attempt is made to repair the bony defect. Despite the fact that this measure is quickly performed, and allows an easy vesico-urethral anastomosis, we seldom find symphysectomy to be necessary in the course of total prostatectomy, and we do not perform this procedure routinely because of the increased incidence of postoperative morbidity (Middleton 1977).

3. Distal Urethral Transection. With the retropubic

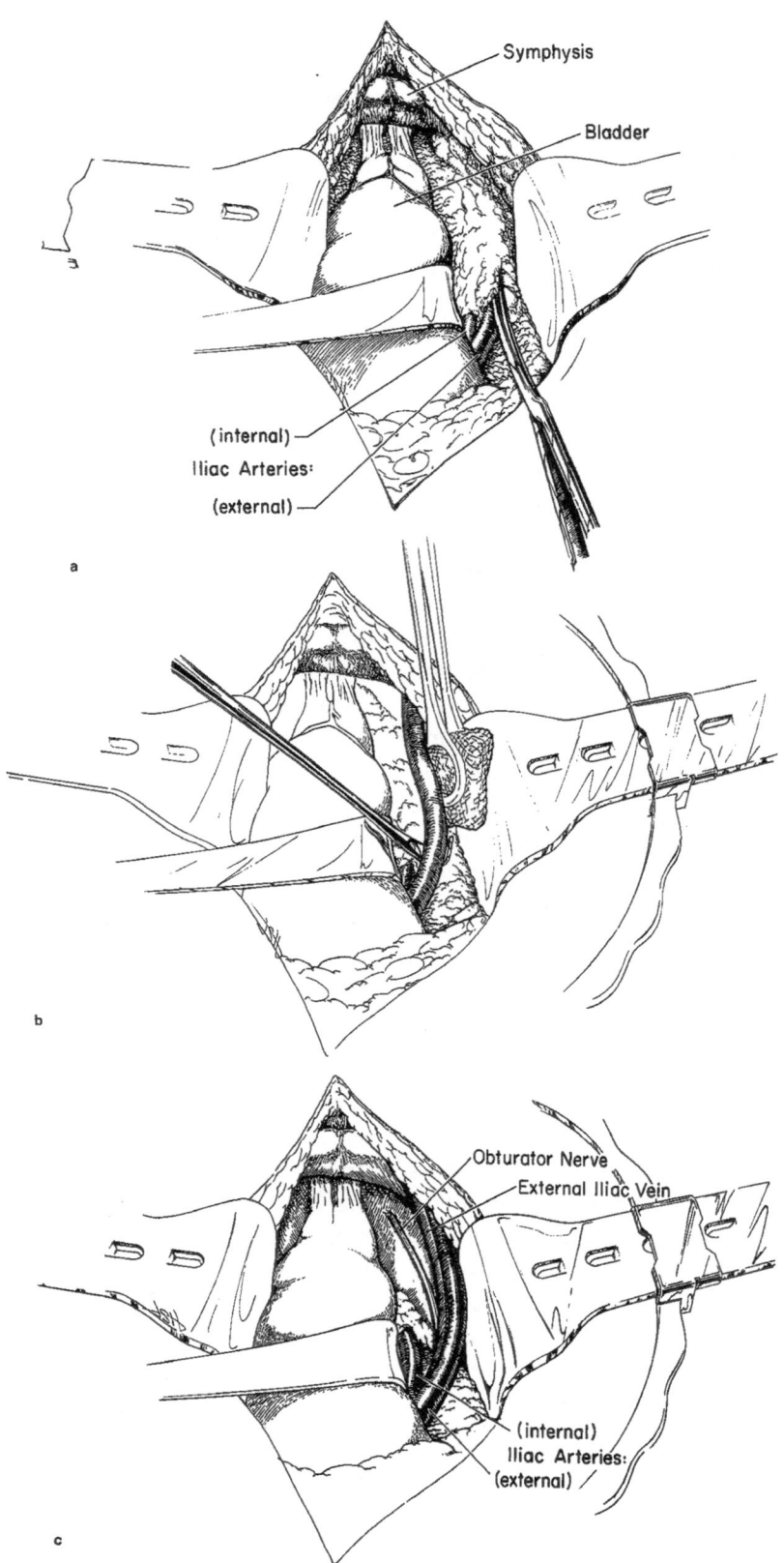

Figure 4. Retroperitoneal lymph node dissection: a. Beginning dissection on the external iliac artery. b. Fatty tissue and lymphatics being swept under the external iliac artery. c. Dissection completed on the right side.

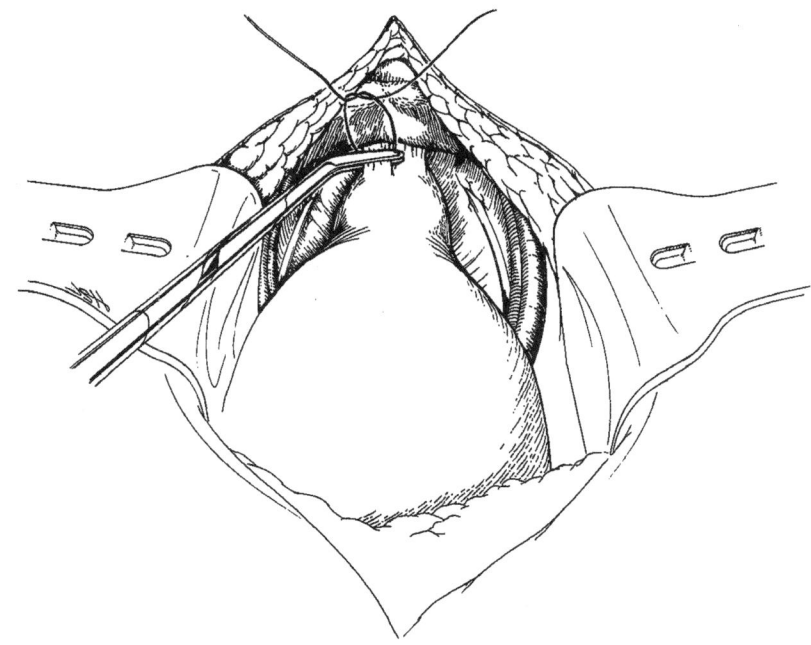

Figure 5. Ligation of puboprostatic ligaments.

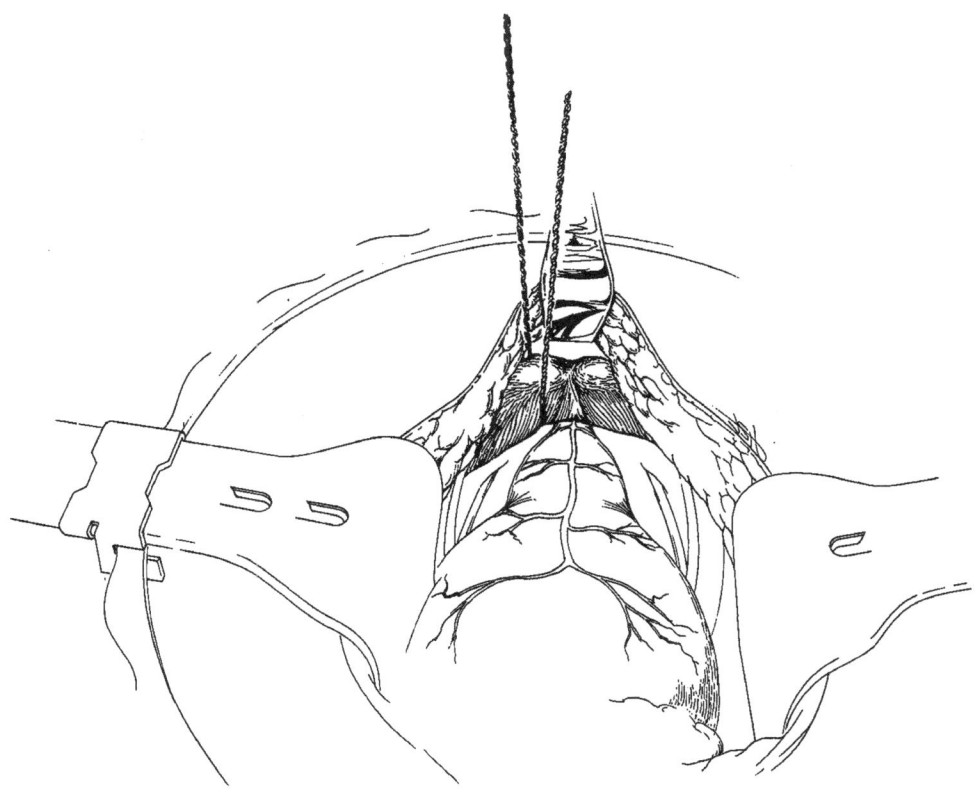

Figure 6. Symphysectomy: Gigli saw in position.

space now fully developed down to the urogenital diaphragm, a space beneath the prostatourethral junction is created by passing an index finger down the lateral surface of the prostate and then beneath the prostate between the prostate and the anterior rectal wall. It is quite helpful to have an assistant place his finger in the rectum prior to this maneuver so that the operator can assess at all times the degree of proximity he is maintaining with the rectum.

With a finger beneath the prostatourethral junction, the urethra is partially transected with a scalpel. The incision is made on the surface of the prostatic capsule 2 mm proximal to the urethra. After this cut is begun, through-and-through sutures of 2-0 chromic are placed in the distal urethral margin (Figure 7). These sutures are tagged and left loose for the time being. Later they are used to identify the urethral margin and complete the urethrovesical anastomosis. With the urethra one-half transected, the exposed Foley catheter is grasped and a loop of catheter pulled out through the urethral incision. An occlusive clamp is then placed across the Foley which is then transected distal to the clamp. The distal stump of catheter is removed from the penis and discarded. The posterior surface of the urethra is then transected (Figure 8).

4. Prostatic "Button". Some surgeons feel that leaving a "button" of prostate is dangerous because of possible apical tissue tumor involvement, the incidence of which has been reported to be as high as 75 percent (Byar et al. 1972). Despite this fact, we believe our approach is justified because (1) only a very minimal amount of prostatic capsule is left, (2) all prostatic glandular tissue is removed with the specimen, and (3) leaving this piece of capsule greatly reduces the chance of urinary incontinence. As an additional safeguard we send a section of the prostate taken from an area immediately proximal to this transsection for pathologic evaluation, and we are prepared to remove additional tissue down to the membranous urethra should tumor be found in the specimen.

5. Exposure of Posterior Portion of Prostate. Following severance of the urethra, anterior traction on the bladder catheter allows access to the posterior prostate. With an assistant's finger again in the rectum for guidance, sharp and blunt dissection allows separation of the prostate from the anterior rectal wall (Figure 9). This dissection is often described as being between the anterior and posterior leaves of Denonvilliers' fascia. Unfortunately two distinct layers are not apparent (Jewett 1976),

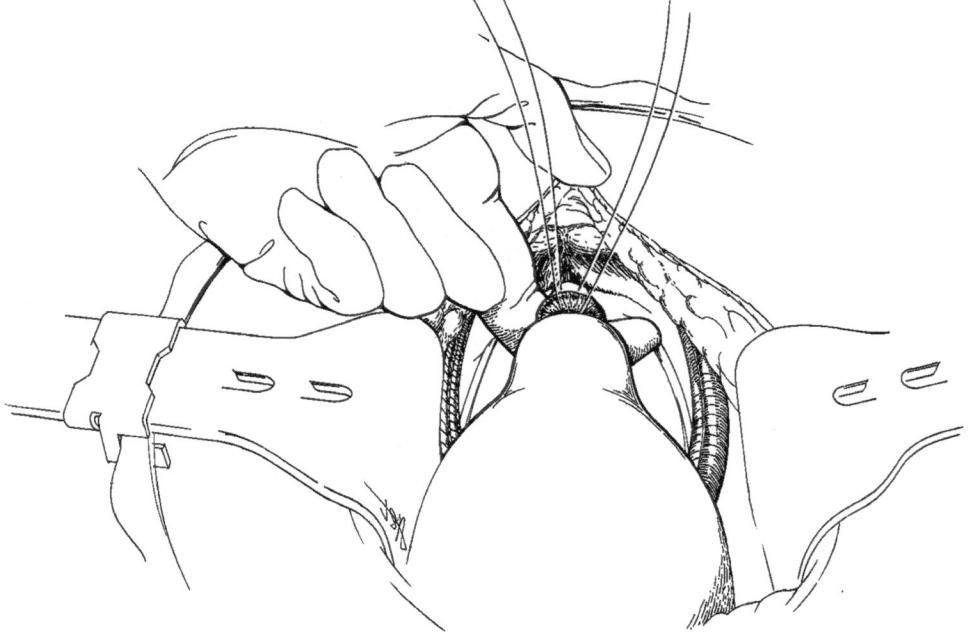

Figure 7. Transection at the prostatourethral junction: Structure half divided and stay sutures placed in the distal urethra.

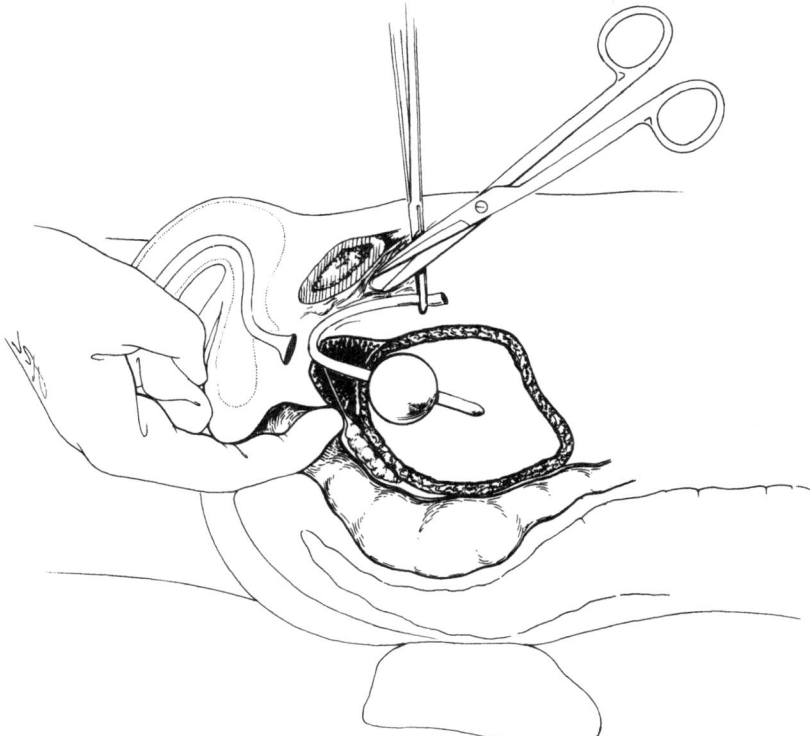

Figure 8. Transection completed at the prostatourethral junction.

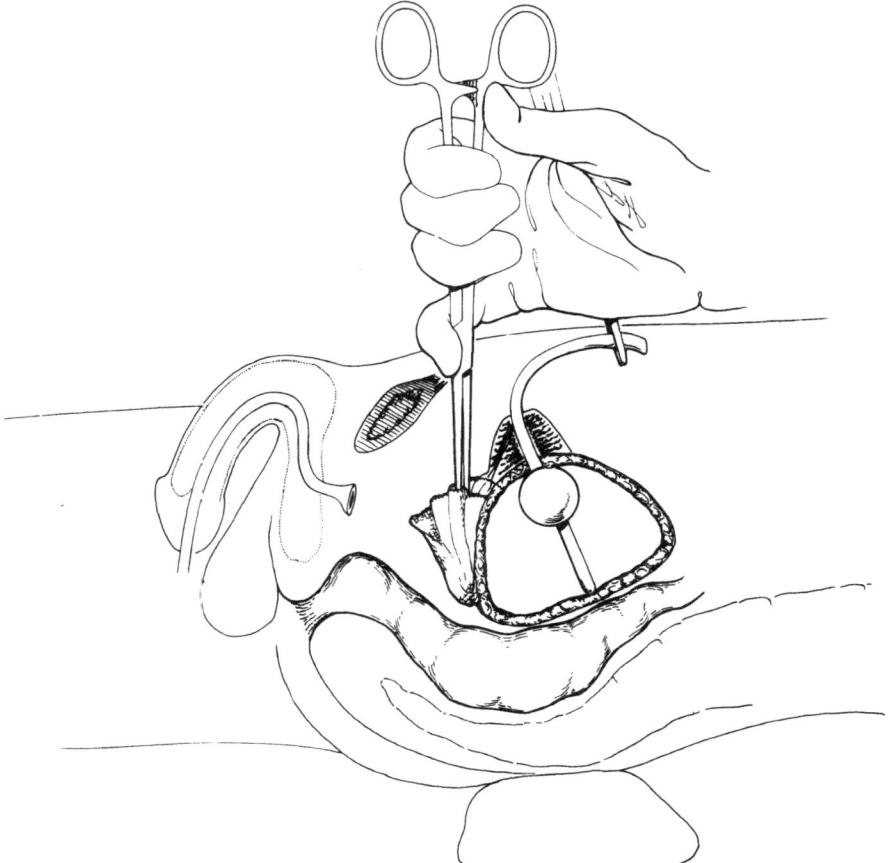

Figure 9. Separation of prostate from anterior wall of rectum.

and the dissection may in fact directly strip the serosal surface of the rectum.

If at this point troublesome bleeding occurs from the area of the urogenital diaphragm, it can be controlled by introducing a No. 20 French 30 cc balloon Foley catheter through the penis into the pelvic cavity. With the balloon inflated, traction applied to the catheter acts to tamponade the bleeding points.

Dissection behind the prostate is continued again by sharp and blunt dissection with a guiding finger still in the rectum, until both seminal vesicles are well visualized.

6. *Transection of Bladder Neck.* Attention is then directed anteriorly, and the bladder neck sharply divided down to and around the urethral catheter (Figure 10). The balloon of this catheter is then punctured and the tip of the catheter is pulled through the bladder neck opening. By grasping both ends of this catheter, which now forms a loop through the prostatic urethra, it is possible to elevate the prostate anteriorly and to complete resection of the bladder neck down to the seminal vesicles (Figure 11). The entire prostate is removed with the bladder neck left intact, if possible. If tumor extends into the prostate in the bladder neck

area, a cuff of bladder adjacent to the bladder neck is sacrificed. If the bladder neck is sacrificed, it is first necessary to open the bladder anteriorly in line with the planned incision. The interior of the bladder is visualized, the ureteral orifices identified, and catheterized if necessary. The ureters are then carefully avoided during the completion of the bladder neck transection.

Transection of the bladder neck area is continued transversely until the seminal vesicles are encountered. Extreme care is necessary, especially if a cuff of bladder is removed, to insure that the transection proceeds in a transverse plane at right angles with the urethral outlet, in order to avoid dissection into the trigone – an error that can result in excessive blood loss and possible ureteral injury. With the prostate retracted anteriorly and caudally, dissection of the seminal vesicles is completed on the anterior surface (Figure 11). The ampulla of the vas deferens is identified, ligated and divided. The lateral vascular pedicles are isolated, ligated and divided. The tips of the seminal vesicles are dissected down to a vascular pedicle, which is in turn ligated and divided. The entire prostate with seminal vesicles attached is then removed and submitted as a pathologic specimen.

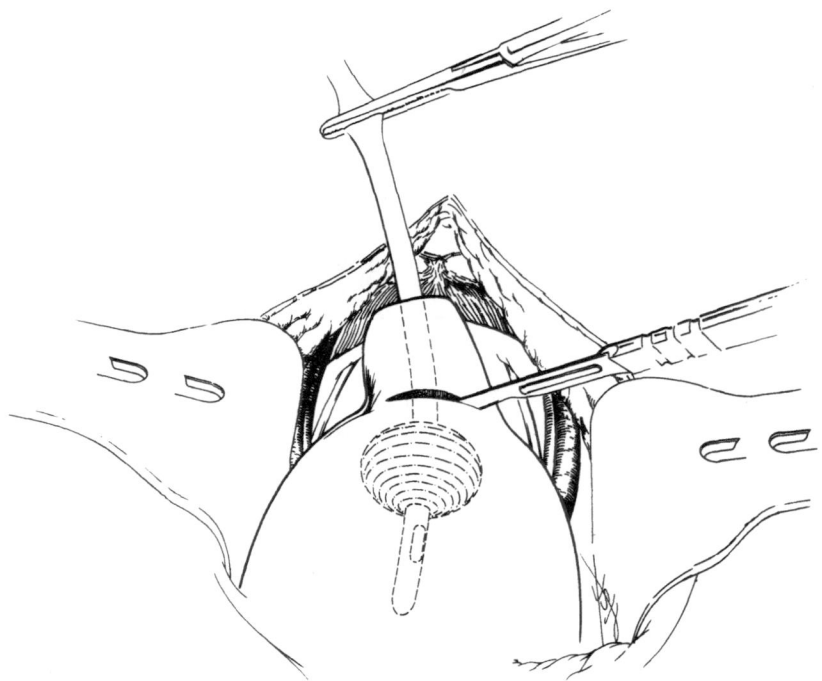

Figure 10. Transection at the prostatovesical junction.

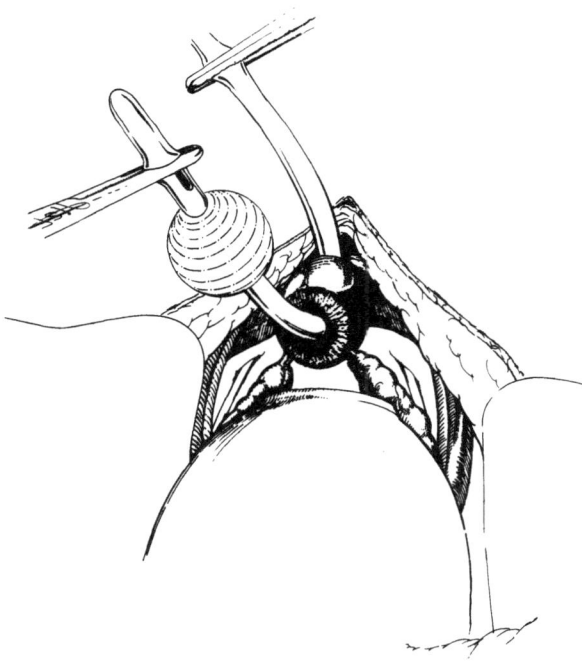

Figure 11. Elevation of transected prostate, allowing dissection of seminal vesicles.

7. Inspection of Prostatic Bed. With the specimen removed, the bladder neck, the anterior rectal wall and the posterior bladder are carefully inspected and bleeding points controlled by coagulation or ligation. If during the course of prostatic removal rectal injury does occur, careful two- or three-layer closure of the tear is carried out with fine chromic suture material under direct visualization. If this suture line appears at all tenuous, a diverting colostomy should also be performed. If the rectum is intact and hemostasis in the pelvis adequate, the catheter traversing the urethra is deflated and the GU diaphragm again inspected and bleeding points suture ligated.

8. Urethral Anastomosis. Using the previously placed urethral sutures as guides a total of six 2-0 chromic sutures are circumferentially placed full thickness through the urethra. The No. 20 French urethral catheter is passed on through the bladder neck into the bladder. The balloon of this catheter is not inflated at this time. The retractor blade holding the bladder cranially is removed and the anastomosis between the urethra and the bladder neck is then completed by passing the six urethral sutures through the vesical wall from inside out in their respective positions. These through-and-

through sutures are tied down with the knots on the outside, beginning with the posterior sutures (Figure 12). During completion of this anastomosis slight traction on the Foley catheter, which is now inflated with 30 cc of saline, aids alignment and approximation. If the bladder neck has been sacrificed because of tumor involvement in this area, it is necessary to close the bladder neck with through-and-through sutures of 2-0 chromic in the 3 o'clock and 9 o'clock positions prior to beginning the urethral anastomosis (Figure 13a, b).

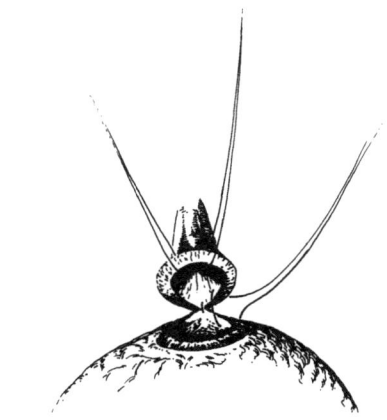

Figure 12. Urethrovesical anasto

9. Anterior Bladder Tube. If the vesicourethral alignment appears difficult because of excessive urethral resection, removal of a long prostate, or because of bladder neck resection, creation of an anterior bladder tube may be beneficial (Figures 14, 15a, b and 16: Tanagho and Smith 1972; Schoenberg and Gregory 1976). In 22 patients[1] treated in this fashion and observed over one to five years, stress incontinence is present in one patient and another requires occasional dilatation for a resultant urethral stricture. In no instance have we had to rely on perineal traction sutures (Vest 1940; Dees 1969), nor have we had to rely postoperatively on Foley traction to complete a tight urethral anastomosis.

10. Closure. Once the bladder-to-urethra anastomosis is completed, the wound is irrigated, a one-inch Penrose drain is positioned near but not on the anastomosis and brought out inferior to the incision. The rectus muscles are approximated loosely

[1] Nine of these patients had surgery performed by Mohan Gursahani, M.D.

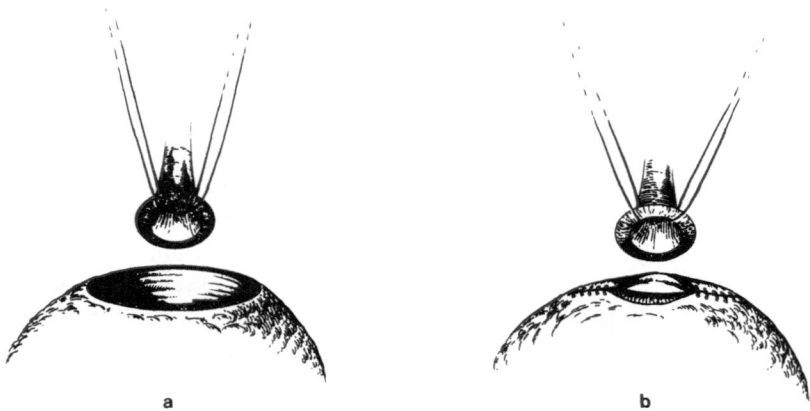

Figure 13. Urethrovesical anastomosis following resection of the bladder neck. a. Bladder neck resected. b. Closure of bladder neck in 3 o'clock and 9 o'clock positions.

in the midline. No attempt is made to reattach these muscles to the symphysis. The rectus fascia is closed with vertical mattress sutures using 2-0 nylon, the subcutaneous tissues are approximated with 3-0 plain and the skin with 4-0 nylon. Nylon retention sutures, placed through-and-through and tied over rubber protectors, are used occasionally, especially in obese patients. The Foley catheter is securely taped to avoid traction. A dense occlusive dressing is placed.

E. Postoperative Care

Routine postoperative orders are written and include the monitoring of urine output hourly. If the output falls, patency in the catheter must be checked by gentle irrigation. Distention of the bladder can be disruptive, and must be avoided.

The catheter is left indwelling for seven days. Before removal, 100 cc of contrast is placed in the bladder under fluoroscopic visualization and the

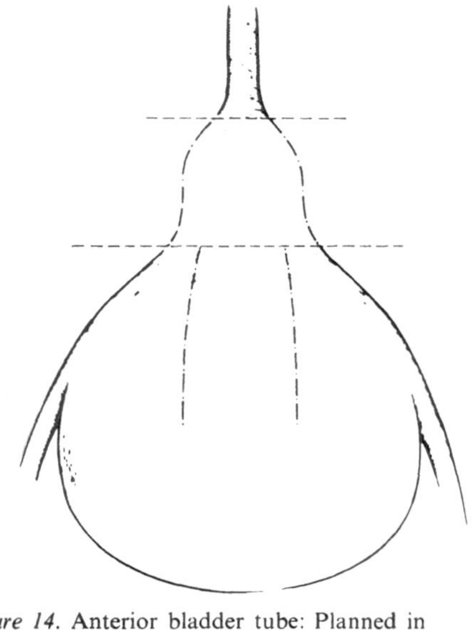

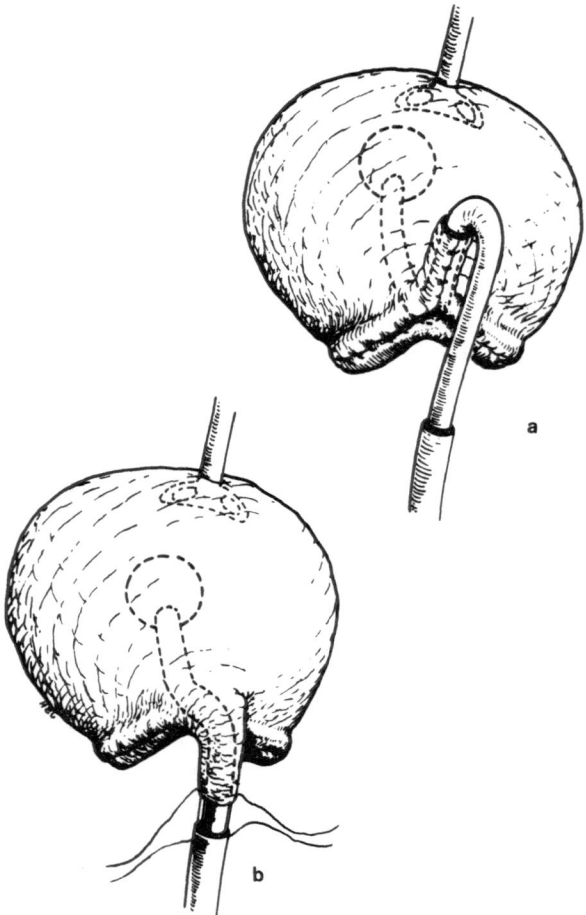

Figure 15. Anterior bladder tube. a. Construction of tube. b. Anastomosis of tube to urethra.

Figure 14. Anterior bladder tube: Planned in

patient asked to void around the catheter, or if this is impossible, immediately after catheter removal. If extravasation is noted, the catheter is repositioned immediately and left in place for an additional five days. Early urethral healing is usual if a prostatic ureteral cuff has been retained. Leaks are more commonly associated with those procedures requiring bladder neck narrowing or the creation of an anterior bladder tube.

Following removal of the catheter, the patient is observed as regards urinary continence and if necessary is encouraged to void in a stop-and-go pattern, thus exercising the perineal muscles. Early incontinence of varying degrees, often of a stress nature and occasionally lasting for up to three months, is treated conservatively using a condom catheter if necessary. After three months, further improvement in continence is unlikely, and at that time an incontinence procedure should be considered. At this time we prefer the American Medical Systems device No. 742 placed in a perineal position.

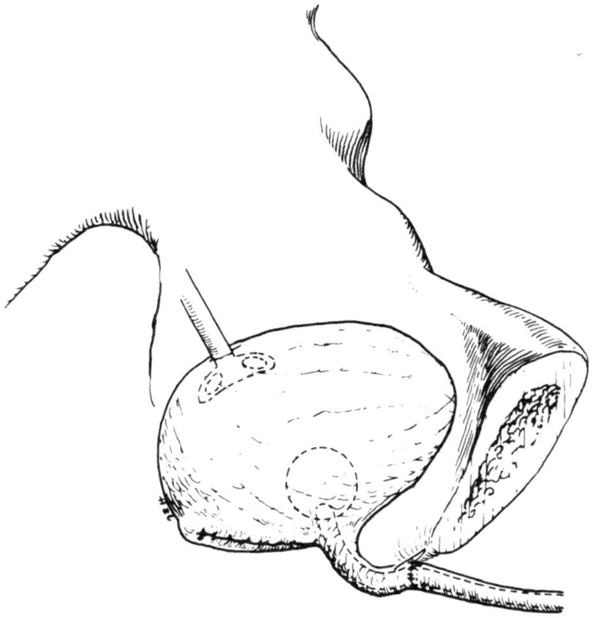

Figure 16. Anterior bladder tube completed.

III. PATIENT FOLLOWUP

A followup IVP is obtained at three months and the patient is seen every six months and monitored by history and by measurement of serum acid phosphatase for the possibility of metastatic spread.

Occasionally following radical prostatectomy the removed nodes, which have been reported negative on frozen section, prove to be positive on permanent section. If only one node is positive, no further therapy is instituted. Patients having two or more positive nodes can be treated with external beam radiotherapy. We have not used radiotherapy on such patients because of the increased likelihood of leg and genital edema when aggressive lymphadenectomy and radiotherapy are combined (Bagshaw 1978), but have instead instituted estrogen therapy with 3 mg of diethylstilbestrol daily.

Impotency is admitted by the majority of patients following radical prostatectomy. We explain the possibility of correcting this disorder by the implantation of a solid rod or inflatable prosthesis. We can perform such surgery one year after total prostatectomy on request of a patient who is clinically well.

REFERENCES

Bagshaw MA: Radiation therapy for cancer of the prostate. In: Genitourinary cancer, Skinner DG and DeKernion JB (eds), Philadelphia, WB Saunders Co, 1978, p 355-379.

Barzell W, Bean MA, Hilaris BS, Witmore WF, Jr: Prostatic adenocarcinoma: Relationship of grade and local extent to the pattern of metastases. J Urol 118: 278, 1977.

Bauer WC, McGavran MH and Carlin MR: Unsuspected carcinoma of the prostate in suprapubic prostatectomy specimens: A clinicopathological study of 55 consecutive cases. Cancer 13: 370, 1960.

Boxer RJ, Kaufman JJ and Goodwin WE: Radical prostatectomy for carcinoma of the prostate. 1951-1976: A review of 239 patients. J Urol 117: 208, 1977.

Byar DP, Mostafi FK and the Veterans Administration Cooperative Urological Research Group: Carcinoma of the prostate: Pragmatic evaluation of certain pathologic features in 208 radical prostatectomies. Cancer 30: 5, 1972.

Carlton CE Jr: Radioactive isotopic implantation for cancer of the prostate. In: Genitourinary cancer, Skinner DG and DeKernion JB (eds), Philadelphia, WB Saunders Co, 1978, p 380-387.

Chu TM, Wang MC, Scott WW, Gibbons RP, Johnson DE, Schmidt JD, Loening SA, Prout GR and Murphy GP: Immunochemical determination of serum prostatic acid phosphatase. Invest Urol 15: 319, 1978.

Culp OS and Meyer JJ: Radical prostatectomy in the treatment of prostatic cancer. Cancer 32: 113, 1973.

Dees JE: Vesicourethral anastomosis in radical perineal prostatectomy. Urology Digest 8: 16, 1969.

Emmett JJ, Green LF and Papantoniou A: Endocrine therapy in carcinoma of the prostate gland. Ten year survival statistics. J Urol 83: 471, 1960.

Foti AG, Cooper JF, Herschman H and Malvaez RR: Detection of prostatic cancer by solid-phase radioimmunoassay of serum prostatic acid phosphatase. N Engl J Med 297: 1357, 1977.

Glenn JF: Surgical therapy of cancer of the prostate. In: Genitourinary cancer, Skinner DG and DeKernion JB (eds), Philadelphia, WB Saunders Co, 1978, p 344-354.

Hanash KH, Utz DC, Cook EN, Taylor WF and Titus JL: Carcinoma of the prostate: A 15 year follow up. J Urol 107: 450, 1972.

Jewett HJ: The present status of radical prostatectomy for stages A and B prostatic cancer. Urol Clin North Am 2: 105, 1975.

Jewett HJ: Radical perineal prostatectomy for prostatic cancer. In: Progress in clinical and biological research, vol 6: Prostatic disease, Marberger H, Haschek H, Schirmer HKA, Colston JAC and Witkin E (eds), New York, Alan R Liss, 1976, p 250-218.

Kohler PR: Current status of lymphography in patients with cancer. Cancer 37: 503, 1976.

Middleton AW Jr: A comparison of the morbidity associated with radical retropubic prostatectomy with and without pubectomy. J Urol 117: 202, 1977.

Nichols RT, Barry JM and Hodges CV: The morbidity of radical prostatectomy for multifocal stage I prostatic adenocarcinoma. J Urol 117: 83, 1977.

Pereiras PV, Meiers W, Kunhardt B, Troner M, Huston D,

Barkin JS and Viamonte M: Fluoroscopically guided thin needle aspiration biopsy of the abdomen and retroperitoneum. Am J Roentgenol 131: 197, 1978.

Schoenberg HW and Gregory JG: Anterior bladder tube in radical retropubic prostatectomy. Urology 7: 495, 1976.

Schroeder FH and Belt E: Carcinoma of the prostate: A study of 312 patients with stage C tumors treated by total perineal prostatectomy. J Urol 114: 257, 1975.

Silverberg E and Holleb AI: Major trends in cancer: A 25 year survey. Cancer 25: 2, 1975.

Tanagho EA and Smith DR: Clinical evaluation of a surgical technique for the correction of complete urinary incontinence. J Urol 107: 402, 1972.

Tomlinson RL, Currie DP and Boyce WH: Radical prostatectomy: Palliation for stage C carcinoma of the prostate. J Urol 117: 85, 1977.

Vest SA: Radical perineal prostatectomy: Modification of closure. Surg Gynecol Obstet 70: 935, 1940.

Vickery AL Jr and Kerr WS Jr: Carcinoma of the prostate treated by radical prostatectomy: A clinicopathological survey of 187 cases followed for 5 years and 148 cases followed for 10 years. Cancer 16: 1598, 1963.

Whitmore WF Jr: Retropubic implantation of L-125 in the treatment of prostatic cancer. In: Progress in clinical and biological research, vol 6: Prostatic disease, Marberger H, Haschek H, Schirmer HKA, Colston JAC and Witkin E (eds), New York, Alan R Liss Inc, 1976, p 223-233.

21. COMBINED RADIOTHERAPY FOR CARCINOMA OF THE PROSTATE

W.G. GUERRIERO

The presently accepted treatment for apparent early stage prostate carcinoma is radical surgery. However, of late, some centers that have extensive experience with irradiation for control of locally advanced prostatic carcinoma have suggested that early prostatic carcinoma may be adequately treated by one of several methods of radiotherapy and even some locally advanced cases may actually be cured by this method of treatment.

The appearance of radiotherapy in the armamentarium available for the treatment of prostatic carcinoma is not a recent event. Young commented on the use of radium implants for prostatic carcinoma in 1922 (Young 1922). The first recorded use of radium was by Pasteau in 1911 (Pasteau 1911). Complications of radium treatment and the success of Young's radical operation eventually led to abandonment of the use of radium. For the same reason, external radiotherapy by the orthovoltage technique never became popular. The dramatic results obtained with hormonal therapy in the 1940s continued to prevent research into the usefulness of irradiation. An additional factor which probably prevented experimentation with radiotherapy was a commonly held misconception that prostatic carcinoma is not radiosensitive. Prostatic adenocarcinoma is actually quite radiosensitive but radioresponse is slow because of the slow growth of the tumor. With the development of supervoltage therapy and the recognition that prostatic carcinoma which has grown through the prostatic capsule is not surgically curable, a resurgence of enthusiasm for radiotherapy occurred – at least for locally advanced prostatic tumor. In the last ten years interstitial treatment by various methods has become popular and those centers performing supervoltage external radiotherapy have increased their experience. A chronology of the history of radiotherapy is seen in Table 1.

I. RADIATION BIOLOGY

In order to understand the rationale for the use of combined interstitial and external radiotherapy for carcinoma of the prostate, one must understand something about radiation biology and the natural history of prostatic carcinoma. Unlike surgery, radiation does not remove the tumor from the patients. Radiation modifies the behavior of the tumor, sometimes actually resulting in death of tumor cells, but frequently only delaying the onset of metastases and extending the symptom-free interval, the patient eventually dying of the carcinoma.

Viable tumor cells are capable of reproduction. Cell death is the loss of proliferative capacity. Following radiotherapy the tumor cell is modified in such a way that it is incapable of reproduction. If the cell cannot divide, it is no risk to the patient. Thus, the loss of proliferative capacity is of primary importance in the survival of the patient after treatment with radiotherapy.

Table 1. Historical perspective of carcinoma of the prostate.

1911	Reports of treatment of prostatic carcinoma with catheter-induced radium (Pasteau 1911)
1922	Deming treated 100 cases of carcinoma of the prostate with radium (Deming 1922)
1941	Huggins and Hodges reported on the effect of estrogens on carcinoma of the prostate (Huggins & Hodges 1941)
1952	Flocks reported the use of interstitial colloidal gold (Au^{198}) (Flocks et al. 1954)
1962	Bagshaw and Kaplan reported success with external radiation (Bagshaw et al. 1965)
1965-67	Others confirmed Bagshaw's report (George et al. 1965; Del Regato 1967)
1972	Whitmore reports the use of I^{125} interstitial irradiation (Whitmore et al. 1972)
1972	Carlton uses combined interstitial and external radiotherapy (Carlton et al. 1972)

Lysis of irradiated cells is a function of the radiation dose and the duration of the intermitotic period. Adenocarcinoma of the prostate has a long intermitotic period. Radioresponse is slow since this depends on interference with cell division. Only after 6 months to 1 year does one appreciate the effect of radiation on prostatic carcinoma.

A specified radiation dose kills a constant fraction of irradiated cells. The larger the tumor, the more difficult it is to completely eradicate the cancer. Smaller tumors are more likely to be completely destroyed by irradiation as only a few cells will be unaffected by the radiotherapy.

Sublethal irradiation doses may modify the behavior of tumors but the host will eventually die of the disease. It is important to give as much irradiation as possible in order to completely destroy the tumor, but sublethal doses may be as effective as lethal doses in clinical cases of prostatic carcinoma. For example, modfication of the behavior of adenocarcinoma of the prostate in a 70 year-old male may result in the patient living his entire life expectance without sign of clinical malignancy but at the time of death, autopsy will show that the patient still has prostatic carcinoma. Thus, one may ask oneself, 'Though it is desirable, is it really important to completely eliminate prostate carcinoma in the elderly patient?'

Tumor response is proportional to the number of rads x time of treatment divided by the tumor volume. The most frequent question which is asked this author is how many rads are given by your method? This is a very difficult question to answer because actual dose varies markedly with time and tumor volume. It frequently is really not as important to know how many rads were delivered to the patient but how rapidly the irradiation was given and how much tumor volume was irradiated.

Neither the rate of tumor regression nor persistency of histologically intact cells in irradiated tissue truly indicates the probability of regrowth of tumor – the only proof of viability is demonstration of the ability of cancer cells to proliferate. Unfortunately at this time no test is presently clinically available which can provide this information (Suit 1975).

II. STAGING OF PROSTATIC CARCINOMA

The most important factor in the survival of patients with prostatic carcinoma is the stage of the patient's tumor when it is first discovered and the malignant potential of the tumor as evidenced by its differentiation – not what type of therapy is offered.

For many years it was thought that prostatic carcinoma began as a single focus of malignancy in the posterior lobe of the true prostate. The tumor might lie dormant for many years before growing to the size of a palpable nodule, and if not removed, eventually, the tumor would penetrate the prostatic capsule, spread to the seminal vesicles and bladder base, and metastasize to bone and lymph nodes by the pelvic vertebral veins and lymphatics. Around this concept of the natural history of prostatic cancer developed a staging system which was a curious mixture of clinical presentation and physical findings. This staging system was used to select those patients who might possibly be cured by radical prostatectomy (Table 2: Whitmore 1956).

Today, as a result of pathologic examination of radical prostatectomy specimens and lymphadenectomy, we realize that our original concept of the natural history of prostatic carcinoma was probably incorrect.

Table 2. Stages of cancer of the prostate.

STAGE A: Clinically Latent Prostatic Cancer – Neither symptoms, signs nor laboratory studies, lead to suspicion of the presence of cancer but microscopic study of tissue from the prostate reveals the presence of previously unsuspected cancer.

STAGE B: Clinically Manifest Early Prostatic Cancer – Symptoms are absent but a suspicion of carcinoma is aroused by the presence of an area of induration apparently confined within the limits of the prostatic capsule and no evidence of metastasis can be found.

STAGE C: Clinically Manifest Locally Advanced Prostatic Cancer – local symptoms from the neoplasm are present to a variable degree and digital rectal examination discloses a variable degree of induration of the prostate, seminal vesicles, and bladder base, but evidence of metastasis cannot be demonstrated.

STAGE D: Clinically Manifest Advanced Prostatic Cancer – the manifestations of the cancer in the prostatic area vary in respect to symptoms and digital rectal findings, but conclusive evidence of metastasis is demonstrated.

McNeal has shown that prostatic carcinoma usually is multifocal or has diffusely spread throughout the prostate when the tumor is examined histologically following prostatectomy (McNeal 1969). The tumor may originate anywhere in the periphery of the true prostate; not just in the posterior lobe (Figure 1). When the tumor is small, the cancer seems to follow the planes of least resistance spreading centrally before penetrating the prostatic capsule. Small tumors are usually well differentiated and grow slowly. Large tumors, which are frequently poorly differentiated, behave more aggressively, spreading without regard to tissue planes. McNeal has suggested that like all other cancer, continuous logarithmic growth is typical of prostatic cancer, but each tumor seems to have its own growth rate. Some tumors grow very slowly, but malignant potential exists in all prostatic carcinoma. Thus, it is only because prostatic cancer is usually well differentiated and appears most frequently in elderly men that its true potential for malignancy is not appreciated.

Confirmation of McNeal's work is found in a paper by Byar and Mostofi (Byar et al. 1972) in which 208 radical prostatectomy specimens were examined. Both sides of the gland were involved with tumor 80.3 percent of the time, and in 91

percent of cases the tumor was found to be multifocal or had diffusely involved the gland. Thus, we see that prostatic cancer is rarely a single focus of malignancy when first discovered and usually involves most of the gland, even when it is felt to be surgically curable by clinical examination.

It is extremely important to clearly understand that if the prostatic capsule has been penetrated, surgery probably has little hope of curing the patient. Jewett has reported that survival of patients with clinically extensive prostatic carcinoma who have been treated with radical prostatectomy is 13 percent at 10 years and 5 percent at 15 years. If the tumor is confined to the gland when examined pathologically, survival is 37 percent at 10 years and 33 percent at 15 years (Jewett 1970). Jewett has also shown that if a discreet nodule is present clinically, local extension is found less than 20 percent of the time, but if more than 1 lobe is involved, extension will be found greater than 50 percent of the time when the specimen is examined histologically. Even when an isolated nodule is present by rectal exam, 77 percent of the pathologic specimens will show diffuse disease throughout the prostate and 20 percent of the patients will have seminal vesicle invasion.

McCullough and Prout have shown that with clinically extensive tumor, pelvic lymph nodes may be involved up to 80 percent of the time. Even when the tumor is confined to the prostate gland, 25 percent of patients will be found to have positive pelvic nodes (McCullough et al. 1974). If these two factors, local extension and pelvic node metastases, are accurately determined not to be present prior to surgery, the patient has an excellent chance of cure by radical prostatectomy (Wilson et al. 1977).

If the patient does not have extension clinically and if he has a negative pelvic node dissection, the chance of microscopic penetration of the capsule is slight and survival should be enhanced. Of the 87 patients studied with negative nodes by Wilson, Dahl and Middleton, only 14 percent had microscopic invasion of the capsule and in only 1 instance was microscopic seminal vesicle invasion found (Wilson et al. 1977).

Most Stage A tumors are small and well differentiated, and in those patients with less than 1 cubic cm of tumor, survival is excellent even without treatment (Byar 1972). However, a number of

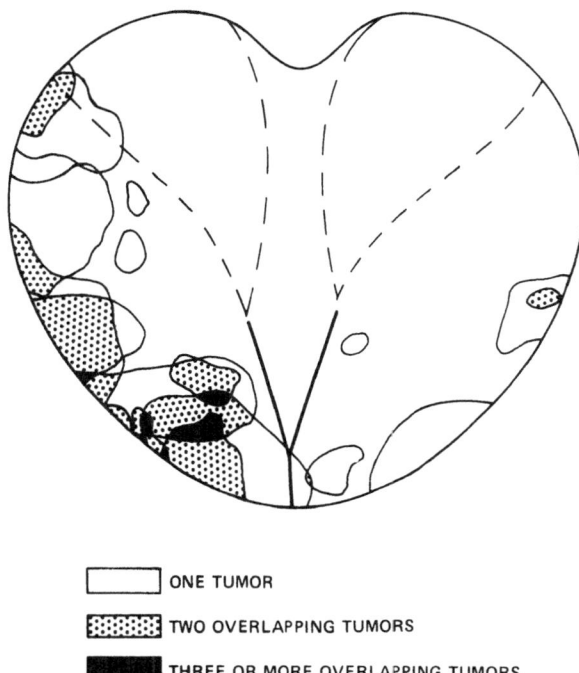

☐ ONE TUMOR

▦ TWO OVERLAPPING TUMORS

■ THREE OR MORE OVERLAPPING TUMORS

Figure 1. Multicentric origin of carcinoma of the prostate.

patients with Stage A tumors have diffuse or multifocal disease. Large and frequently poorly differentiated Stage A tumors appear to be highly malignant and deserve treatment. Stage A tumors may, of course, be treated with radical surgery, but most surgeons are hesitant to operate on these patients because of technical difficulties presented by the previous transurethral prostatic resection and the increased risk of incontinence. We feel radiotherapy is a better choice for these patients.

In Correa and Mason's study (Correa et al. 1974) of 8 patients with diffuse disease undergoing radical prostatectomy, 5 patients died of prostatic carcinoma or with prostatic carcinoma still present at the time of death. The degree of differentiation of these tumors also appears to be quite important, for Bauer and Carlin (Bauer et al. 1960) found that survival was poor in their Stage A patients treated with estrogen if the tumor was less than well differentiated.

Less than 15 percent of Stage A patients appear to have nodal metastases. These patients are the ones who have diffuse or multifocal disease and histologically the tumor is usually poorly differentiated (Guerriero et al. 1978).

The natural history of prostatic carcinoma is extremely important in the prognosis of the patient. Problems exist with radical prostatectomy as performed for Stage A and B disease. With the addition of pelvic lymphadenectomy for staging, statistics for radical prostatectomy should improve, but of course this is at the expense of fewer patients being selected for treatment with surgery. On the other hand, large-volume, poorly differentiated tumors are frequently highly malignant and not effectively treated with radical prostatectomy and small-volume, well differentiated tumors usually have a good prognosis regardless of treatment.

The vast majority of patients who have prostatic carcinoma who are not candidates for surgery because they have extensive disease or positive pelvic lymph nodes are the best candidates for radiotherapy.

III. IRRADIATION OTHER THAN COMBINED INTERSTITIAL IRRADIATION

Methods for irradiation of prostate carcinoma other than combined interstitial irradiation are interstitial implantation of colloidal gold (Flocks 1954), external supervoltage radiotherapy (Bagshaw 1965), and interstitial irradiation with implantation of I^{125} (Whitmore 1972).

A. Interstitial Colloidal Gold

The first successful method of prostatic radiotherapy was the interstitial implantation of colloidal gold. Flocks treated over 1,000 prostates with colloidal gold between 1952 and 1969. Having used colloidal gold with and without radical prostatectomy, he reported control of patients but not many cures with Stage C disease (Flocks 1969). Some patients with small tumors, however, were felt to be cured by this method of treatment. Minimal complications were reported at the usual dosage levels of 40-50 millicuries and irradiation levels of 8,000-9,000 rads. Flocks determined that approximately 6,500 rads were necessary to control most tumors (Taylor 1977). He felt that isolated nodules could be treated without excision of the prostate by injection of a suspension of colloidal gold and reported that 9 out of 10 patients so treated were alive ten years later. Large tumors, however, appeared to require surgical removal with the use of colloidal gold as an adjunct to prevent local recurrence (Flocks 1964). Complications appeared to be severe early in his series but were less with experience. Interestingly, his complications included bladder stones, which have not been seen to my knowledge with other forms of irradiation therapy and may have occurred as a result of bladder neck contracture. Flocks stated that cure was not possible with lymph node metastasis despite the initial hope that colloidal gold would be picked up by lymphatics and carried to the nodes. Survival data from Flocks' series are found listed in Table 3 (Flocks 1969).

B. External Supervoltage Therapy

External supervoltage therapy for carcinoma of the prostate was initially reported by Bagshaw in 1962 (Bagshaw and Kaplan 1962). External radiotherapy has several advantages: no surgical procedure is needed, a uniform tumor dose is assured, and extended fields may be designed for metastatic

Table 3. Au[198] colloidal gold interstitial radiotherapy.

	5 years	10 years	15 years
Stage B (Au[198] alone)	80%	80%	–
Stage C (Au[198] + prostatectomy)	54%	35-40%	15%

disease. There are, however, some disadvantages. Namely, the amount of irradiation appears to be limited by the radiosensitivity of adjacent structures such as the rectum, and staging of the tumor is inadequate without lymphadenectomy. For this reason, Bagshaw has modified his series and is now performing lymphadenectomy for staging before initiating external radiotherapy treatment (Bagshaw et al. 1975). He has reported that 90 percent of tumors treated regress in size and that progressive enlargement of tumors at 3-6 months following completion of therapy probably means active tumor. Seventy-two percent of external radiotherapy treatment failures appear to occur within 24 months. In his series, local failure occurred only 5 percent of the time, local and distant disease progression 33 percent of the time, and distant metastases alone were found in 62 percent of those patients who were felt to have failure of radiotherapy treatment. Thirty percent of patients developed impotence (Ray et al. 1973). Five and ten year uncorrected actuarial survival from Bagshaw's series reported in 1975 is given in table 4 (Bagshaw et al. 1975).

Table 4. Survival rates with external supravoltage therapy.

	Patients	5 years	10 years
Stage A, B	100	72%	44%
Stage C	150	51%	38%

C. Interstitial Iodine Seeds

Whitmore and Hilaris at Memorial Sloan Kettering Institute have reported the use of interstitial irradiation alone utilizing I[125] seeds (Hilaris 1974). The usual preoperative staging procedures are performed and then a bilateral retroperitoneal node dissection for staging. A radiotherapist then inserts I[125] seeds into the prostate through long needles. The I[125] is contained within titanium capsules, 4.5 mm by 0.75 mm, marked with gold to make them radiopaque and spaced 0.5 to 1 cm apart. The expected dose of radiotherapy given to the prostate is greater than 8,000 rads in two months or 16,000 rads in one year. The criteria for selection of patients for this treatment include a life expectancy greater than five years, biopsy-proven prostatic carcinoma, Stage B or small Stage C cancer, and no significant bladder outlet obstruction.

Obturator nodes appear to be the first sign of involvement with tumor. Lymph nodes when positive appear to be lateralized to the site of the tumor with bilateral involvement being common. High grade tumors appear to be more prone to lymph node metastasis. Lymph node metastases were found in 10 percent of tumors suspected to be localized and increased with tumors of increasing size and stage. Local failures (increased size of local tumor) occurred in only 10 percent of the patients (Whitmore 1978).

Seventy-five percent of patients with lymph node metastasis appear to have bone metastasis at five years, and 30 percent with negative nodes have had bone metastasis at 5 years, which is at variance with the experience of those using combined radiotherapy. Of most interest has been a very low incidence of impotence, a finding which is noted also using the combined radiotherapy method.

IV. COMBINED INTERSTITIAL AND EXTERNAL RADIOTHERAPY FOR CARCINOMA OF THE PROSTATE

Beginning in 1965 patients with prostatic carcinoma at Baylor College of Medicine Affiliated Hospitals were offered combined treatment of their tumor with external supervoltage radiotherapy and insertion of radioactive gold seeds (Au[198]). Prior to treatment, patients underwent staging lymphadenectomy to determine exactly what extent of disease was present prior to treatment. The schema for this protocol is found in Figure 2. Those patients with tumor felt to be confined to the prostate by rectal examination were offered radical prostatectomy. As experience with radiotherapy has accumulated, most of our patients have selected node dissection and radiotherapy.

The staging system we have used for our patients treated with combined radiotherapy is seen in Table

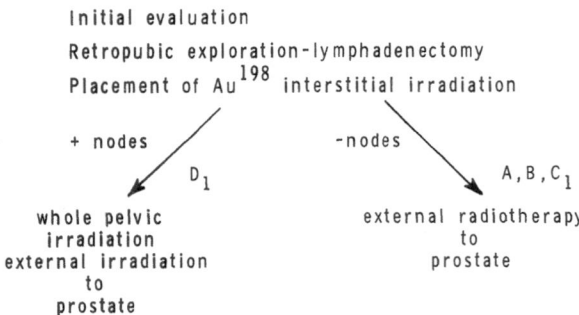

Initial evaluation

Retropubic exploration-lymphadenectomy

Placement of Au^{198} interstitial irradiation

+ nodes   -nodes

D_1 A,B,C_1

whole pelvic   external radiotherapy
irradiation   to
external irradiation   prostate
to
prostate

Figure 2. Treatment of carcinoma of the prostate with combined radiotherapy.

5. This is a modification of the system popularized by Jewett and reflects the use of radiotherapy rather than surgery for treatment. Patients are initially staged by rectal palpation, excretory urography, serum acid phosphatase, and radioactive bone scan to determine if the patient is a candidate for radiotherapy treatment. After exploration, lymphadenectomy and implantation of gold seeds in the prostatic tumor, fields for external radiotherapy are selected. In reporting our results we stage our patients as a result of the pathologic report of the lymphadenectomy and our clinical impression at the time of surgical exploration. Our goals in treatment are as follows: Those patients with Stage A or B tumor are treated for cure. It is hoped that small Stage C tumors will be cured or prove to be radioresponsive and some of these patients will have long term control of their malignancy. Stage D_1 tumors are given whole pelvic irradiation in addition to external radiotherapy to the prostate with the goal of irradiating residual pelvic tumor and delaying the onset of bone metastases.

Radiotherapy appears to be most effective in

Table 5. **Staging** of prostatic carcinoma for radiotherapy.

A_1	Clinically occult carcinoma, small volume, less than 3 TUR chips involved, focal
A_2	Clinically occult carcinoma, multifocal or diffuse, greater than 3 chips involved
B	Clinically apparent carcinoma confined to the prostatic capsule by rectal exam
C_1	Extensive carcinoma, less than 6 cm in size, penetrating prostatic capsule
C_2	Extensive carcinoma, greater than 6 cm in size, penetrating prostatic capsule
D_1	Positive pelvic nodes
D_2	Bony metastasis or distant nodal metastasis; Visceral metastasis

treating small tumors. Experience has shown that tumors greater than 6 cm in size cannot be effectively treated with radiotherapy. For this reason, we divide Stage C into Stage C_1 and C_2. Patients with C_2 tumors almost certainly have far advanced malignancy. Nodal metastases are present in this group greater than 85 percent of the time. It is our feeling that these patients are not likely to be controlled by any method of local therapy.

If the patient has a prostatectomy for benign prostatic disease and more than 3 chips (1 cubic cm of tumor) are found, the patient is treated with radiotherapy. In those patients who have less than 3 chips positive for tumor, a re-resection is recommended. If no further tumor is found, no treatment of the carcinoma is offered. Up to 26 percent of the time tumor has been found on re-resection of prostatectomy specimens (McMillan and Wettlaufer 1976). In the case of patients in whom occult carcinoma with greater than 1 cm of tumor is present, only if a significant volume of prostate is still palpable by rectal examination after prostatectomy is it necessary to insert radioactive seeds into the gland. If the pathologist determines that the tumor is less than well differentiated and/or widely disseminated throughout the gland, a lymphadenectomy is necessary as the chance of lymph node metastasis is great. Whether seeds are inserted then is a matter of election of the radiotherapist.

If the tumor appears to be well differentiated and small in volume, it is unlikely that nodal metastasis will be present. For this reason, staging lymphadenectomy does not appear to be too important in well resected, small Stage A tumors unless the tumor is less than well differentiated. For these reasons, those patients with small volume Stage A tumor frequently receive only external radiotherapy.

Radioactive gold seeds can be used in a sophisticated manner to increase the flexibility of radiotherapy as a method of treating prostatic carcinoma. The use of radioactive seeds maximizes the number of rads which can be given to the tumor. Twenty to forty millicuries of radiation are usually provided by the gold seeds when needed. Placing the seeds also provides an aiming point for the radiotherapist but this is a minor advantage. Most of the radiation dose in our program is given by supervoltage external radiotherapy – usually with a linear accelerator. Because most of the treatment is given by external means, the patient can be effectively treated to *his* tolerance. We expect to deliver at least 4,500 rads by external radiotherapy for a cumulative dose of greater than 6,500 rads into the tumor, but in some patients much more is given.

V. PELVIC LYMPHADENECTOMY

At the time of lymphadectomy, all nodes are removed from the obturator fossa and from the external and internal iliac chain (Figure 3). No periaortic node dissection is done, as prostatic carcinoma is felt to spread in continuity from pelvic to periaortic nodes and is probably incurable when it has reached the periaortic level. The presacral nodes are not examined. Recently, Morales has reported that up to 15 percent of patients with negative obturator and iliac nodes will have positive presacral nodes (Golimby et al. 1978).

In our experience and that of others (Whitmore et al. 1972), obturator nodes seem to be the first to be involved with tumor. Most patients with small volume obturator node metastasis appear to have a relatively good prognosis. All patients with positive nodes have extension of their external radiotherapy fields to encompass these nodes. Usually no frozen

sections are done at the time of surgery as we have found frozen sections to be unreliable for micrometastasis. If one side appears to be grossly involved, a frozen section is obtained to confirm the diagnosis and no node dissection is done on the contralateral side. If only one side is positive, it usually is the side with the greatest tumor involvement in the prostate.

We cannot say whether node dissection improves the patient's prognosis, but, as can be seen in Table 6, survival with small volume positive nodes (Stage D_1) is good.

Table 6. Radiotherapy for carcinoma of prostate one year survival by stages.

Stage	No. patients	Overall survival
A_2	42	98%
B	82	85%
C_1	91	86%
D_1	80	79%

We have had several patients with positive serum acid phosphatase tests and positive nodes but negative bone scans who have been followed for greater than two to three years without development of bone metastasis. In some of these patients, the acid phosphatase has decreased following whole pelvic radiotherapy. Some of these patients have continued to have an elevated acid phosphatase and some have received estrogens. None of these patients to date have developed a positive bone scan.

Following lymphadenectomy the endopelvic fascia may be divided and the prostate mobilized as needed to permit the radiotherapist access to the cancer. Mobilization is minimized as much as possible in order to preserve potency. The number of radioactive seeds inserted and their location is decided by the radiotherapist, depending on the volume of tumor present and whether the carcinoma is localized to a particular portion of the gland.

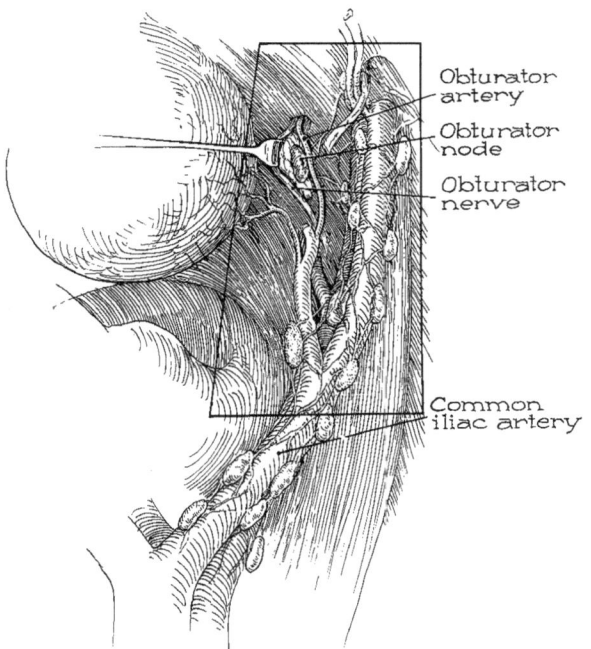

Figure 3. Surgical margins for pelvic lymphadenectomy.

Obturator artery
Obturator node
Obturator nerve
Common iliac artery

VI. POSTOPERATIVE CARE

Following lymphadenectomy and placement of gold seeds, the patient remains in the hospital for approximately 5-7 days. Several weeks following surgery the radiotherapist begins treatment which may be given over a period of one month. Followup is as for patients with radical prostatectomy except that at one year the patient undergoes extensive reevaluation and needle biopsy of the prostate. If needle biopsy is positive at one year, additional seeds may be inserted into the prostate gland at the discretion of the radiotherapist. The patient is usually not given additional external radiotherapy.

VII. RESULTS

Five-, seven- and ten-year results with this method of treatment are listed in Tables 7 and 8. As of 1976, 295 patients had been staged surgically and followed for longer than one year. Many other patients have been treated with external radiotherapy alone. As of 1976, a total of 542 patients had been treated with radiotherapy in our center for prostatic carcinoma. In the last three to five years, the number of cases being placed in the series has rapidly increased. The average age of patients treated by this method is 64 years. Our criteria for lymphadenectomy and surgical staging with follow-up radiotherapy have included an expected survival of greater than 5 years, physical condition adequate to undergo lymphadenectomy and prostatic exploration, and prostatic carcinoma less than 6 cm in size. As can be seen in Table 7, few patients are available for review at the ten-year level; however, patients treated 7-10 years ago have done quite well and in most series treated with radical prostat-

Table 7. Results of combined interstitial and external radiotherapy for carcinoma of the prostate.

Stage	5 years alive/No. patients followed		7 years alive/No. patients followed		10 years alive/No. patients followed	
A	11/11	(100%)	2/2	(100%)	1/1	(100%)
B	35/37	(94%)	21/23	(91%)	1/1	(100%)
C_1	25/29	(86%)	8/9	(88%)	2/2)	(100%)
D_1	14/17	(82%)	4/4	(100%)	0/1	(0%)
Total	85/94	(90%)	35/38	(92%)	4/5	(80%)

Table 8. Results of combined interstitial and external radiotherapy for carcinoma of the prostate.

Stage	Patients alive NED/ Total treated	
A	7/11	(64%)
B	19/37	(51%)
C_1	18/29	(62%)
D_1	6/17	(35%)
Total	50/94	(53%)

ectomy dramatic declines in survival occurred at 7 years. In addition, we have as yet not seen many patients developing metastases who did not have them at the time of initial treatment. Another way of looking at this data is to examine the patients with C_1 and D_1 disease (Table 9). Survival in these patients is dramatic. In surgical series most of these patients are dead within five years. Little difference in survival is noted in any of our patients regardless of stage.

Of significance in our series is the fact that a large number of our tumors are well differentiated as are

Table 9. Combined radiotherapy for carcinoma of the prostate (NED = No evidence of disease).

Stage	Years surviving	Total No. patients	Deaths	Survival	Alive/Alive NED	Alive NED
A		11	0	100%	7	64%
B	5 years	37	2	94%		
	7 years	23	2	91%		
	10 years	1	0	100%		
	Total	37	4	89%	33/19	57%
C_1	5 years	29	4	86%		
	7 years	9	1	88%		
	10 years	2	0	100%		
	Total	29	5	82%	24/18	75%
D_1	5 years	17	3	82%		
	7 years	4	0	100%		
	10 years	1	1	0%		
	Total	17	4	76%	13/6	54%

those in most surgical series. In addition, we are primarily dealing with small volume carcinoma. Figure 4 illustrates differentiation as to stage in our series. Only 11 percent of our patients appear to have poorly differentiated carcinoma. It is important to note, however, that these patients are surviving regardless of stage the same number of months as those who have well to moderately differentiated carcinoma. This may reflect the fact that radiotherapy is more effective for poorly differentiated carcinoma than for well differentiated tumor. As we have already mentioned, longterm followup is extremely important in evaluating the results of treatment of prostatic carcinoma. In Table 9 are seen nine Stage C_1 patients treated more than 7 years ago. Three of these nine patients are alive with disease and can be expected to expire with cancer. Only two patients have died, both free of disease. Twenty-three patients with stage B tumor have been followed for more than 7 years. The overall survival of this group is 91 percent. Seventy percent are either alive without evidence of disease or dead

with no evidence of disease. These patients could best be compared with surgical series in which the patients have been surgically staged.

Our obvious objective in the treatment of prostatic carcinoma is to cure the patient's disease. It is our opinion that this goal is obtainable with radiotherapy in patients with small volume tumor (Stages A_2, B and maybe C_1) but not in those patients with large volume tumor such as the C_2 patients. Based on radiation biology, one of the expected responses with radiotherapy is a delay in the onset of metastasis. This has been seen clinically in other tumors such as breast carcinoma. In our series, we feel that a similar response is being found. Certainly the 82 percent five-year survival of D_1 disease is probably a reflection of this. Whitmore, Bagshaw and others have emphasized the apparent radioresponsiveness of prostatic carcinoma. Ninety percent of patients treated by them and also by us evidence shrinkage of the tumor when examined 6-12 months post irradiation. Ray and Bagshaw have emphasized that enlargement of the tumor after six months is a bad prognostic sign. We rarely see, however, loss of control of the primary tumor. Most of our patients with advanced disease have onset of bone metastasis and not enlargement of the primary.

VIII. COMPLICATIONS

Complications with combined radiotherapy have been few. Of most concern have been several cases of pulmonary emboli and persistent extremity lymphedema. To understand the complications presented by our method of treatment, one must separate those which are felt to occur as a result of the surgery from those which can be ascribed to the radiotherapy. Lymphedema, persistent lymphatic drainage, and wound infections have occurred in less than 10 percent of our patients and generally resolve with proper treatment or time. These complications can be said to be the result of the surgical procedure, lymphadenectomy. Irritative symptoms, such as proctitis, cystitis, and urethritis, occur after radiotherapy and are usually mild and transient but sometimes can be troublesome. Rectal stenosis requiring colostomy occurred in two patients, both early in our series. One patient eventually died of

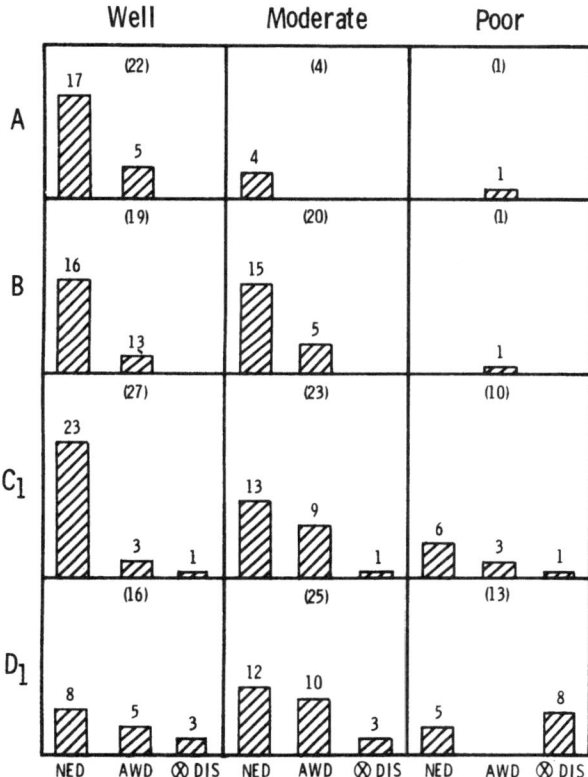

Figure 4. Stage and differentiation of prostatic cancer patients treated with combined radiotherapy. NED = No evidence of disease. AWD = Alive with disease. XDIS = Dead with disease.

multiple small bowel fistulae.

The confusion seen in other series as to the incidence of impotence in patients treated with radiotherapy is not resolved by an analysis of our data. On careful questioning, we have found only 2 percent of our patients to have moderate to severe lack of potency, but 25 percent could not be questioned about this problem or their responses were felt to be unsatisfactory. Whitmore has also suggested that interstitial radiotherapy may result in less loss of potency than external radiotherapy but the reasons for this are unknown (Whitmore 1978).

IX. POST-THERAPY NEEDLE BIOPSY

Evaluation of patients following treatment is somewhat difficult. As mentioned previously, 90 percent of patients have shrinkage of the local tumor. Radioactive bone scans, acid phosphatase determinations, intravenous pyelograms, CBC, BUN and creatinine are performed in our patients at yearly intervals. One year following treatment the patient undergoes needle biopsy of the prostate in order to determine if tumor is still present. The effect of radiation on the tumor is noted in all cases. It is sometimes difficult for the pathologist to determine whether the change that is present in the cells is tumor or irradiation, but it is felt that an experienced pathologist can usually make this differentiation. An additional problem with needle biopsy done post treatment in these patients is that frequently little tissue is palpable by rectal examination and the irradiated prostate is hard to hit with the needle. Multiple cores must be taken. A negative biopsy is felt to be significant if definable prostate is obtained. In Table 10 are listed the results of needle biopsy on the patients in our series. As can be seen, approximately 65 percent of all

patients have negative needle biopsies one year following treatment. As has been shown by Perez (1976), if the biopsy is performed earlier than one year, the incidence of positive biopsies is increased. This is illustrated in Figure 5. If the patient is found to have a positive biopsy and the radiotherapist feels additional treatment can be given, this is done.

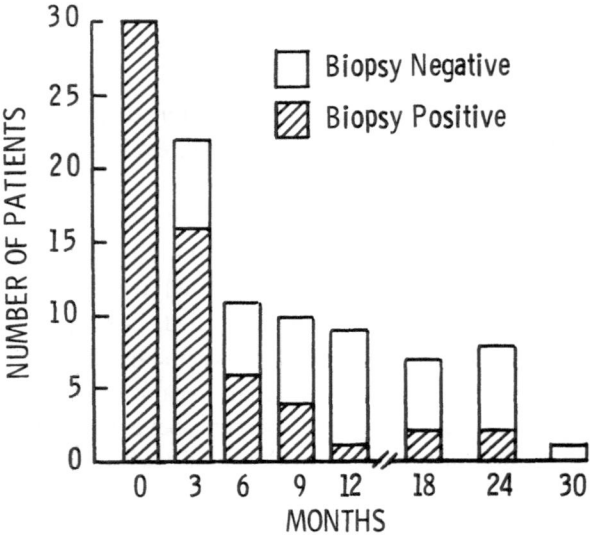

Figure 5. Biopsy results post radiotherapy.

However, if maximum treatment is already being provided to the patient, no further treatment is offered and the patient returns to followup status. No patient with a positive needle biopsy has received estrogens unless evidence of bone metastasis is found. To date, patients with positive needle biopsies who have demonstrated good response clinically have done as well as those patients with negative needle biopsy. Thus, the significance of a positive needle biopsy is unknown. Of most importance appears to be whether the patient has an initial response to treatment.

It is our hope that irradiation therapy will offer a significant alternative to the patient considering radical surgery for small volume prostatic carcinoma. We feel that radiotherapy has already proved its place for the patient with extensive disease and is particularly applicable to the elderly patient who is a poor surgical risk in which, though the prostate cancer may not be cured with radiotherapy, the behavior of the tumor may be so modified that the patient lives out his limited life expectancy with no clinical evidence of prostatic carcinoma.

Table 10. Radiotherapy for carcinoma of prostate followup biopsy results.

	Negative/Total	
Stage A	13/21	62%
Stage B	28/43	65%
Stage C_1	28/45	62%
Stage D_1	12/27	44%

REFERENCES

Bagshaw MA, Kaplan HS: Radical external radiotherapy of localized prostatic carcinoma. Presented at the 10th International Congress of Radiology, September 15-18, 1962.

Bagshaw MA, Kaplan HS and Sagerman RH: Linear accelerator supervoltage radiotherapy. Radiology 85: 121, 1965.

Bagshaw MA, Ray GR, Salzman JR and Meares EM Jr: Extended-field radiation therapy for carcinoma of the prostate: a progress report. Cancer Chemother Rep 59: 165, 1975.

Bauer WC, McGavran MH and Carlin MR: Unsuspected carcinoma of the prostate in suprapubic prostatectomy specimens – a clinicopathological study of 55 consecutive cases. Cancer 13: 370, 1960.

Byar DP, Mostofi FK, The Veterans Administration Cooperative Urological Research Group: Carcinoma of the prostate: prognostic evaluation of certain pathologic features in 208 radical prostatectomies – examined by the step-section technique. Cancer 30: 5, 1972.

Byar DP, the Veterans Administration Cooperative Urological Research Group: Survival of patients with incidentally found microscopic cancer of the prostate: results of a clinical trial of consecutive treatment. J Urol 108: 908, 1972.

Carlton CE Jr, Dawoud F, Hudgins P and Scott R Jr: Irradiation treatment of carcinoma of the prostate: a preliminary report based on 8 years of experience. J Urol 108: 924, 1972.

Correa RJ Jr, Anderson RG, Gibbons RP and Mason JT: Latent carcinoma of the prostate – why the controversy? J Urol 111: 644, 1974.

Del Regato JA: Radiotherapy in the conservative treatment of operable and locally inoperable carcinoma of the prostate. Radiology 88: 761, 1967.

Deming CL: Cancer of the prostate and seminal vesicles – results in one hundred cases of cancer of the prostate and seminal vesicles treated with radium. Surg Gynecol Obstet 34: 99, 1922.

Flocks RH, Kerr HD, Elkins HB and Culp DA: Treatment of carcinoma of the prostate by interstitial radiation with radioactive gold (Au^{198}): a preliminary report. J Urol 71: 628, 1954.

Flocks RH: Interstitial irradiation therapy with a solution of Au^{198} as part of combination therapy for prostatic carcinoma. J Nucl Med 5: 691, 1964.

Flocks RH: Present status of interstitial irradiation in managing prostatic cancer. JAMA 210: 328, 1969.

George FW, Carlton CE Jr, Dykhuizen RF and Dillon JR: Cobalt-60 telecurietherapy in the definitive treatment of carcinoma of the prostate: a preliminary report. J Urol 93: 102, 1965.

Golimby M, Al-Askari S, Brown J and Morales P: Extended pelvic lymphadenectomy in prostate cancer. Presented at the Seventy-Third Annual Meeting of the American Urological Association, Inc, Washington, DC, May, 21-25, 1978.

Guerriero WG, Barrett MT, Bartholomew T, Hudgins PT and Carlton CE Jr: Combined interstitial and external radiotherapy in the definitive management of carcinoma of the prostate. 1978.

Hilaris BS, Whitmore WF JR, Batata MA and Grabstald H: Radiation therapy and pelvic node dissection in the management of cancer of the prostate. Am J Roentgenol Radium Ther Nucl Med 121: 832, 1974.

Huggins C and Hodges CV: Studies of prostatic cancer – effect of castration on estrogen and of androgen injection on serum phosphatase in metastatic carcinoma of the prostate. Cancer Res 1: 293, 1941.

Jewett HJ: The case for radical perineal prostatectomy. J Urol 103: 195, 1970.

McCullough DL, Prout GR Jr and Daly JJ: Carcinoma of the prostate and lymphatic metastases. J Urol 111: 65, 1974.

McMillen SM and Wettlaufer JN: The role of repeat transurethral biopsy in stage A carcinoma of the prostate. J Urol 116: 759, 1976.

McNeal JC: Origin and development of carcinoma of the prostate. Cancer 23: 24, 1969.

Pasteau D: Traitement du cancer de la prostate par le radium. Rev Mal Nutr 363, 1911.

Perez CA: Radiation therapy in the management of carcinoma of the prostate. Curr Probl Cancer 1:30, 1976.

Ray GR, Cassady JR and Bagshaw MA: Definitive radiation therapy of carcinoma of the prostate – a report on 15 years experience. Radiology 106: 407, 1973.

Suit HD: Radiation biology: a basis for radiotherapy. In: Textbook of radiotherapy, second edition, Fletcher GH (ed), Henry Kimpton Publishers, Great Britain, 1975, p 75.

Taylor WJ: Radiation oncology – cancer of the prostate. Cancer 39: 856, 1977.

Whitmore WF Jr: Symposium on hormones and cancer therapy: hormone therapy in prostatic cancer. Am J Med 21: 697, 1956.

Whitmore WF Jr, Hilaris B and Grabstald H: Retropubic implantation of iodine 125 in the treatment of prostatic cancer. J Urol 108: 918, 1972.

Whitmore WF Jr: Radioiodine seeds in the treatment of prostatic cancer. Presented at the 1978 Regional Subject Oriented Seminar of the American Urological Association, St. Louis, Missouri, April 27-29, 1978.

Wilson CS, Dahl DS and Middleton RG: pelvic lymphadenectomy for the staging of apparently localized prostatic cancer. J Urol 117: 197, 1977.

Young HH: Technique of radium treatment of cancer of the prostate and seminal vesicles. Surg Gynecol Obstet 34: 93, 1922.

INDEX

Absent penis, 85
Accessory glands, 5-8
  nerve supply, 19-20
Ampulla, 12-13, 22
Amputated penis, 101-104
Anatomy of male reproductive organs, 8-20
Androgens, 6
  deficiency, 20
  replacement therapy, 20
  transport, 38
Artificial insemination, 63
Avulsion of the genital skin, 98
  stent for repair, 99
  grafts for, 99
Azoospermia, 26, 40, 47

Balanitic epispadias, 88
Basal cells (table), 13
Benign prostatic hyperplasia (BPH), 178-194
  sequelae and symptoms, 179
  treatment by prostatectomy, 184-194
  (See also Prostatectomy)
Bifid penis, 82
Bladder, 12, 25
  nerve supply, 19
Bladder neck, 62
  transection of in prostatectomy, 246
Blastemal cells, 5
Blood testis barrier, 13
Blood toxins, role in varicocele formation, 56-7
Bulbo-urethral glands, 12, 14, 23
Burns, 105-108

Calculi, 199
Carcinoma of the penis, 215-225
  staging, 216
  pre-malignant lesions, 216
  penectomy as treatment for, 215
    partial, 217-8
    total, 218
  lymphadenectomy for, 219-224
Carcinoma of the prostate, 237-249
  evaluation for, 238-39
    digital rectal exam, 238
    prostatic biopsy, 238
    lymphangiography, 239
    percutaneous lymph node aspiration, 239
  surgical procedures for, 237, 240-49
    bilateral retroperitoneal lymph node dissection, 240
    total retropubic prostatectomy, 237, 240-49

Carcinoma of the testicle, 226-34
  treatment
    orchiectomy, 226-8
    retroperitoneal lymphadenectomy, 226, 229-34
  typing, 228
  staging, 228-9
Castration, 27
Chemical injuries, 105
Chordee
  with epispadias, 89-90
  without hypospadias, 70
    repair (Allen-Spence procedure), 71
Circumcision, 80
  injuries associated with, 110
Coelomic epithelium, 5-6
Collateral circulation of the testicle, 34
Congenital anomalies and pathophysiology, 25-7
  correction for, 79-97
Contractures, as a result of perineal burn, 108
Corpora cavernosa, 23, 114, 125, 136
Corpus cavernosography, 23, 156-7, 216
Corpus spongiosum, 11, 139
Counterimmunoelectrophoresis, 238
Cremasteric artery, 35
Cryptorchidism, 48, 83

Deferential artery, 35
Diphallus, 31-83

Ejaculation, 22, 62
  physiology, 24-5
Ejaculatory duct, 11-14, 25
Electric injuries, 105
Elephantiasis, 112
Embryogenesis, 12
Embryology of the male reproductive organs, 5-8
Emission, 62
Ephedrine, 64
Epididymal obstruction, 40-41
Epididymectomy, 195-7
  scrotal approach, 196-8
Epididymis, 13, 18, 22, 26, 27, 38, 196
Epididymitis
  etiologies, 195
  surgery of, 196-8
Epididymovasostomy, 38-45
Epispadias, 87-90, 95
Epithelial tag, 70
Epithelium, 13
Erection, 21-24

Estrogen, 6, 20
Exstrophy-epispadias complex, 87-96
External genitalia, 8

Fetal prostate, 6
Fetal testes, 5
Fibrosis, 125
Flaccidity, 115
Fossa navicularis, 70
Fournier, 112
Fracture of the penis, 104
Fructose, 62

Genital tubercle, 70
Genito-urinary duct system, 7
Germ cells, 5
Germinal cell hypoplasia, 56
Golgi apparatus, 14
Gonad, 6
Gonadal blastema, 5, 6
Gonorrhea urethritis, 196
Granuloma (See Sperm granuloma)

Hidradenitis suppurativa, 110
Homograft, 108
Hormonal control of male reproductive function, 21
Human chorionic gonadotropin (HCG)
    therapy for varicocele 57, 60
Human fetus, 7
Hyalinization, 48
Hydrocele, 27, 204-7
Hydrocelectomy, 204-10
    excision operation, 208
    extrusion procedure, 210
Hypertrophy of the bladder wall, 179
Hypospadias
    associated anomalies, 69
        chordee without hypospadias, 70
        glanular or balanic, 70
        penile, 70
    penoscrotal, scrotal, or perineal, 70
    incidence of, 69
        associated with microphallus, 84
    repair
        optimum time, 71
        chordee without hypospadias (Allen-Spence procedure), 71
        Flip-flap (Mustarde procedure), 72
        rolled penile skin tube (King procedure), 73
        one-stage pedicle graft (Hodgson II procedure), 73
        one-stage free graft (Devine-Horton procedure), 74
        two-stage technique (Belt-Fuqua procedure), 74
        other second-stage techniques (Byars procedure, Cecil-Culp
            procedure), 75
    urinary diversion with, 76

Impotency, 114
    associated with prostatectomy, 249
Increased intrascrotal temperature, 56
Inguinal orchiectomy, 226-8
Intersexuality, 47

Kleinfelter syndrome, 47-8

Lateral spermatic ligament, 33-4

Leydig cells, 8, 13
    in steroidogenesis, 22
Lord extrusion procedure, 210
Lymphadenectomy for penile carcinoma, 219-24
Lymphangiography, 239
Lymphatics
    of bladder, 18
    of male reproductive organs, 18
    of penis, 17

Mafenide acetate, 101
Maldescended testes
    obstructed, 31
    functionally dystopic, 31
    ectopic, 31
Male reproductive organs, 5-27
    nerve supply, 18
    physiology, 20-27
    physiological functions (table), 22
Malignancy after orchiopexy, 32
Meatal stenosis, 69, 80-81
Meatotomy, 81
Mesonephros, 5
Microphallus, 83-84
Microsurgery
    for epididymovasostomy, 38, 41-44
    optical aids for, 160
Microvascular repair, 101
Minnesota Multiphasic Personality Inventory (MMPI), 123
Mucosa of vas deferens (table), 13
Mullerian cysts, 199
Mullerian ducts, 6-7, 12
Mullerian systems, 5

Natural erection, 115
Necrotizing gangrene, 112
Nerve supply
    of accessory glands, 19-20
    of bladder, 19
    of male reproductive organs, 18
    of penis, 19
Nocturnal penile erections, 123
Nocturnal penile tumescence, 114, 127
Nodular hyperplasia, 178

Oligospermia, 47
Optical aids for microsurgery, 160
Orchiectomy, 170
    inguinal, 226-8
    scrotal, 228
Ornade, 65

Paraphymosis, 79-80
Patch material, 130
Pectiniform septum, 11
Pelvic structures (figure), 9
Penectomy, 170
    for carcinoma, 215, 217-8
Penile angulation, 126
Penile epispadias, 88
Penile gangrene, 101
Penile prosthesis
    semi-rigid, 114
    inflatable, 115
    implantation, 115, 120, 122

in Peyronie's disease, 127, 131-2
in prostatectomy, 260
Penile torsion, 86
Penis, 8, 12
    anatomy, 11-15, 215
    nerve supply, 19
    vasculature, 15, 17, 23
    lymphatics
        drainage system, 215-6
        supply, 17
Penopubic epispadias, 88
Percutaneous lymph node aspiration, 239
Peyronie's disease
    history, 125
    systemic therapy, 127
    local therapy, 127-8
    surgical excision of plaque, 129-132
Phimosis, 79
Pituitary gonadotrophins, 20
Plaque, 125
    surgical excision, 129-132
Postpubertal castration, 27
Prepubertal castration, 27
Preputial glands, 14
Priapism, 135
Primary blastema, 5
Primordial germ cells, 6
Principal cells (table), 13
Prostate, 9, 11-12, 14-15, 18, 23-25, 27
    fluid, 27
    glands, 6
    secretions, 24
    vascular supply, 17
Prostatectomy, 178-192
    indications for, 180
    operative techniques for
        retropubic, 182
        transvesical (suprapubic), 186
        perineal, 187
        transurethral resection (TURP), 190
    treatment for carcinoma of prostate, 237-249-49
Prostatic massage, 27
Prostatic urethral (table), 12
Prosthesis (See Penile prosthesis, Testicle prosthesis)

Radiation injury, 109
Radioimmunoassay, 229-238
REM sleep activity, 123
Reproductive function, hormonal control of, 21
Retractile testes, 31
Retrograde ejaculation, 62
Retrograde venous flow in varicocele formation, 56-7
Retroperitoneal lymphadenectomy, 63
    for carcinoma of the testicle, 226, 229-34
Retropubic lymph node dissection, 237-8

Scrotal anomalies, 86-7
Scrotal mass, 226
Scrotal orchiectomy, 228
Scrotum
    anatomy, 207
    musculature, 15
Subaceous glands, 14
Semen, 24, 26
Seminal emission (table), 23

Seminal vesicles, 9, 12-13, 22, 24-26, 198-201
Seminal vesicular retention cysts, 199
Seminal vesiculectomy, 198-204
    indications for, 199
    perineal approach, 200
    transcoccygeal approach, 200-201
    extravesicular transperitoneal approach, 201
    transvesical approach, 201-2
Seminal vesiculitis, 198-199
Seminiferous tubules, 13, 38
Seminoma, 228-9
"Sentinel node," 216
Sertoli cell, 13, 22
Sertoli Cell Only syndrome, 48
Shunts, 135
Silver sulfadiazine, 101
Sperm granuloma, 154
Sperm maturation, 39
Sperm transport, 22, 39, 145
Spermatic cord, 14, 19
Spermatic vein ligation, 57
Spermatic vessel triangle, 34
Spermatoceles, 196
Spermatocytogenesis, 22
Spermatogenesis (table), 22
    hormonal regulation, 24
Spermatozoa, 22
Sterilization, 143
Subcervical urethral glands of Albarran, 14
Subcutaneous (Dartos) pouch, 35
Subsymphyseal epispadias, 88
Swelling in the penile shaft, 126
Syphilis, 196

Testicular function (table), 24
Testicular prosthesis, 36
Testicular rupture, 105
Testis, 6, 13, 19, 22, 25-27
Testis biopsy, 47-8, 54
Thermal injuries, 105
Thigh pockets, 100
Transsexual, 170
Trigone prostate, 10
Tuberculosis, 196
Tumors
    epididymal, 196
    germ cell/non-germ cell, 228
    seminal vesicular, 199
Tunica albuginea, 11, 114, 125
Tunica vaginalis, 14
Turgidity, 115

Ureter, 12, 25
Urethra, 8, 12, 24
Urethral folds, 70
Urethral glands, 14
Urinary bladder, 9
Urinary diversion with hypospadias, 76
Urinary incontinence, 224, 248
Urinary tract anomalies with bilaterally undescended testes, 32
Urogenital diaphragm, 14

Vaginoplasty, 170
Varicocele, 55-62
    treatment by supplemental human chorionic gonadotropin

(HCG), 57, 60
  treatment by varicocelectomy, 57-59
    high inguinal approach, 58
    retroperitoneal procedure, 59
    scrotal approach, 59
Vas deferens, 9, 12-13, 18-19, 22, 25-26, 144-45
Vas flushing, 149
Vascular supply
  of male reproductive organs, 15-18
  of penis, 17
  of prostate, 17
    and bladder, 16
Vasectomy, 143-54
Vasography, 54

Vasovasostomy, 157-164
  anastomoses, 158
  testing for spermatozoa, 164
Venous valvular incompetence, 56
Vesicular fluid, 26
Vesiculectomy (See Seminal vesiculectomy)

Webbed penis, 85
Wolffian ducts, 5-7

Xenograft, 108

Y-V plasties, 63